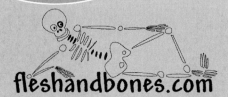

Immunology

For Medical Students

Commissioning Editor: Louise Crowe
Project Development Manager: Siân Jarman
Project Manager: Frances Affleck
Designers: Judith Wright and George Ajayi
Illustrations Manager: Bruce Hogarth

Immunology
For Medical Students

Roderick Nairn
PhD
Professor and Chair
Department of Medical Microbiology and Immunology
Senior Associate Dean, Academic Affairs
Creighton University School of Medicine
Omaha
Nebraska, USA

Matthew Helbert
MBChB MRCP MRCPath PhD
Consultant Clinical Immunologist and Honorary Senior Lecturer
St Bartholomew's Hospital
London, UK

Illustrations by Ethan Danielson

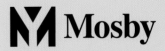

EDINBURGH LONDON NEW YORK OXFORD PHILADELPHIA ST LOUIS SYDNEY TORONTO 2002

MOSBY
An imprint of Elsevier Limited

First published 2002
  Reprinted 2003, 2004, 2005 (twice), 2006

ISBN 0 323 03576 0

British Library Cataloguing in Publication Data
A catalogue record for this book is available from the British Library

Library of Congress Cataloging in Publication Data
A catalog record for this book is available from the Library of Congress

Note
Medical knowledge is constantly changing. As new information becomes available, changes in treatment, procedures, equipment and the use of drugs become necessary. The authors and the publishers have taken care to ensure that the information given in this text is accurate and up to date. However, readers are strongly advised to confirm that the information, especially with regard to drug usage, complies with the latest legislation and standards of practice.

The
publisher's
policy is to use
**paper manufactured
from sustainable forests**

Printed in China

PREFACE

We have recognized the need for an immunology book that is primarily focused on the needs of medical students for as long as we have been teachers of immunology. This book has been written to fill this need. Immunology can fall into different medical school courses or modules. Often, the immunology is taught in the Host Defense course, which integrates basic and clinical immunology (including allergy, immunopathology, etc.). Some medical schools, however, teach basic immunology and clinical immunology in two separate courses. This book should be useful for either curriculum organization.

We have concentrated on a simple, straightforward treatment of the subject. The book is relatively short and contains the topics we considered important to understand the human immune system and its role in protecting us from disease. This reflects our acknowledgement of the time constraints on today's medical student. With new topics and a growing amount of information considered to be essential, there are increasing demands on students. It is therefore important to have a concise, readable, textbook and that has been our primary aim. Most chapters contain the information needed for a typical 50-minute large class or small-group teaching/learning session. This, of course, means that details dear to the hearts of some immunologists are not covered!!

We are aware of two specific problems that medical students have with immunology. First, the immune system is complex, because it has evolved to respond to the wide range of pathogens. Many students find themselves bogged down in the complexities of the molecules and cells of the immune system, without having an understanding of how these components work together to fight infection. We begin our book with two overview chapters which explain what the immune system does and then how the components fit together. We recommend that students begin by reading these chapters. Further on in the text, there are more short, integrating overview chapters. These are not just for revision, but are there to make sure that the student understands how the material that they have read fits into the overall system. The second problem is that medical students do not always immediately see the relevance of immunology to day-to-day clinical practice. We have included clinical correlations throughout the text, which explain how understanding the science of immunology can translate into understanding real clinical problems.

The book is a concise description of the science of immunology, a topic that defies a final complete description, because there is much still to be learned. Hopefully, we will have succeeded in inducing an interest and appreciation of the relevance of immunology to medical students, to form the basis for a lifetime of learning about the immune system and its potential for use in improving the human condition. Most medical students today could still be practicing medicine in 40–50 years. Approximately, 50 years ago immunology was still in its infancy. For example, we did not know the chemical structure of antibody molecules in any detail, and treatments such as organ transplantation had not been carried out. The next 50 years will likely bring equally important advances in the field. History suggests that we would be foolish to try to predict what they will be. We hope that you enjoy participating in these advances in immunology and their application to human disease as much as we have in those that we have been privileged to observe in our careers.

2002   R.N. & M.H.

ACKNOWLEDGEMENTS

Many thanks to my wife, Morag, for deciphering the many drafts of my chapters, and to my family for their forbearance while this book was being written, to my mentors and colleagues for their insights and guidance, and especially all at Harcourt for their faith in the book and for expertly shepherding the project to completion. The book is dedicated to Morag and Carolyn, Muriel, James and Alastair.

R.N.

I am indebted to Lindsay and Caroline, who have given me tremendous insights to understanding immunology patients. Writing this book would not have been possible without Pat's immense patience.

M.H.

HOW TO USE THIS BOOK

Immunology for Medical Students is organized to be read comprehensively. The flow of the book is from genes and molecules to cells and organs, and finally to the immune system as an integrated system protecting the body from infection and regulating the health of the body.

- Section 1 introduces the basic concepts and is essential for an understanding of the language of immunology.
- Section 2 continues with a discussion of the antigen-recognition molecules, that is, antibodies, T cell receptors and the molecules encoded by the major histocompatibility complex.
- Section 3 deals with immune physiology, the role of the cells and organs of the immune system in the response to a pathogen.
- Section 4 discusses the innate immune system.
- Section 5 considers hypersensitivity, allergy/asthma, autoimmunity, immunodeficiency, transplantation, etc.

Throughout the book the core knowledge objectives are listed as Learning Points at the ends of chapters to aid in review. There are also four integrating overview chapters (e.g., Review of antigen recognition, Review of innate immunity), and these focus the student on the major points. Each section is relatively freestanding. For example, Section 5, Immune system in health and disease, could be used in a clinical correlations course, independent of the remainder of the book. *Immunology for Medical Students* will be most useful in the comprehensive Host Defense type courses growing in popularity in medical schools.

The icons used throughout are illustrated overleaf. You should become familiar with them immediately in order to follow the illustrations. We have selected several pathogens (listed in the figure overleaf) to use throughout the book as examples. As a reminder, some basic aspects of the structure and mechanism of action of these organisms are described. You should re-acquaint yourself with these organisms, undoubtedly encountered in microbiology or infectious disease courses, and use the figure as a convenient reference as you encounter these pathogens in the examples in this book.

CLINICAL BOX

Clinical boxes, throughout the text, put immunology into a clinical context. The clinical material selected is current and relevant.

TECHNICAL BOX

Technical boxes show how advances in the field have expanded our knowledge of how the immune system works, and provided new means of preventing disease.

ICONS

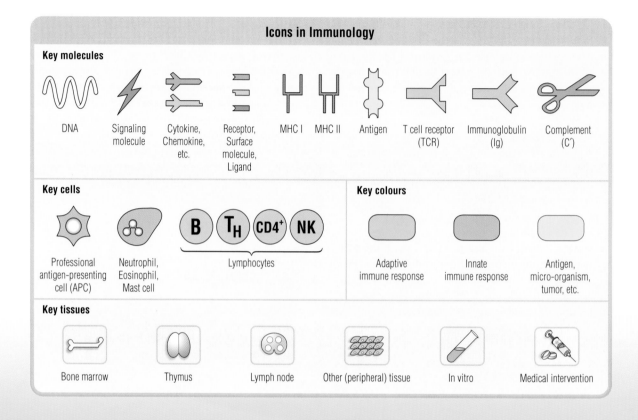

Icons in Immunology

Key molecules

DNA | Signaling molecule | Cytokine, Chemokine, etc. | Receptor, Surface molecule, Ligand | MHC I | MHC II | Antigen | T cell receptor (TCR) | Immunoglobulin (Ig) | Complement (C′)

Key cells

Professional antigen-presenting cell (APC) | Neutrophil, Eosinophil, Mast cell | B T_H CD4⁺ NK — Lymphocytes

Key colours

Adaptive immune response | Innate immune response | Antigen, micro-organism, tumor, etc.

Key tissues

Bone marrow | Thymus | Lymph node | Other (peripheral) tissue | In vitro | Medical intervention

This Figure shows some of the different types of infection the immune system has to cope with. The mechanisms used by the immune system in response to each of these infections is described in detail in different chapters of this book.

Pathogen	Type of organism	
Human immunodeficiency virus (HIV)	RNA virus	HIV infection requires intimate sexual contact or exposure to blood. HIV has a small genome which frequently mutates, allowing escape from the immune response. Most infected individuals do not develop adequate immunity to clear the virus. Infection frequently results in the acquired immunodeficiency syndrome (AIDS). No vaccine exists.
Influenza virus	RNA virus	Influenza causes global epidemics. Casual contact can result in infection of the respiratory tract causing influenza. Influenza is also a small virus and new epidemics reflect the emergence of mutant strains which are not recognized by the populations' immune system. Vaccines exist but have to be changed every year to overcome mutations.
Epstein–Barr virus (EBV)	DNA virus	EBV infects the pharynx causing glandular fever or "infectious mononucleosis". B lymphocytes of the immune system are also infected and their uncontrolled growth can sometimes lead to lymphoma (a type of malignancy). EBV has a large genome which does not mutate frequently. The genome encodes proteins which help EBV evade the immune system.
Hepatitis B virus (HBV)	DNA virus	HBV infects liver cells. In many individuals, there is only transient liver damage. In others, there is chronic, severe liver damage, possibly as a result of the immune response to HBV.
Bordetella pertussis	Bacterium	*B. pertussis* infects the airways and causes whooping cough, which can be life threatening. A very effective vaccine exists and whooping cough has become rare in the developed world.
Escherichia coli	Bacterium	*E. coli* is a normally harmless bacterium living in the colon. If it enters the bloodstream in small numbers, phagocytes usually destroy such bacteria. When *E. coli* survives in the bloodstream, septic shock may occur.
Mycobacterium tuberculosis	Bacterium	*M. tuberculosis* also infects the airways. It is able to survive inside phagocytes. Because of this intracellular site it is difficult for the immune system to clear infection and tuberculosis may result. Tuberculosis is a major threat to global health, in part because patients with AIDS are particularly unable to clear mycobacterial infection.
Schistosoma	Helminth	This worm invades the gut and urinary tract. A special part of the immune system, involving mast cells, has a role in eradicating such infections.

CONTENTS

Section One

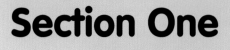

Introduction

Basic concepts and components of the immune system

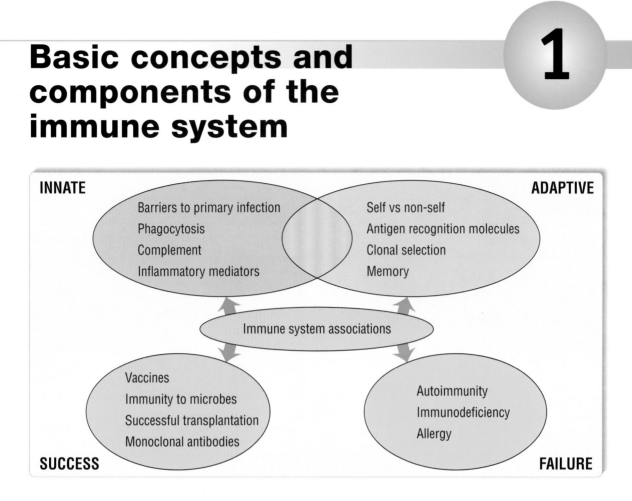

This chapter will briefly introduce the major components of the human immune system, what they do and how they accomplish their host defense role. We inhabit a world dominated by microbes, many of which can cause harm. The immune system is the body's primary defense system against invasion by microbes. Studies of the immune system are aimed at answering the following questions.

- How does our body defend itself from pathogenic, i.e. disease-causing microbes?
- How is a pathogen that succeeds in breaching the body's defenses eliminated?
- How does our body remember a prior exposure to a pathogen and respond faster and more effectively when the pathogen is re-encountered?

The human body has evolved in such a way that there are natural barriers to prevent entry by microbes (see also Ch. 2 and Section IV). For example, the skin and mucous membranes are part of the **innate** or **non-adaptive immune system**. However, if these barriers are broken (e.g., after cutting a finger), then microbes, including potential **pathogens** (harmful microbes), can enter the body and then begin to multiply rapidly in the warm, nutrient-rich systems, tissues and organs.

One of the first features of the immune defense system that a foreign organism would encounter after being introduced through a cut in the skin is the **phagocytic white blood cells** (leukocytes, e.g., macrophages), which congregate within minutes, and begin to attack the invading, foreign, microbes (see Chs 2 and 20). Later on, neutrophils (Fig. 1.2) would be recruited into the area of infection. These phagocytic cells bear molecules (pattern-recognition molecules) that detect structures commonly found on the surface of bacteria. Phagocytosis, the ingestion of particulate matter into cells for degradation, is a fundamental mechanism by which many creatures defend themselves against invading foreign organisms (Ch. 20). Various other protein components of serum, including the **complement** components (Ch. 19), may bind to the invader organisms and facilitate their phagocytosis, thereby limiting the source of infection/disease. Other small molecules, known as **interferons**, mediate an early response to viral infection by the innate system.

The innate immune system is often sufficient to destroy invading microbes. If it fails to clear infection rapidly then it activates the **adaptive** or acquired **immune response**, which takes over. The connection between the two systems is mediated by messenger

BOX 1.1
A young baby with her mother in India

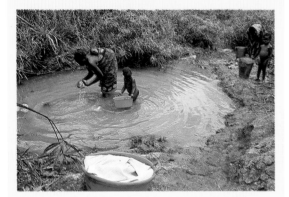

Fig. 1.1 A young baby. (With permission from Andy Crump, TDR, WHO and the Science Photo Library.)

This baby was born a few weeks ago. Her mother is able to provide her with food, warmth and shelter. However, she has left the safe environment of the uterus and is now exposed to a wide range of harmful bacteria, viruses, fungi and worms. Her mother is barely able to protect her from these pathogens, particularly in the environment of the developing world where drinking water is often contaminated with human feces. Over the next 5 years she has a 1 in 8 chance of dying from infections. The largest threat is from water-borne infections causing severe diarrhea. Measles virus infects through the respiratory tract and kills up to 1 in 20 children in the developing world. In addition, this child will encounter parasites that are transmitted through insect bites and worms that can burrow through the skin.

What is remarkable is that seven out of eight children born in this hostile environment survive. What is the nature of the systems that protect children from such a wide range of infections?

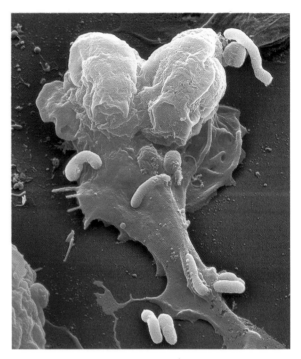

Fig. 1.2 Scanning electron micrograph of a macrophage (red) engulfing bacteria (yellow). (With permission from Juergen Berger, Max-Planck Institute and the Science Photo Library.)

Adaptive immune responses are highly effective but they can take 7–10 days to mobilize completely. A very important aspect of the adaptive immune response is the molecular mechanism used to generate specificity in the response. The immune system as a whole distinguishes *self* from *non-self*. It is able to cope with the great diversity in non-self structures by anticipating these different structures (foreign antigens) and creating a diverse repertoire of antigen receptors or **antigen-recognition molecules**. These receptors bind to small areas of the molecular structures of the non-self entities (e.g., foreign pathogens) called **antigenic determinants** or **epitopes**. The genetic mechanisms used for generation of this diverse range of antigen-recognition molecules are described in Chapters 6–8, 14 and 15. Several versions of these antigen receptors are employed by the immune system; these are **antibodies** (B cell antigen receptors), **T cell antigen receptors** and the protein products of a genetic region referred to as the **major histocompatibilty complex (MHC)**. All vertebrates appear to possess an MHC. The MHC genes of humans are referred to as human leukocyte antigen (HLA) genes and their products as HLA molecules (Ch. 8).

Antibodies are the most highly studied of the antigen-recognition molecules. In addition to being antigen receptors on B cells, they are also found as soluble antigen-recognizing molecules in the blood (**immunoglobulin** or **antibody**). Both the B and T cell

molecules known as **cytokines**. The interferons are part of the cytokine family.

The effector cells of the adaptive immune defense system are also white blood cells: the **T** and **B lymphocytes** (Chs 2, 12, 14 and 15). The B and T cells of the adaptive immune system are normally at rest, but they become activated (see Chs 2 and 11) on encountering a foreign (non-self) entity referred to as an **antigen**.

Bone marrow   Thymus   Lymph node

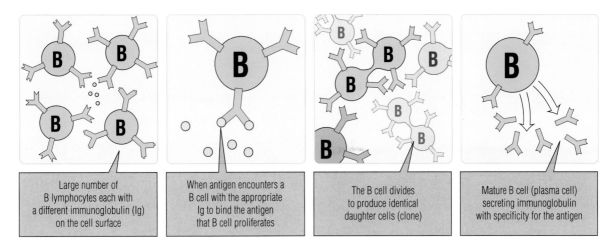

| Large number of B lymphocytes each with a different immunoglobulin (Ig) on the cell surface | When antigen encounters a B cell with the appropriate Ig to bind the antigen that B cell proliferates | The B cell divides to produce identical daughter cells (clone) | Mature B cell (plasma cell) secreting immunoglobulin with specificity for the antigen |

Fig. 1.3 Clonal selection with B cells.

antigen receptors are **clonally distributed** (see Fig. 1.3 for B cells and antibodies), which means that a unique antigen receptor is found on each lymphocyte. When a foreign antigen enters the body, it eventually encounters a lymphocyte with a matching receptor. This lymphocyte divides and, in the case of B cells, the daughter clones produce large amounts of soluble receptor. In the case of T cells, large numbers of specific effector cells bearing the appropriate receptor on their cell surface are generated. B and T cell antigen receptors differ in one very important way: B cell antigen receptors can interact directly with antigen, whereas T cell antigen receptors only recognize antigen when it is presented to them on the surface of another cell by MHC molecules (Chs 2, 7 and 8).

In addition to recognizing non-self antigens, the cells of the immune system also recognize alterations of self that result from certain disease processes, e.g., modified self antigens found on tumor cells, and may eliminate the tumor cell once it is recognized (Fig. 1.4 and

Ch. 33). The ability to recognize self antigen can, if unregulated, lead to disease, for example some forms of diabetes mellitus.

A critically important feature of the adaptive immune response is that it displays memory of a prior encounter with a microbe (or antigen). This is the basis of protection from disease by vaccination with an attenuated form of the pathogen, but it is also the way in which the body is protected from re-infection. For example, we are regularly exposed to influenza viruses. If we re-encounter the same antigenic form of influenza virus, or even an antigenically similar (i.e., cross-reactive) form, the response is faster and greater in magnitude (Fig. 1.6) and infection is limited or prevented. Unfortunately, since influenza virus is one of a class of organisms capable of radically changing its genetic structure (and antigenic make-up), there are always *new* viruses around to cause new infections.

Several overall characteristics of the innate and adaptive immune systems are summarized in Figure 1.8.

The medical successes associated with advances in knowledge about the host defense system include improvements in public health arising from vaccination against communicable diseases (Chs 4 and 23), success with organ transplantation such as with kidneys and hearts (Chs 8 and 32), treatments to alleviate hereditary defects in the immune system (Ch. 30), drugs to control the symptoms of allergy (Ch. 25) or hypersensitivity (Chs 24, 27–29) and a variety of technological developments coupled to the ability to manufacture antibodies with precise specificities (**monoclonal antibodies**): these are used for everything from pregnancy tests to diagnosing cancer (Chs 4 and 5).

Information obtained about the immune system has had an important role in our understanding and treatment of communicable diseases. Therefore, this is a

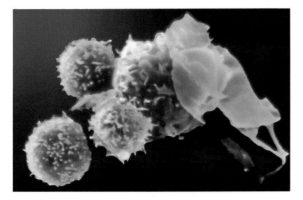

Fig. 1.4 Scanning electron micrograph of T cells (blue) and a tumor cell (red). (With permission from BSIP Lecaque and the Science Photo Library.)

subject deserving of study in medical school. Moreover, the potential for studies of the immune system to result in therapies for diseases such as cancer, or dis- eases with an autoimmune component (e.g., diabetes mellitus, rheumatoid arthritis, multiple sclerosis), strongly recommends it to the attention of future physicians.

BOX 1.2
Young person with jaundice

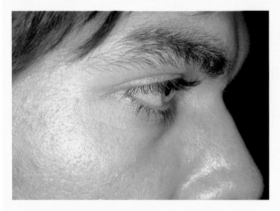

Fig. 1.5 Jaundice. (Reproduced with permission from Savin, J.A., Hunter, J.A.A. and Hepburn, N.C. 1997. *Skin signs in clinical diagnosis. Diagnosis in color.* Mosby-Wolfe; London.)

This medical student has been infected with hepatitis B virus, following a needlestick injury from an infected patient. Hepatitis B is also spread sexually, and in the developing world it is a leading cause of death in adults. Hepatitis B virus multiplies in the liver. The immune response to hepatitis B virus causes inflammation (hepatitis) and in most patients this process can eliminate the virus. If the virus persists, however, cirrhosis or even cancer (hepatoma) can develop.

However, hepatitis B infection is preventable. In recent years, hepatoma is no longer the problem it was in some parts of the world. This has been achieved through vaccines preventing transmission of hepatitis B. This book will help you to answer the question: How can such a safe, simple intervention have such a major impact on health?

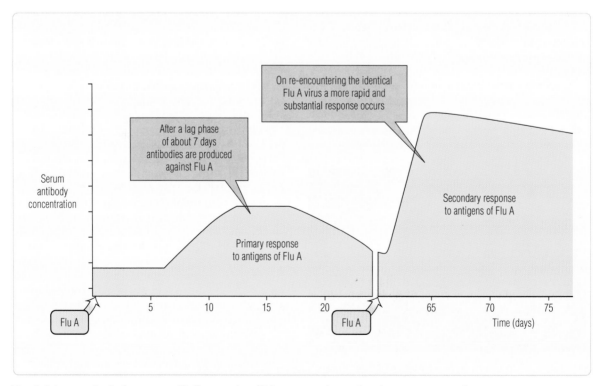

Fig. 1.6 Immunological memory of influenza virus (flu) exposure (secondary immune response).

Bone marrow   Thymus   Lymph node

BOX 1.3
A man sneezing

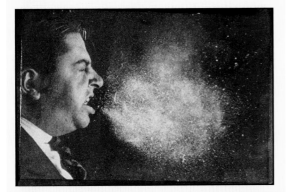

Fig. 1.7 Sneezing spreads influenza virus. (With permission of the American Association for the Advancement of Science.)

Everyone knows what it is like to have influenza. The majority of people have attacks every few years or so. In the 1990s, influenza killed approximately 1 out of 200 people that it infected. In 1918, there was an influenza epidemic that killed over 20 million people around the world. By the end of this book you should be able to answer questions such as: How is it that we fail to build up life-long immunity to influenza and why are some outbreaks of infectious agents such as influenza virus so lethal? What can be done to protect people against influenza?

BOX 1.4
Man with kidney failure

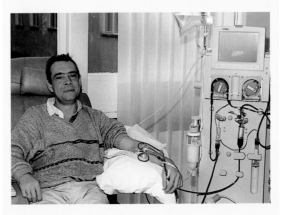

Fig. 1.9 Kidney failure. (Courtesy of Dr. H.R. Dalton, Royal Cornwall Hospital, UK.)

This man has irreversible kidney failure. Three times a week he must attend hospital for dialysis. As a consequence, he is unable to work. His relationship has broken up as a result of his constant ill health. He recently read that his treatment costs more than $40 000 (£25 000) per year. Every year, several thousand people die in car accidents. Many of these people have perfectly healthy kidneys that could be transplanted into our patient. He wants to know why he is waiting so long for a transplant. He is worried about the medication that he will need to take after the transplant. He has heard that these drugs will suppress his immune system and that they will predispose him to certain infections. Would you be able to answer his questions about his treatment? This book will help you to respond to questions like this from your patients.

Fig. 1.8
Comparison of some overall features of the innate and adaptive immune systems*

	Innate	Adaptive
Characteristics	Non-specific response	Very specific
	Fast response (minutes)	Slow response (days)
	No memory	Memory
Components	Natural barriers, phagocytes and secreted molecules	Lymphocytes and secreted molecules
	Pattern-recognition molecules	Antigen-recognition molecules

* See also Figs 2.1, 19.1 and 20.14.

LEARNING POINTS

Can you now:

- List the main characteristics of the innate and adaptive immune systems?
- List at least three examples of antigen-recognition molecules?
- Define clonal distribution with respect to antigen receptors on B and T cells?
- Contrast antigen recognition by T and B cells?
- Contrast the primary and the secondary immune response to an antigen?
- List at least three reasons why the study of the immune system is important to you as a physician in training?

Bone marrow   Thymus   Lymph node

Basic concepts

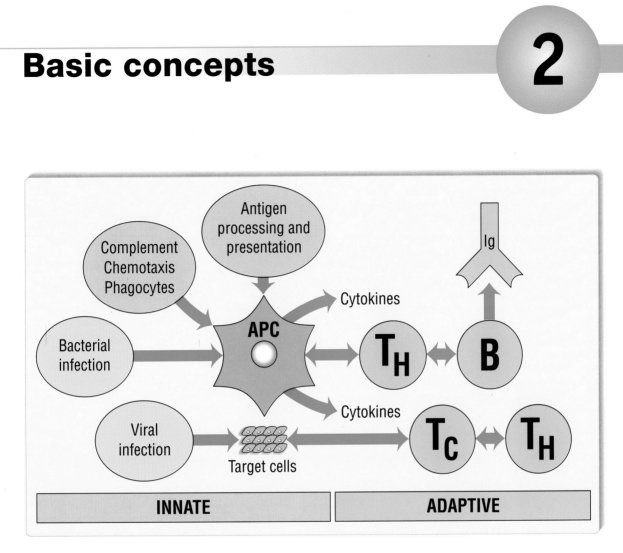

The essential features of the host defense system are an innate component that functions as a first-line of defense, and an adaptive component that takes longer to mobilize but confers specificity and exhibits memory. Figure 2.1 contrasts the main features of the two components. As shown in the overview figure above, the two components are not independent but are functionally interrelated in various critical ways, for example through the actions of soluble effector molecules called **cytokines** and other serum proteins, such as the **complement** components (Ch. 19).

INNATE IMMUNITY

An innate immune system exists in some form in most organisms. There are several important principles about the operation of the innate system. First, it is

Fig. 2.1
Contrasting aspects of innate and adaptive immune responses

Feature	Innate	Adaptive
Response time	Rapid (minutes/hours)	Slow (days/weeks)
Pathogen (non-self) recognition mechanisms	Few	Very many
Memory	No	Yes
Improvements to pathogen-recognition molecules made during response	No	Yes

fast! Unlike the adaptive system, which may take days to mobilize, aspects of the innate system are extremely quickly mobilized. For example, phagocytic cells, particularly macrophages resident in tissues, will recognize infection via pattern-recognition molecules that detect structural motifs on invading bacteria. Another pattern-recognition molecule is the mannan-binding lectin (MBL) of the complement system, which recognizes molecules containing mannose on the surface of bacteria and helps to activate the complement cascade (Fig. 2.3, below, and Ch. 19). This use of non-pathogen-specific recognition molecules is another feature of the innate system.

The innate system utilizes phagocytic cells, chiefly neutrophils and macrophages, and a limited number of molecules such as the serum proteins of the complement system, which can interact directly with certain microbes to protect the host. Other cells important in the innate response are the **natural killer** (NK) cells (Ch. 21), which can detect certain virally infected cells and lyse them. Another group of important soluble molecules that are part of the innate defense system are the interferons (Ch. 19). Viral infection triggers interferon production by the infected cell. Interferon will inhibit the replication of many viruses and is not pathogen specific.

Many innate system components, for example complement, interferon and other mediator molecules or cells (such as macrophages), can affect cells of the specific adaptive system. This is another important concept. The innate and adaptive systems are interconnected and overlapping. The adaptive system is usually triggered by the innate system and it only comes into play if the innate system fails to overwhelm the invaders, or if the invading organism has found a way to avoid interaction with the innate system. The innate and adaptive systems will be compared and contrasted throughout the book, and the mechanisms that pathogens use to avoid detection by the immune system will also be the subject of a later discussion.

ADAPTIVE IMMUNITY

An innate immune defense system is widespread in nature but an adaptive system is first observed in the evolutionary tree at the level of vertebrates. The adaptive immune system is capable of specifically distinguishing self from non-self. This is accomplished by creating an anticipatory defense system of recognition molecules that interact with foreign, non-self antigen. Vertebrate genomes contain a number of genes encoding a large number of antigen-recognition molecules. These gene families include antigen receptors capable of recognizing any given antigen (Fig. 2.2), including self-antigens (unfortunately!). In addition, there is a

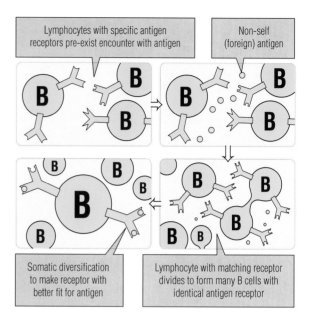

Fig. 2.2 Lymphocytes with specific antigen receptors exist before an encounter with antigen.

molecular mechanism that enables some of the receptors (antibodies) to be modified at the somatic level to create a better fit (more specific binding) as needed, to protect the host against a particular foreign antigen, e.g., pathogenic microbe.

The capacity of vertebrates to generate an anticipatory defense system against non-self entities was increased by duplication of genes in the germline that encoded proteins that had *binding sites* and could function as receptors (Fig. 2.3). The products of these gene duplications are the gene families that encode the antigen-recognition molecules (antibodies, T cell receptors, MHC proteins) we know and study today. The nature of the original function of the primordial recognition molecules is not known.

In addition to generating diversity via gene duplications, which are inherited in the germline, diversity in the adaptive response is created by somatic mutations. These occur in somatic not germ cells and so will only affect the **phenotype** and are not transmitted to offspring. Somatic mutations modify the genes for certain receptors and improve their fit with antigen. The adaptive immune response involves synthesizing receptors for antigens prior to exposure to antigen, i.e., the protective molecules pre-exist the encounter with the harmful microbe; they may then be modified during the immune response to become more precisely chemically complementary to the non-self entity.

A major step forward in understanding how this system works came with the idea that each lymphocyte expressed a unique antigen receptor. Once an antigen encounters a lymphocyte bearing the receptor

Bone marrow   Thymus   Lymph node

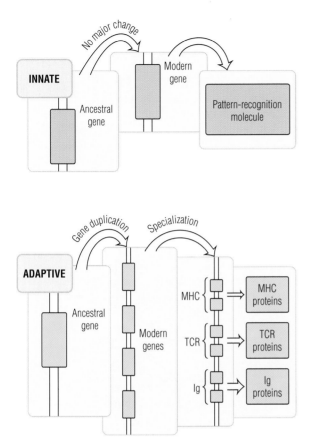

Fig. 2.3 Evolution of antigen-recognition molecules and pattern-recognition molecules. TCR, T cell receptor.

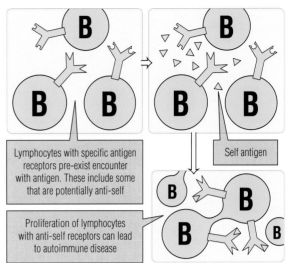

Fig. 2.4 Proliferation of anti-self response.

that best fitted the antigen, this pre-existing cell divides and gives rise to many daughter cells (clones). Thus, the lymphocyte is clonally expanded making available more of the receptor specific for the antigen encountered (Fig. 2.2). In other words, the repertoire of receptors is expressed clonally on lymphocytes and "on binding antigen" a pre-existing clone is selectively expanded to generate more of the precise receptor required to interact with the antigen encountered (Fig. 2.2).

One complication of an anticipatory system with pre-existing receptors, however, is that anti-self receptors can be generated (Fig. 2.4), and the cells carrying these potentially damaging receptors must be deleted or inactivated. When mistakes occur and potentially anti-self cells are allowed to remain active then autoimmune (anti-self) disease can occur (Ch. 27). Similarly immune tolerance by tissue the body "views" as foreign is a goal of the transplant surgeon – and of some parasites.

This model for understanding the development of the capacity to recognize and respond specifically to non-self is known as the **clonal selection theory** (Fig. 1.3). Aspects of the theory will be further developed in Chapters 6, 7, 14 and 15.

COMPONENTS OF THE IMMUNE SYSTEM

The major features of an adaptive immune response are *specificity*, *diversity* and *memory*. The response is specific in that it discriminates among different molecular entities; it is diverse in that it has the capacity to respond to almost any antigen that may be encountered, and it has memory in that it can recall previous contact with antigen and show a stronger response the second time. The last feature is the principle of vaccination, illustrated in Box 2.1.

The immune system uses cells (Fig. 2.6) and soluble molecules as effectors to protect the host. There are a number of different cell types, all leukocytes, which have specialized to have different functions. For example, phagocytic cells such as neutrophils and macrophages are used non-specifically to destroy invading microbes. Mature cells can occur in blood or in tissues, e.g., lymphocytes in blood and dendritic cells in tissue. Lymphocytes (B and T cells) provide *specific* immunity. The products of B cells, antibodies, are soluble molecules, sometimes referred to as the humoral immune system. Extracellular pathogens are eliminated chiefly by antibodies, whereas intracellular pathogens require T cells (and macrophages) for elimination. The function of T cells is sometimes referred to as **cell-mediated immunity** in contrast to **humoral** or antibody-mediated immunity. **Antigen presenting cells** (APCs), such as dendritic cells in the

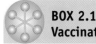

BOX 2.1
Vaccination with hepatitis B

Hepatitis B viral (HBV) infection can cause short-term illness, typically jaundice, or chronic illness such as cirrhosis, liver cancer or death. About 5000 people die from chronic hepatitis B in the US every year and approximately 1.25 million people are infected in the US. Hepatitis B is spread through contact with the bodily fluids of an infected person. A vaccine is available. The vaccine is a recombinant protein (hepatitis B surface antigen: HBsAg) expressed from a plasmid in yeast cells.

The typical vaccination schedule is three intramuscular injections. The second dose is given 1–2 months after the first dose, and the third dose is given 4–6 months after the first dose. There is an alternative two-dose schedule for adolescents that appears to be just as effective. In order to assess protection, blood samples are taken after vaccination to ensure that sufficient antibody to HBsAg is present in the vaccine recipient's blood. A level of ≥ 10 milli-international units per ml (10 mIU/ml) of antibody to HBsAg is thought to be necessary for protection. Figure 2.5 shows a graph of conversion to protected status after the three-dose schedule. If an individual does not have ≥ 10 mIU/ml of antibody to HBsAg then the vaccine schedule is repeated.

Figure 2.5 also illustrates the difference in antibody response between a primary and secondary (or subsequent) exposure to antigen. The initial, primary, response is relatively slow and low level. On subsequent immunization the response is faster and of greater magnitude.

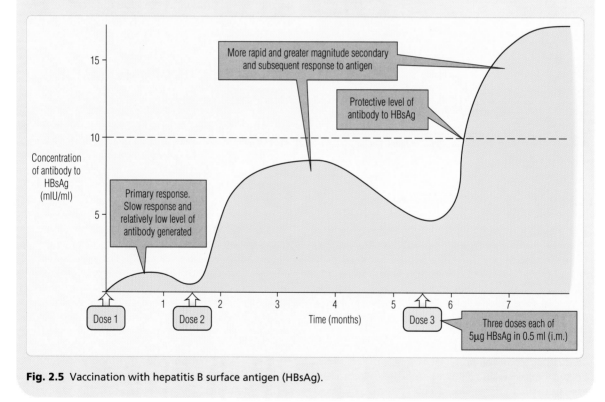

Fig. 2.5 Vaccination with hepatitis B surface antigen (HBsAg).

skin and macrophages (Fig. 2.7) are critical in initiating the activation of B and T cells.

Antigen processing and presentation is presented in Chapter 10. Briefly, APCs, such as macrophages, take up antigens and subject them to proteolytic degradation in various compartments of the cell. These events are called antigen processing and they are required because, although B cell antigen receptors bind directly

Bone marrow   Thymus   Lymph node

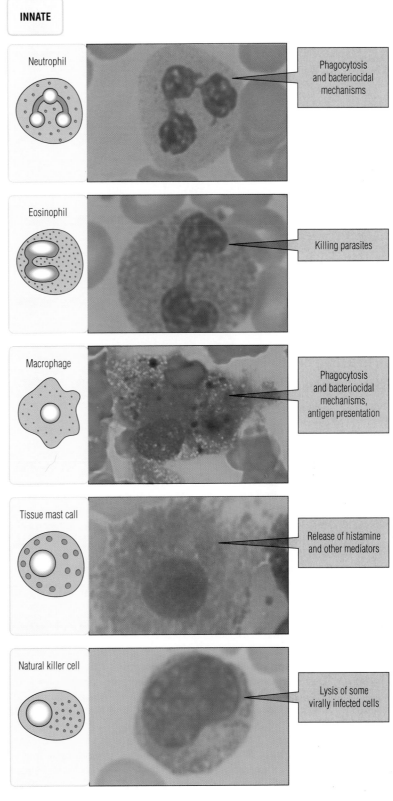

Fig. 2.6 Major cells of the immune system.

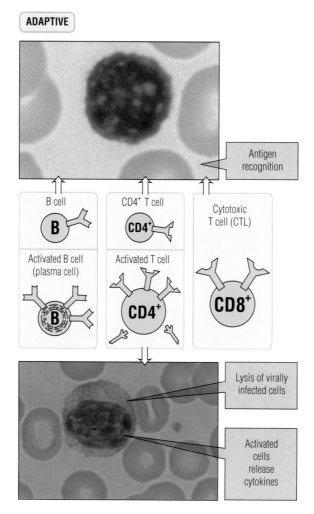

Fig. 2.6 *continued*

to antigen, T cell receptors for antigen only recognize *processed* antigen that is displayed on APCs. The peptide antigens are displayed in the peptide-binding groove of MHC molecules (Ch. 8).

Some organisms try to evade the immune system but the innate immune system has developed methods of fighting back (see Box 2.2).

ACTIVE AND PASSIVE IMMUNITY

Two further divisions of immunity exist. **Active immunity** is where the individual plays a direct role in responding to the antigen, e.g., after an encounter with influenza virus (Box 4.1). This contrasts with **passive immunity**, where immunity is transferred from one individual to another by transferring immune cells or serum from an immunized individual to an unimmunized individual, e.g., when anti-hepatitis B antibody is provided after a needlestick injury (Box 4.2). The antibodies to hepatitis B are developed in another individ-

ual and administered to confer protection more rapidly than can be achieved by the injured individual making the necessary antibodies themselves.

PHASES OF AN IMMUNE RESPONSE

There are several steps or phases in an active immune response (Fig. 2.8). First is the **cognitive phase** where antigen is recognized. Antigen encounters a cell bearing a receptor that fits the antigen. This cell is activated and proliferates (Ch. 11). Secondly, more and more of the same clone of cells is produced—this is the **activation phase**. The cells undergo various changes, known as differentiation, to enable a response. For example, various developmental steps occur (Ch. 14) in a B cell leading to a whole new cell, called a plasma cell, which synthesizes and secretes large amounts of antibody molecules. At this point, the antibodies help to elimi-

Bone marrow   Thymus   Lymph node

nate the antigen. This phase is a third phase, referred to as the **effector phase**. Various steps take place to down-regulate the response once the antigen is eliminated.

These steps are designed to regulate the response and prevent it continuing after the antigen or microbe is neutralized or eliminated.

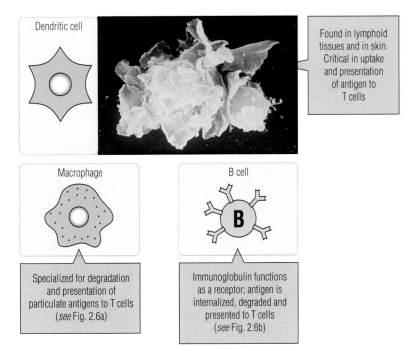

Dendritic cell

Found in lymphoid tissues and in skin. Critical in uptake and presentation of antigen to T cells

Macrophage

Specialized for degradation and presentation of particulate antigens to T cells (*see* Fig. 2.6a)

B cell

Immunoglobulin functions as a receptor; antigen is internalized, degraded and presented to T cells (*see* Fig. 2.6b)

Fig. 2.7 Antigen-presenting cells.

BOX 2.2
Dealing with sneaky pathogens

There are many ways in which organisms evolve to evade the immune system and equally numerous ways in which the immune system has developed to fight back. The innate immune system includes two populations of cells which combat special types of evasion mechanisms.

Parasitic worms have adapted to live inside the host at mucosal surfaces, notably the gut. These surfaces are out of reach of many immune system mechanisms and the large, multicellular worms are difficult to attack. Mast cells and eosinophils are innate immune system cells which reside or are recruited to mucosal surfaces and can recognize worms. In doing so, they stimulate secretion of mucus and smooth muscle contraction in the affected organ. The worm looses its grip and is expelled from the host.

At the other extreme, some viruses have evolved mechanisms for evading recognition by T cells. For example, herpes viruses can switch off expression of MHC molecules in infected cells. Because T cells use MHC molecules to detect antigen, herpes virus infection can go unrecognized. Natural killer cells have evolved to gauge the level of MHC expression on cells. If MHC expression on a cell is reduced, they are able to kill the cell. Natural killer cells thus overcome the evasion mechanism used by herpes viruses.

Mast cells, eosinophils and natural killer cells are all described in detail in Chapter 21.

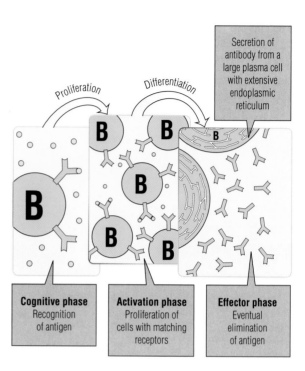

Proliferation

Differentiation

Secretion of antibody from a large plasma cell with extensive endoplasmic reticulum

Cognitive phase
Recognition of antigen

Activation phase
Proliferation of cells with matching receptors

Effector phase
Eventual elimination of antigen

Fig. 2.8 Phases of an immune response.

LEARNING POINTS

Can you now:

- Describe at least three characteristics of the innate and adaptive immune response systems?
- Describe at least three ways in which the innate and adaptive systems are interrelated?
- Explain the concept of an anticipatory immune defense system?

- Describe the phases of an immune response and the critical role of clonal selection in achieving a specific response?
- Describe the fundamental properties of an adaptive immune response system?
- List the major cells involved in the innate and adaptive immune response?

Bone marrow   Thymus   Lymph node

Section Two

Antigen-recognition molecules

Introduction to antigen recognition

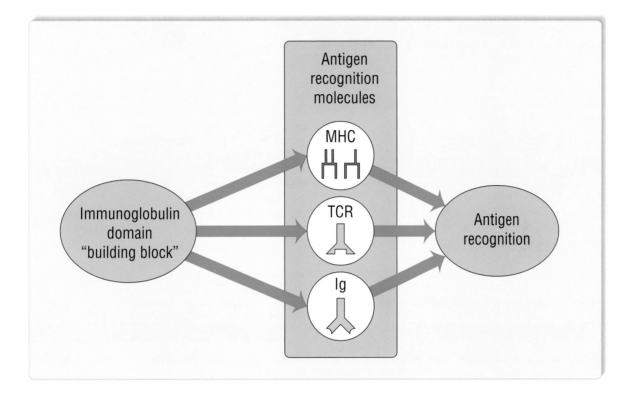

As described in Chapters 1 and 2, there are two main systems that allow humans to identify foreign (non-self) materials.

These are:

- the innate immune system
- the adaptive immune system.

The innate or non-adaptive immune system is characterized by the presence of phagocytic cells and blood proteins such as the complement proteins. These proteins are serum proteins that form protein cascades, each activated component activating the next to give a response that amplifies. Complement can bind to bacteria making holes in their membrane and can also attract phagocytes to foreign material. Complement also helps to eliminate **immune complexes** (antibody–antigen) and prevent them damaging the body. In addition to complement, pattern-recognition molecules found in the blood are also part of the innate system. For example, the liver makes a mannan-binding lectin (MBL) that recognizes mannose residues on glycoprotein and glycolipid molecules found in the bacterial capsule. Binding of MBLs to a bacterial capsule triggers the complement cascade and may help in direct killing of the bacterium (Ch. 19) or in the recruitment of phagocytes. In general, our own cells are not attacked by complement proteins because they possess proteins that inactivate complement. This is an example of how attack/defense systems like the immune system are regulated in an attempt to prevent damage to self.

The innate immune system relies on pre-existing molecules and cells, which non-specifically attack invaders, and this system protects us well against a wide range of infections. Most of the time, the innate system protects against infection by removing the infectious agent. However, it is unable to respond *specifically* to microbes or other foreign material (antigen). Microbes evolve much more rapidly than vertebrates, thus enabling them to evade non-adaptive defense systems by changing their structure. This is one reason why vertebrates developed an adaptive immune system. This system depends on gene rearrangement to generate a large number of pre-existing receptors (repertoire), expressed on lymphocytes, that can identify essentially any antigen.

ANTIGEN-RECOGNITION MOLECULES

There are three groups of molecules that specifically recognize foreign antigen for the adaptive immune system. The first two are cell-surface located receptors found on B and T cells. The B cell receptor is also secreted from differentiated B cells (plasma cells) to create a soluble antigen receptor, known as **antibody**. The third group of antigen receptors is encoded in the major histocompatibility complex (MHC). This cluster of genes is known as human leukocyte antigen (HLA) in humans. The MHC molecules function to present antigenic peptides to T cells.

B and T cell receptors (BCR and TCR)

As described in Chapter 2, adaptive immunity depends on clonal selection for its efficient operation. Each B or T cell expresses a unique antigen receptor on its cell surface. On encountering foreign antigen, the cell expressing a receptor that best fits the antigen divides and produces daughter cells (**clones**) that each have the same receptor. Diversity of receptors is generated by gene rearrangement (Chs 6 and 7). This allows a vast repertoire of receptors to be made from a limited number of genes that rearrange and combine to give the diversity needed. Thus, the B and T cell antigen receptors are inherited as gene fragments. The gene fragments are joined together to form a complete antigen receptor gene only in individual lymphocytes as they develop. The process of rearranging and joining fragments of antigen receptor genes creates a diverse array of receptors. Theoretically, the number of different antibody molecules that could be made by the B

lymphocytes in an individual could be as high as 10^{11}. This is why we believe that there are sufficient B and T cell antigen receptors to identify all the antigens, e.g., microbes, in our environment. Keep in mind that receptors for every antigen in a microbe need not exist so long as one or a few exist. The immune system only needs to identify one of the many potential antigens in a microbe to protect the host by interfering with the ability of the microbe to grow and divide.

The genes encoding B cell antigen receptors also undergo a process during the immune response called **hypermutation** to create receptors that are an even better fit for the foreign antigen. This process of rapid mutation of sequences that encode the binding site for antigen creates many more unique receptors and an even more specific and diverse repertoire.

The antigen receptors of B and T cells in addition to being generated via similar genetic mechanisms are also similar with respect to their protein structures. The **immunoglobulin fold**, where parallel strands of amino acids fold into a compact globular domain, is common to several receptor families, including the antigen receptors found on immune cells.

Major histocompatibility complex molecules

The third group of antigen receptor molecules is represented by the proteins encoded by the MHC genes. There are two main classes of molecule, which were initially named because of their role in tissue (histo-) graft rejection (compatibility). Class I MHC molecules are found essentially on all cells, and class II are found chiefly on B cells, macrophages and dendritic cells. Their function is to present peptides to T cells. Molecules in

---

BOX 3.1
The advantages of HLA diversity: HLA and HIV-1

One argument put forward as an explanation for the extensive polymorphism of the HLA genes is that the more different HLA class I molecules there are, the more peptides can be presented to cytotoxic T cells, and the less likely it will be that a pathogen could escape the immune response by expressing no epitopes that could be bound by an MHC molecule. Therefore, by extrapolation, individuals who are heterozygous for the HLA genes should be at a survival advantage compared with homozygotes. Some evidence for this hypothesis has been obtained recently. A study of several hundred patients infected with human immunodeficiency virus type 1 (HIV-1) showed that, although HIV-1-infected patients

homozygous or heterozygous at the class I HLA loci (*HLA-A*, *HLA-B* and *HLA-C*) could all progress to AIDS (acquired immunodeficiency syndrome), those patients that were homozygous for the HLA class I loci progressed more quickly towards AIDS and death. In addition, it was observed that there was a faster progression to AIDS and death with an increase in the number of homozygous HLA class I loci.

This study provides some evidence for a selective advantage of MHC diversity in surviving longer with HIV/AIDS. By extension to the human population at large, it seems likely that the considerable diversity (polymorphism) of the MHC genes contributes a selective advantage for the human species (Ch. 8).

   🦴 Bone marrow   Thymus   Lymph node

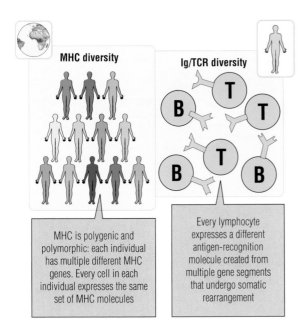

MHC diversity

Ig/TCR diversity

MHC is polygenic and polymorphic: each individual has multiple different MHC genes. Every cell in each individual expresses the same set of MHC molecules

Every lymphocyte expresses a different antigen-recognition molecule created from multiple gene segments that undergo somatic rearrangement

Fig. 3.1 Diversity mechanisms of major histocompatibility complexes (MHC) compared with immunoglobulin (Ig) and T cell receptors (TCR).

the two classes have similar structures and are also part of the family of molecules that utilizes the immunoglobulin fold (the immunoglobulin supergene family).

The structure of the MHC molecules is described in greater detail in Chapter 8, and their function in Chapter 10. Briefly, the T cell receptor can only recognize a foreign antigen if it is presented as a complex with an MHC molecule. The T cell receptor contacts residues on the foreign peptide and the MHC molecule. This is a different kind of antigen recognition from that involving the B cell antigen receptor, which binds directly to the antigen. The dual recognition requirement distinguishes T cell receptor molecules from B cell receptor molecules. The physiological function of MHC molecules is to capture and display antigens from cell-associated microbes, such as viral proteins made in the host cell, for identification as foreign by T cells.

The genes that encode MHC molecules are the most variable genes we know of in the human genome. They are said to be extensively polymorphic (existence of multiple alleles or forms of the same gene). Their diversity, however, exists in the population as a whole, not in the individual. A comparison of MHC diversity with immunoglobulin and T cell receptor diversity is provided in Figure 3.1. In each human, there are approximately six different class I and II MHC gene products. Given that their parents likely have completely different HLA genes, most people have 12 different class I and II MHC molecules on the surface of certain of their lymphoid cells. Unlike B cell or T cell receptors, which differ in every lymphocyte in an individual, all the MHC alleles are the same in an individual, but they are different between individuals. Thus, in the population as a whole, some MHC molecules will exist that can bind antigenic peptides from a given microbe but, potentially, any given individual may not bind a peptide from that microbe. This means that some individuals in the population may be more susceptible to a given microbe-induced disease than others. For example, if the structure of your MHC molecules makes it impossible for you to recognize and bind *any* peptide antigen from a given virus you will not be able to activate a T cell response to cells infected with that virus. Consequently, you would be susceptible to the virus-induced disease. However, the broad specificity of the peptide-binding groove in MHC molecules (described in Chs 8 and 10) makes it unlikely that there would be no peptide(s) from any given microbe that would fit the peptide-binding groove of an individual's MHC molecules.

LEARNING POINTS

Can you now:

- List the main categories of antigen-recognition molecule?
- Explain how T and B cell receptor diversity is achieved?
- Explain MHC polymorphism and why it is advantageous?

Antigens and antibody structure

4

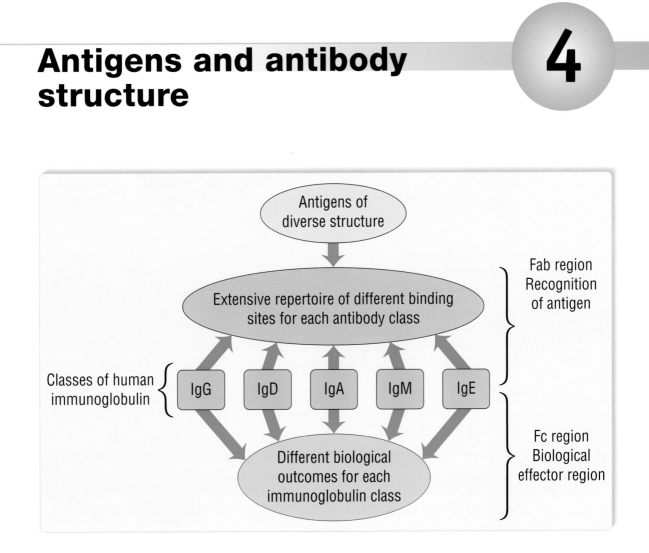

The first part of this chapter describes the various types of antigen and which antigens elicit the best immune responses. The second part describes the general structure of **antibodies (immunoglobulins)**. In Chapter 5 we explore in more depth the nature of antibody–antigen interaction and in Chapter 6 we explain how antibody diversity is generated.

Antigens that cause a strong immune response can have an extensive variety of chemical structures. Antibodies are the antigen-specific proteins produced by B lymphocytes in response to contact with antigen. Antibodies circulate in the blood and lymph as plasma components. Each individual has the capacity to synthesize a vast number of different antibody molecules, each capable of specifically interacting with an antigen.

ANTIGENS

Antigens and immunogens

In Chapter 1, antigens were introduced as foreign (non-self) molecules. At this point, some further definition is required to distinguish antigens, which by themselves may or may not cause an immune response, and immunogens, which always do. An immunogen is a substance that by itself causes an immune response, e.g., production of an antibody. Effective immunogens are foreign to the host, fairly large (generally with a molecular weight greater than about 6000) and chemically complex (e.g., proteins made up of 20 different amino acid residues are better immunogens than nucleic acids made up of four different nucleotide bases). Antigens, by comparison, are compounds capable of being bound by immunological receptors, e.g., antibodies, but they do not necessarily elicit an immune response by themselves. For example, a relatively simple chemical compound, such as penicillin, cannot by itself induce an antibody response. These simple molecules are known as **haptens**. If the hapten is coupled to a macromolecule (e.g., a protein), antibodies can be generated that bind very specifically to the hapten (Fig. 4.1).

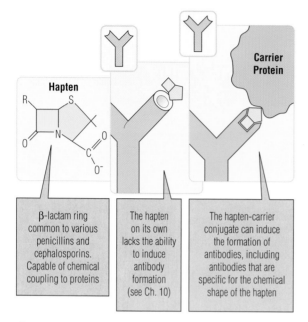

Fig. 4.1 Hapten–carrier conjugate.

β-lactam ring common to various penicillins and cephalosporins. Capable of chemical coupling to proteins	The hapten on its own lacks the ability to induce antibody formation (see Ch. 10)	The hapten-carrier conjugate can induce the formation of antibodies, including antibodies that are specific for the chemical shape of the hapten

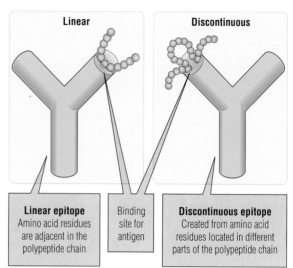

Linear epitope Amino acid residues are adjacent in the polypeptide chain	Binding site for antigen	**Discontinuous epitope** Created from amino acid residues located in different parts of the polypeptide chain

Fig. 4.2 Linear and discontinuous epitopes.

Epitopes (antigenic determinants)

The terms antigen, antigenic determinant and epitope are sometimes used interchangeably. However, an **epitope** is generally used to refer to an area on a much larger antigen molecule (e.g., a viral protein) with which an antibody can react. A viral protein may contain a large number of epitopes capable of interacting with many different specific antibodies. There are two different types of epitope (Fig. 4.2):

- discontinuous or conformational epitopes resulting from bringing together amino acid residues from non-contiguous areas of the polypeptide chain into a three-dimensional (3D) shape
- continuous or linear epitopes, which are contiguous areas of sequence, e.g., amino acids 12–22 in a polypeptide chain.

Immunological receptors on T cells recognize linear epitopes because of the way in which processed antigen is presented to them (associated with MHC molecules; see Ch. 10). Antibodies, as indicated in Figure 4.2, can recognize both types of epitope.

Adjuvants

On occasion, an antigen may induce a weak or low immune response. Substances called adjuvants provide a variety of stimuli to the immune system and, if given along with the antigen, enhance the amount of response produced to that antigen. This is discussed in more detail in Chapter 23.

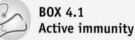

BOX 4.1
Active immunity

Vaccination, or active immunization, has greatly reduced the incidence of a number of infectious diseases (e.g., smallpox, polio). The key principle (Ch. 2) is that prior exposure to a pathogen induces a protective response if the pathogen is ever encountered again. Active immunization may involve the use of antigens prepared by recombinant DNA techniques, for example a hepatitis B surface antigen (HBsAg) very successfully protects individuals from this infection. Hepatitis B virus (HBV) is a major cause of hepatitis, which is associated with considerable morbidity and mortality. There are a very large number of chronic carriers of this virus, and eliciting antibodies by immunization with a vaccine of this type confers resistance to infections (see also Boxes 2.1 and 22.3).

ANTIBODIES

Antibody isolation and characterization

Antibodies are immunoglobulins that react specifically with the antigen that stimulated their production. They make up about 20% of the plasma proteins and were initially detected by analytic techniques, such as electrophoresis, in the "gamma globulin" fraction of serum (Fig. 4.3). Serum is the liquid phase that is separated from clotted blood. It differs from plasma (the liquid

Bone marrow   Thymus   Lymph node

BOX 4.2
Passive immunity

During the process of making an arrest of a known intravenous drug user who had broken into a house, a police officer is stabbed by a needle in the individual's pocket. Contaminated needles can be a source of hepatitis B infections. The police officer had not been vaccinated against hepatitis B virus, and consequently was given human IgG containing antibodies to hepatitis B virus (anti-hepatitis B immunoglobulin; HBIG). This antibody preparation is obtained from vacinee volunteers who have high levels of antibody and confers instant protection without requiring the body to develop a response (passive immune therapy). The protection lasts only as long as the infused antibody persists. Pooled human serum with high concentrations of antibody to hepatitis B surface antigen (HBsAg) is used to protect individuals who are not immunized and who are accidentally exposed. Follow-up therapy usually includes hepatitis B vaccine to stimulate active immunity (Box 4.1).

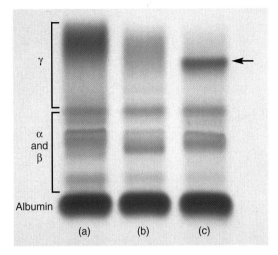

Fig. 4.4 Gel electrophoresis of serum from different patients. (a) Patient with polyclonal expansion of B cells and increased protein in the γ-globulin area. (b) Normal serum from a control sample. (c) Monoclonal expansion of B cells with an immunoglobulin spike (arrow) from a patient with a B cell malignancy. (With permission from the Department of Medical Illustration, St Bartholomew's Hospital, London.)

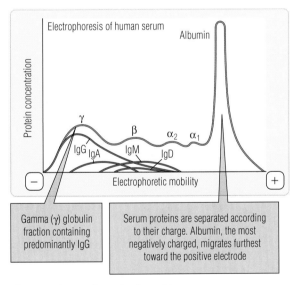

Fig. 4.3 Electrophoresis of total human serum.

phase that may be separated when blood is drawn and prevented from clotting) in lacking the protein fibrinogen. The antibody-bearing fraction of plasma or serum is referred to as immunoglobulin. The immunoglobulins in serum are a highly heterogeneous spectrum of proteins, not a single molecular species (Fig. 4.3), since normal serum immunoglobulins are the heterogeneous products of many clones of B cells (polyclonal Ig;

Ch. 2). Antibodies that arise in response to a single complex antigen (e.g., a bacterial protein with multiple epitopes), are heterogeneous in chemical structure and specificity because they are formed by several different clones of B cells, each expressing an immunoglobulin capable of binding to a different epitope on the antigen (see Chs 6 and 14). This made biochemical studies of immunoglobulins very difficult initially because pure molecules of one specificity could not easily be isolated. One finding that helped in this regard was the observation that after electrophoresis of serum the immunoglobulin region in patients with a B cell malignancy was often a band covering a very narrow range of electrophoretic mobility (Fig. 4.4). In this disease, a single clone of B cells may proliferate and these multiple cells secrete a homogeneous immunoglobulin that accumulates in the serum at relatively high concentration. These immunoglobulins became a source of relatively pure protein for biochemical studies early in the investigation of their structure. Today, **monoclonal antibodies**, homogeneous antibodies from a single clone of B cells, can be prepared in virtually unlimited quantities (Box 4.3). This has been useful for studies of immunoglobulin structure and function, for clinical investigations and for therapy.

Antibody structure

All antibodies have the same basic molecular structure (Fig. 4.6). They are made up of light (L) and heavy (H)

BOX 4.3
Production of monoclonal antibodies

The heterogeneity of a typical antibody response made antibodies hard to study or use therapeutically. Monoclonal antibodies are homogeneous immunoglobulins. They can be prepared with almost any desired specificity. Hybridoma technology makes it possible to derive homogeneous immunoglobulins of any desired specificity for use in biomedical research and for therapy. The production of hybridomas is illustrated in Figure 4.5. The aim is to produce immortalized cells which only secrete immunoglobulin directed against the antigen used in immunization. It is important to be sure that myeloma cells which have not fused with immunized B cells do not survive. To do this, the myeloma cells that are used have a mutation resulting in lack of a specific metabolic enzyme, without which they die in some culture media. After fusion, the cells are grown in these media and both non-immortalized B cells and non-fused myeloma cells will die. Only myeloma cells which have fused with B cells, and received the correct metabolic enzyme survive. Colonies of hybrid cells are grown up and screened for the production of antibody of the desired specificity. Screening for antibody-positive colonies usually involves an enzyme-linked immunosorbent assay (ELISA), described in Chapter 5. Monoclonal antibodies have found a variety of clinical uses, e.g., measurements of substances such as hormones. In vivo, monoclonal antibody anti-CD3, which reacts with human T cells, has been used as a treatment in transplant rejection (Ch. 33). Similarly, monoclonal antibodies that react with tumor cells have been used in diagnosis and treatment of cancer (Ch. 24).

Mouse monoclonal antibodies used in humans can generate complications because of the host response to the foreign (mouse) antibodies. In an attempt to overcome this problem, "humanized" monoclonal antibodies have been generated by molecular genetic techniques. Briefly, the gene segments for human constant regions are combined with the gene segments encoding the mouse monoclonal variable regions to create a chimeric antibody with mostly human sequences; this minimizes the part of the antibody that could be recognized as foreign by humans. This concept is developed further in Chapter 9.

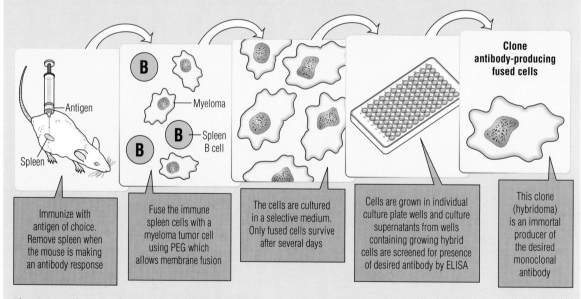

Immunize with antigen of choice. Remove spleen when the mouse is making an antibody response

Fuse the immune spleen cells with a myeloma tumor cell using PEG which allows membrane fusion

The cells are cultured in a selective medium. Only fused cells survive after several days

Cells are grown in individual culture plate wells and culture supernatants from wells containing growing hybrid cells are screened for presence of desired antibody by ELISA

This clone (hybridoma) is an immortal producer of the desired monoclonal antibody

Fig. 4.5 Production of monoclonal antibodies (PEG, polyethylene glycol).

chains, which refers to their molecular weights; the light chains have a molecular weight of approximately 25 000 and the heavy chains have a molecular weight of approximately 50 000–70 000. In the basic immunoglobulin, there are two heavy and two light chains linked together by intermolecular disulfide bonds as shown in Figure 4.6. There are five different classes of human heavy chain with slightly different

Bone marrow   Thymus   Lymph node

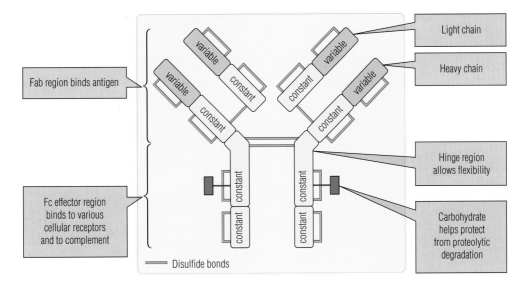

Fig. 4.6 Basic antibody structure.

Fig. 4.7
Selected properties of human immunoglobulins.

	IgG	IgA	IgM	IgE	IgD
Heavy chain symbol	γ	α	μ	ϵ	δ
Mean serum conc. (mg/ml)*	0.5–10	0.05–3	1.5	0.0005	0.03
Serum half-life (days)	21	7	7	2	2
Activates complement	+	–	++	–	–
Placental transfer	+	–	–	–	–
Cell binding via F_c receptors	Mononuclear cells, and neutrophils	Mononuclear cells, and neutrophils	–	Mast cells and basophils	–

*Varies considerably with subclass. For example, IgG1 is the most prevalent IgG subclass (~65%).

structures. These are designated by lower case Greek letters: γ (gamma) for IgG, α (alpha) for IgA, μ (mu) for IgM, δ (delta) for IgD, and ϵ (epsilon) for IgE (Fig. 4.7). Light chains are divided into two types, κ (kappa) or λ (lambda). Both types of light chain are found in all five classes of immunoglobulin but any one antibody contains only one type of light chain. Any one IgG molecule consists of identical H chains and identical L chains organized into the Y-shaped structure shown in Figure 4.6. Both IgG and IgA can also be divided on the basis of physicochemical and biological properties into subclasses. For example, human IgG molecules can be subdivided into IgG1–IgG4. The molecular structures (amino acid sequences) of members of two different subclasses (e.g., IgG1 and IgG3) are more similar to each other

than are the structures of two immunoglobulins from different classes (e.g., IgG and IgA).

The basic immunoglobulin contains parts with distinctive functions. This was shown by a number of biochemical studies. If the basic immunoglobulin molecule (IgG) is subjected to proteolytic cleavage then several fragments are produced (Fig. 4.8). For example, if the enzyme papain is used to cleave IgG, then two major types of fragment are obtained. One fragment binds antigen and is referred to as Fab (fragment antigen-binding). The other fragment, known as Fc (fraction crystallizable), does not bind antigen but fixes complement (Ch. 19) and possesses various biological effector functions, such as the ability to bind to receptors found on macrophages and various other cells. If pepsin is used the two Fab fragments remain linked

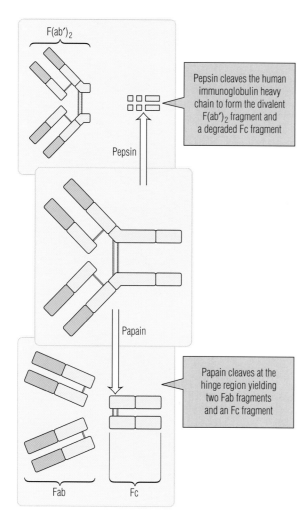

Fig. 4.8 Proteolytic digestion of immunoglobulin. Fab, antigen-binding fragment; Fc, complement-fixing fragment.

Pepsin cleaves the human immunoglobulin heavy chain to form the divalent F(ab')₂ fragment and a degraded Fc fragment

Papain cleaves at the hinge region yielding two Fab fragments and an Fc fragment

$(F(ab'))_2$ but the Fc fragment is digested to small fragments and the effector functions are lost. These findings suggested that different parts of the immunoglobulin molecule have different functions, one for binding antigen and one responsible for other biological functions.

Further biochemical studies, initially involving amino acid sequencing of the L and H chains of a number of different antibody molecules, demonstrated that the L and H chains can be differentiated into regions that are highly variable in sequence (V_L and V_H) and regions that are essentially constant (C_L and C_H). If, for example, several different λ-chains from different immunoglobulins are subjected to amino acid sequencing there will be a region of considerable similarity in sequence, but also a region of about 110 amino acid residues at the N-terminus of the L chain where substantial sequence differences are observed between different λ-chains (Fig. 4.9). The same is true for H chains. The C regions carry out the biological effector functions, such as the ability to bind complement proteins and the V regions bind antigen. The variable regions are critical for the ability to respond to a vast number of different antigen structures.

Additional 3D structure determination has revealed that the immunoglobulins are composed of folded repeating segments called **domains**. An L chain consists of one variable domain and one constant domain,

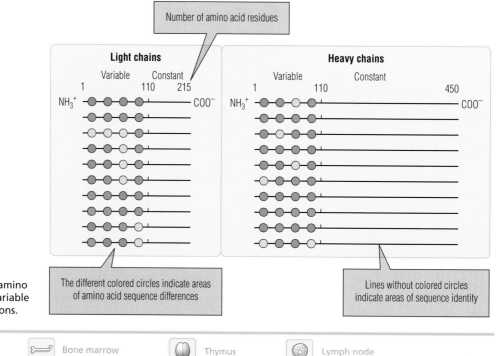

Fig. 4.9
Immunoglobulin amino acid sequences: variable and constant regions.

Number of amino acid residues

The different colored circles indicate areas of amino acid sequence differences

Lines without colored circles indicate areas of sequence identity

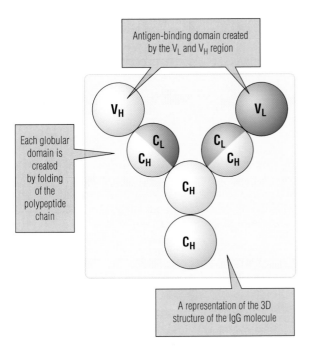

Fig. 4.10 Three-dimensional domain structure of an immunoglobulin molecule.

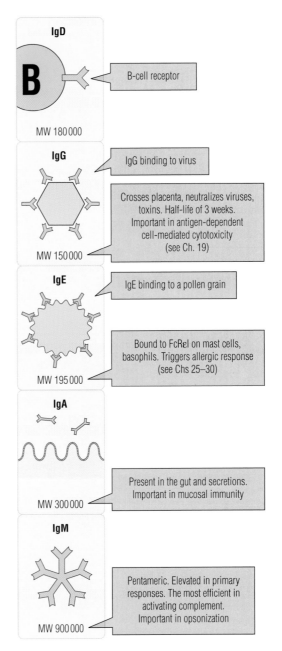

Fig. 4.11 Biological properties of immunoglobulin classes.

and an H chain consists of one variable and three or more constant domains. Each domain is approximately 110 amino acid residues long and is connected to other domains by short segments of more extended polypeptide chain, as shown in Figure 4.10. Other molecules of the immune system have similar domains, giving rise to the term **immunoglobulin supergene family** to describe this group of related proteins.

Selected features and biological properties of the immunoglobulin classes

Antibodies can occur as soluble proteins in the circulation or be displayed on the surface of B cells. The primary function of all antibodies is to bind antigen. This can result in the inactivation of a pathogen, for example by agglutinating bacteria (clumping them together) and preventing their entry to host cells. If bacteria are coated with antibody, this can enhance the likelihood that they will be engulfed by phagocytic cells (opsonization). Antibodies can also activate complement (Ch. 19) and initiate a lytic reaction that destroys the cell to which the antibody is bound. The five classes of antibody have different functions consequent upon differences in structure (Fig. 4.11).

- **IgM.** This is the predominant antibody early in an immune response. It has a pentameric structure, composed of five H_2L_2 units (each similar to an

IgG), held together by a joining (J) chain. It has ten potential antigen-binding sites and because of this it is the most efficient antibody at agglutinating bacteria and activating complement.
- **IgG.** This is the most prevalent antibody molecule in serum (Fig. 4.7). It also survives intact in serum for the longest time (has the longest half-life), and it is able to cross the placenta to allow maternal protection of the newborn. There are four subclasses of human IgG (IgG1–IgG4), and each

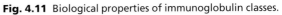

of these has slightly different properties. For example, IgG2 is generally the antibody subclass found to predominate in responses against polysaccharide antigens of encapsulated bacteria.

- **IgA**. This is the main immunoglobulin in secretions such as saliva, milk and tears, and it is heavily represented in the mucosal epithelia of the respiratory, genital and intestinal tracts. The IgA found in secretions (sIgA) consists of two molecules of IgA, a joining (J) chain and one molecule of secretory component. The secretory component appears to protect the molecule from proteolytic attack and to facilitate its transfer across epithelial cells into secretions.
- **IgD**. Less is known about IgD. It is chiefly found on the surface of B cells as a receptor molecule and is involved in cell activation.
- **IgE**. Binding of IgE to an Fc receptor on mast cells and basophils in the presence of antigen triggers an allergic reaction (Chs 25 and 26) by the activation of the mast cell and release of mediators such as histamine. IgE originally evolved to protect against parasitic infections.

As shown in Figure 4.7, immunoglobulins interact with a variety of cell types via the presence of receptors (Fc receptors of various kinds) on the cell. This recruits the cells and their products (e.g., inflammatory macrophages and cytokines) to become a part of the protective host response to foreign antigens.

LEARNING POINTS

Can you now:

- Compare and contrast antigenicity and immunogenicity?
- Define antigen, antigenic determinant, epitope and hapten, and give examples?
- Draw the basic structure of the immunoglobulin molecule indicating the location of the major structural features, for example, variable regions, hinge regions, constant domains?
- Recall what useful fragments of immunoglobulin may be produced by proteolytic digestion, e.g., the antigen-binding fragment (Fab)?
- Recall the structural features and biological properties of the different immunoglobulin classes and subclasses?

Bone marrow   Thymus   Lymph node

Antibody–antigen interaction

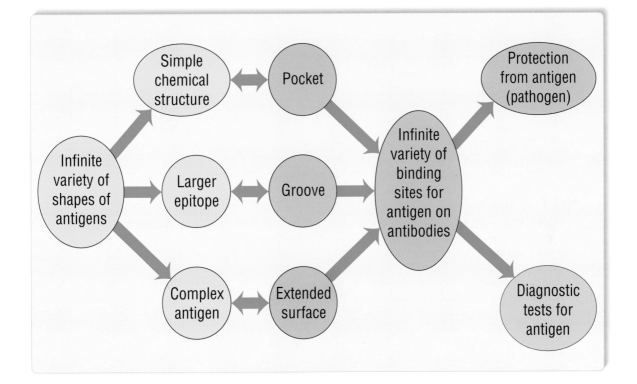

The most striking feature of antibody–antigen interaction is its specificity. Otherwise, antibody–antigen interactions are much like other receptor–ligand interactions. Similar physicochemical forces are involved in the interaction between an antibody and an antigen as between an enzyme and its substrate (or competitive inhibitor), or between a receptor (insulin receptor) and a ligand (insulin). These forces derive from:

- electrostatic interactions between charged side-chains
- hydrogen bonds
- van der Waals forces
- hydrophobic interactions.

The sum of these typically weak non-covalent interactions can be a relatively strong interaction.

The extraordinary specificity of antibodies has led to their widespread utilization in diagnostic testing. In the latter part of this chapter we describe several of the most important applications of antibody–antigen interaction in diagnosing disease.

THE ANTIGEN-BINDING SITE OF ANTIBODIES

A variety of experimental approaches have been used to define the structure of the antibody-binding site for antigen. By far the most detailed and valuable information has come from X-ray crystallographic studies of antigen–antibody complexes. One conclusion from analyses of the three dimensional (3D) structure of several antigen–antibody complexes is that the size and shape of the antigen-binding site can vary greatly. For example, the combining site of a human IgG specific for vitamin K is a long, shallow crevice (Fig. 5.1). However, a mouse antibody specific for the bacterial cell wall component phosphorylcholine, which is a chemical compound smaller than vitamin K, has a combining site with a larger, more open conformation than is found in the antibody specific for vitamin K. For small chemical compounds, like phosphorylcholine or vitamin K, the site on the antibody for binding antigen is analogous to an enzyme active site. For antibodies prepared against intact larger protein molecules

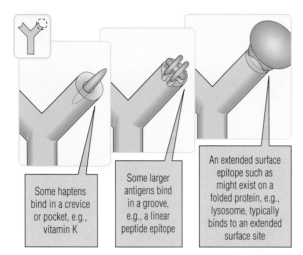

Fig. 5.1 Antigen-binding sites vary in size and shape according to the type of molecule or epitope they bind.

Some haptens bind in a crevice or pocket, e.g., vitamin K

Some larger antigens bind in a groove, e.g., a linear peptide epitope

An extended surface epitope such as might exist on a folded protein, e.g., lysosome, typically binds to an extended surface site

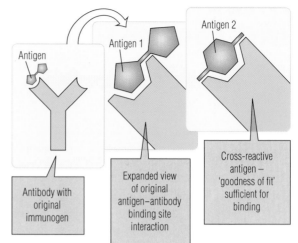

Fig. 5.2 Schematic representation of antibody cross-reactivity.

Antibody with original immunogen

Antigen

Antigen 1

Antigen 2

Expanded view of original antigen–antibody binding site interaction

Cross-reactive antigen – 'goodness of fit' sufficient for binding

(e.g., lysozyme) where the antibody will be specific for an epitope, a part of the protein antigen, the combining site on the antibody may be an extended surface, rather than a cleft or crevice (Fig. 5.1). In all cases, there is chemical complementarity between the residues of the antigen and the residues of the combining site of the antibody. The walls of the combining site are formed from the amino acid residues of regions of the variable segments of the heavy and light chains (V_H and V_L), known as the hypervariable (hV) regions or complementarity-determining regions (CDRs) (Ch. 6). Antibody specificity results from the precise molecular complementarity between chemical groups in the antigen and chemical groups in the antigen-binding site of the antibody molecule.

Cross-reactivity

Occasionally an antibody binds to more than one antigen. This is referred to as cross-reactivity or multi-specificity. The antibody is specific for antigen 1, but a different molecule, antigen 2, fits well enough to create a stable binding interaction (Fig. 5.2). This happens because there are a sufficient number of chemical interactions between the antigen and the antibody to create a stable structure, regardless of the total "goodness of fit". Cross-reactivity can have clinical consequences (see Box 5.1).

DIAGNOSTIC TESTS BASED ON ANTIBODY SPECIFICITY

A variety of diagnostic tests used in studying human disease are based on the specificity of antibodies. The advent of **monoclonal antibodies** has made several of these tests more reliable and useful because of the enhanced specificity and reproducibility of a test using "tailor-made" monoclonal antibodies. Monoclonal antibodies are derived from a single clone and all have the same specificity (see Box 4.3). The remainder of this chapter gives examples of how different tests are utilized and the general principle of each test. In general, these tests are used both qualitatively and quantitatively and can be used to determine the presence of either antigen or antibody.

ELISA (enzyme-linked immunosorbent assay)

The ELISA is a very sensitive and simple test for antigen that utilizes a covalent complex of an enzyme linked to an antibody, either to detect antigen directly or to bind to an antibody/antigen complex (see Fig. 5.4). The enzyme chosen is one that is capable of catalyzing a reaction to generate a colored product from a colorless substrate (e.g., alkaline phosphatase or horseradish peroxidase) (Fig. 5.4). The amount of antibody bound to antigen is then proportional to the amount of colored end-product that can be visualized (in a qualitative test) or measured in a spectrophotometer by optical density scanning (quantitative test). ELISA-type assays are used to screen for the presence of antibodies to HIV protein in a patient's blood sample, for example (see Box 5.3).

Immunofluorescence

Immunofluorescence utilizes antibodies to which fluorescent compounds (fluorochromes) have been

Bone marrow   Thymus   Lymph node

BOX 5.1
Drug allergy/IgE cross-reactivity

Adverse immunological reactions to drugs, particularly antibiotics, can be a significant medical problem. For example, people die from anaphylactic reactions to penicillin (Ch. 28). Penicillin can form a hapten–carrier conjugate with a self-protein that can then act as an immunogen and generate an IgE antibody (see Fig. 4.1). Unfortunately, the anti-penicillin IgE antibodies also cross-react with a number of other antibiotics. This can complicate the treatment of bacterial infections in these patients since they are unable to take the antibiotics necessary to combat the infection.

Penicillin is a so-called β-lactam antibiotic. These antibiotics contain the four-membered β-lactam ring structure, as shown in Figure 5.3. Other antibiotics with similar chemical structures include the cephalosporins and the carbapenems.

Some anti-penicillin IgE antibodies can react with other antibiotics with similar structures. The precise specificity may vary, but there is enough "goodness of fit" (cross-reactivity) to allow significant binding to these other antibiotics and to create treatment problems.

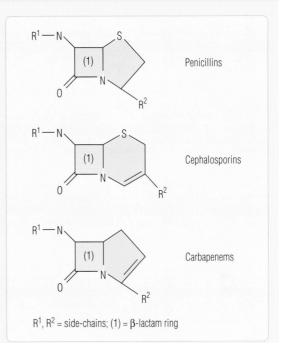

Fig. 5.3 Structures of penicillin and related antibiotics. The β-lactam ring is the shaded area.

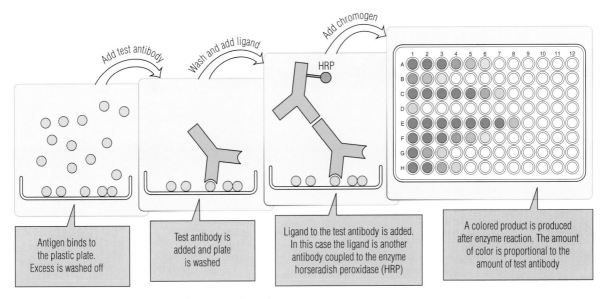

Antigen binds to the plastic plate. Excess is washed off

Test antibody is added and plate is washed

Ligand to the test antibody is added. In this case the ligand is another antibody coupled to the enzyme horseradish peroxidase (HRP)

A colored product is produced after enzyme reaction. The amount of color is proportional to the amount of test antibody

Fig. 5.4 Enzyme-linked immunosorbent assay (ELISA).

 Blood vessel   Gut   Peripheral tissue

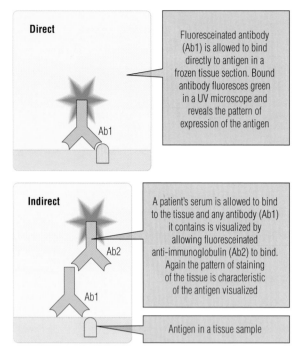

Direct

Ab1

Fluoresceinated antibody (Ab1) is allowed to bind directly to antigen in a frozen tissue section. Bound antibody fluoresces green in a UV microscope and reveals the pattern of expression of the antigen

Indirect

Ab2

Ab1

A patient's serum is allowed to bind to the tissue and any antibody (Ab1) it contains is visualized by allowing fluoresceinated anti-immunoglobulin (Ab2) to bind. Again the pattern of staining of the tissue is characteristic of the antigen visualized

Antigen in a tissue sample

Fig. 5.5 Direct and indirect immunofluorescence using fluorescein isothiocyanate (FITC). Other fluorochromes can be used with different colors.

BOX 5.2
Specific serologic test for syphilis

The spirochete *Treponema pallidum* causes syphilis. It can be diagnosed in the pathology laboratory using darkfield or immunofluorescence microscopy. This bacterium is a flexible, spiral rod (Fig. 5.6). To obtain the picture shown in this Figure, a fluorescent treponemal antibody absorbed test (FTA-ABS) was carried out. A test serum was first absorbed with non-pathogenic treponemes to remove cross-reacting antibodies. Next, the absorbed test serum was reacted with *T. pallidum* organisms on a microscope slide. Then, as per the indirect immunofluorescence assay described in Figure 5.5, any antibodies bound to the *T. pallidum* were detected with FITC-conjugated anti-human IgG antibodies under the fluorescent microscope.

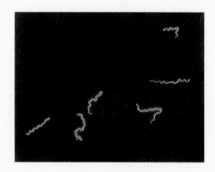

Fig. 5.6 *Treponema pallidum* visualized by a fluorescent treponemal antibody absorbed test. (Illustration produced with the help of Dr S. A. Cavalieri, Department of Pathology, and Dr R. A. Bessen, Department of Medical Microbiology and Immunology, Creighton University School of Medicine, Omaha, Nebraska, USA.)

covalently attached without appreciable loss of antibody activity or specificity. One fluorescent compound that is widely used by immunologists is fluorescein isothiocyanate (FITC), which couples to free amino groups on proteins. It emits a greenish light when exposed to ultraviolet light. Fluorescence microscopes, equipped with ultraviolet (UV) sources, are used to examine specimens that have been exposed to fluorescent antibodies. This test is used extensively to detect antigens in cells or tissue sections. It is also used to screen for autoantibodies to cell or tissue antigens (Ch. 27). Either the test antibodies are directly linked to the fluorescent compound (direct test) or a ligand that can identify the antibody is linked to the fluorescent compound (indirect test) (Fig. 5.5). Often the fluorescent ligand is a second antibody specific for the test antibody, e.g., goat anti-human immunoglobulin. An example of a clinical use of the indirect immunofluorescence assay is provided in Box 5.2.

Fluorescence-activated cell sorting

The fluorescence-activated cell sorter (FACS) is an instrument used to enumerate and/or separate live cells that express an antigen. The cells are stained with antibody that is specific for the cell surface antigen. The antibody is coupled to specific fluorescent reagents such as FITC (several other different colored fluors are available) and then passed through the instrument. The number of stained cells can be counted (e.g., the number of CD4+ T cells) and/or the stained cells can be separated from unstained cells by applying an electric charge to the stained cells and deflecting them into a collection tube (Fig. 5.7; see Ch. 31 for an example).

Immunoblotting (Western blotting)

Immunoblotting is used to characterize antigens in complex mixtures biochemically. For example, it can be used to detect individual antibodies to HIV proteins in serum samples in order to confirm an HIV-positive status indicated by an ELISA test (see Box 5.3).

Bone marrow   Thymus   Lymph node

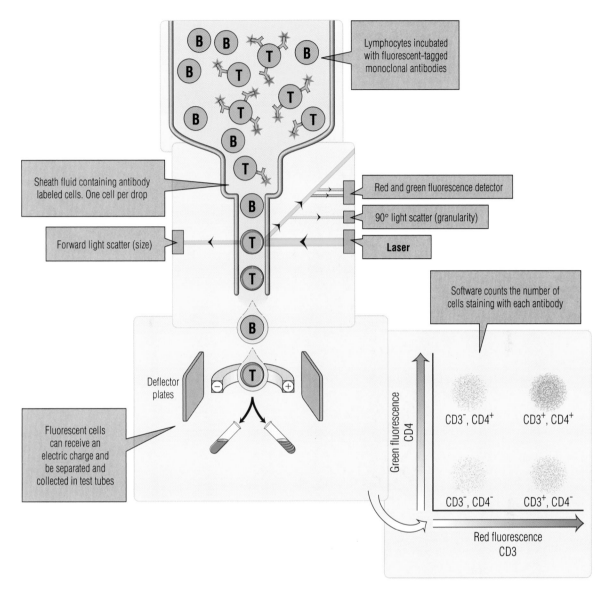

Fig. 5.7 Fluorescence-activated cell sorter (FACS).

In Western blotting (Fig. 5.8), complex protein samples are solubilized in a strong, denaturing, charged detergent (sodium dodecyl sulfate; SDS) and separated according to size in a polyacrylamide gel (SDS–polyacrylamide gel electrophoresis). The larger the molecular weight of the protein, the less distance it migrates into the gel. The separated proteins are then transferred electrophoretically to a nitrocellulose mem-brane (blotting). Next, the blot is reacted with anti-body, washed and a ligand such as a conjugate of the enzyme horseradish peroxidase coupled to protein A (HRP–Prot A) is added to detect the bound antibody. After a substrate for HRP is added, which generates a colored insoluble product, the protein antigen can be visualized as a colored band on the nitrocellulose membrane.

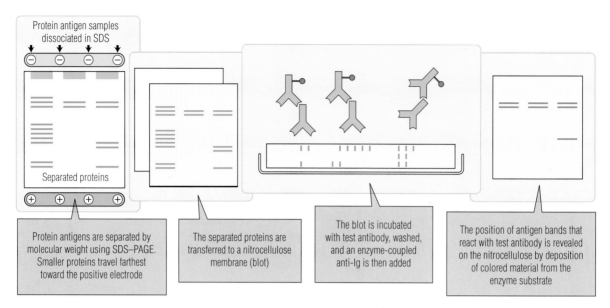

Protein antigen samples dissociated in SDS

Separated proteins

Protein antigens are separated by molecular weight using SDS–PAGE. Smaller proteins travel farthest toward the positive electrode

The separated proteins are transferred to a nitrocellulose membrane (blot)

The blot is incubated with test antibody, washed, and an enzyme-coupled anti-Ig is then added

The position of antigen bands that react with test antibody is revealed on the nitrocellulose by deposition of colored material from the enzyme substrate

Fig. 5.8 Western blotting. SDS–PAGE, sodium dodecyl sulfate–polyacrylamide gel electrophoresis.

BOX 5.3
Unexpected HIV-positive test

C.R. is a 35-year-old Caucasian woman who presents at your clinic complaining of being run down. She has had frequent low-grade fevers over the past 6 months or so, and on examination has swollen lymph nodes in her neck. She is married with two children, one eight and the other 10-years-old. None of the other members of her family has her symptoms.

On physical examination she has white plaques (thrush) on her throat and tongue. Further examination shows that her white blood cell count and serum Ig levels are normal. An ELISA test (see Fig. 5.4) for antibodies to HIV is positive, and this is confirmed by the Western blot test (see Figs 5.8 and 5.9). As shown in Figure 5.9, C.R.'s serum contains antibodies that react with HIV proteins. Further analysis revealed that C.R.'s husband was HIV-positive, but asymptomatic, and neither of their children was found to be positive for HIV antibodies. Further extensive investigation

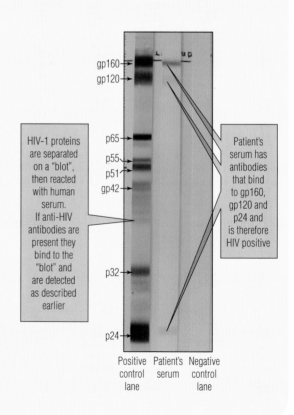

HIV-1 proteins are separated on a "blot", then reacted with human serum. If anti-HIV antibodies are present they bind to the "blot" and are detected as described earlier

Patient's serum has antibodies that bind to gp160, gp120 and p24 and is therefore HIV positive

gp160
gp120
p65
p55
p51
gp42
p32
p24

Positive control lane | Patient's serum | Negative control lane

Fig. 5.9 A Western blot to confirm HIV-positive status. (Illustration produced with the help of Dr S. H. Hinrichs, Department of Pathology/Microbiology, University of Nebraska Medical Center, and Dr S. A. Cavalieri, Department of Pathology, Creighton University School of Medicine, both Omaha, Nebraska, USA.)

Bone marrow   Thymus   Lymph node

BOX 5.3
Unexpected HIV-positive test (*contd.*)

revealed that C.R.'s last child was delivered by Caesarean section and C.R. had received three units of blood during the surgery to offset blood loss. The transfused blood had tested negative for HIV antibodies when it was consigned to the hospital's blood bank. However, further investigation showed that the blood donor had subsequently provided HIV-positive blood and been eliminated as a blood donor. The blood that C.R. had received had been obtained from this HIV-positive donor early in the infection with HIV, and prior to his development of

antibodies to HIV. C.R. had been infected with HIV from the blood transfusion. C.R. and her husband were treated with anti-retroviral therapy. Her husband has remained asymptomatic but C.R. continues to experience recurrent infections with opportunistic organisms such as the *Candida albicans* which was responsible for her thrush. She is routinely treated for these infections and she has a good likelihood of long-term survival if her viral load continues to be controlled, and HIV escape mutants resistant to the drug therapy do not develop.

LEARNING POINTS

Can you now:
- Describe antigen–antibody interaction as a subset of receptor–ligand interactions?
- Draw the structure of the antigen binding site of antibodies for various types of antigen?
- Explain antibody cross-reactivity in terms of "goodness of fit" of the antigen in the combining site?
- Describe a range of diagnostic tests that are based on antigen–antibody interaction, indicating the general principle of each test?
- List at least three examples of diseases where immunological tests are useful in diagnosis?

Antibody diversity

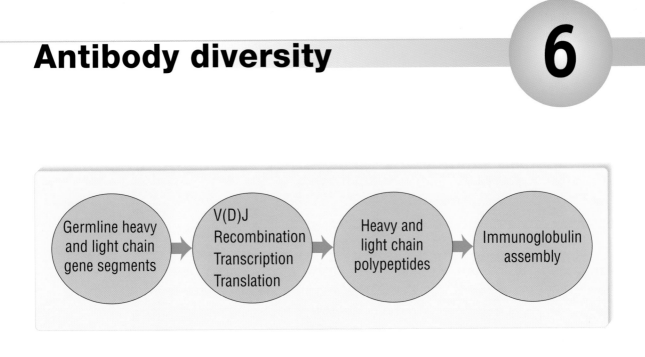

The human body appears to be capable of generating an almost infinite number of antibody (immunoglobin) molecules—perhaps at least one for every antigen in the Universe! Some calculations suggest that there could be as many as 10^{11} different antibody molecules available in the human antibody repertoire (or collection of antibodies of different specificity). The purpose of this chapter is to describe the various mechanisms used in B cells to achieve this diversity. Similar mechanisms are used in T cells to generate T cell receptor (TCR) diversity, but so far they have not been detected in other genes. These various mechanisms are collectively referred to as the "generation of diversity".

IMMUNOGLOBULIN GENES

As described in Chapter 4, immunoglobulins have two kinds of polypeptide chain, heavy and light. Each chain has a variable (V) and a constant (C) region. Instead of being encoded by a single contiguous DNA sequence, immunoglobulin polypeptide chains are encoded by sets of gene segments (Fig. 6.1) that are rearranged during B cell development (Fig. 6.2) to assemble a functional gene encoding either a light or a heavy chain (Fig. 6.3). These gene segments include leader (L), "joining" (J) and diversity (D) genes in addition to V and C genes. Each set of segments is an array of different versions of that "piece" of the gene. For example, there are five different J_κ gene segments. Figure 6.1 illustrates the organization of the human light and heavy chain gene segments and enumerates the different gene segments for immunoglobulins.

During the development of B cells (Ch. 14), the immunoglobulin gene segments are rearranged and brought next to each other to form a contiguous functional gene (Fig. 6.3). The process of rearrangement is known as **somatic recombination** and occurs even in the absence of antigen to create a repertoire of potential antibody (antigen receptor) molecules. Once complete light and heavy chain genes have been assembled, then the immunoglobulin light and heavy chains can be synthesized and the polypeptide chains assembled as an immunoglobulin molecule. This molecule is either expressed at the surface of the B cell or secreted from a differentiated B cell known as a plasma cell (Fig. 6.3 and Ch. 14).

The V regions of the chains constitute the antigen-binding site and the C regions contribute specialized effector functions, such as binding to cellular receptors or complement proteins. Antibody diversity is created by recombining different gene segments to create different V regions. This considerably reduces the number of genes that would otherwise be needed to encode the very large number of different antibody molecules.

Assembly of variable regions by somatic recombination

After the initial gene rearrangements have occurred (Fig. 6.2) the entire gene is transcribed, including the **exons** (coding sequences) and the **introns** (non-coding sequences), into a primary RNA transcript (Fig. 6.3). RNA splicing then takes place, whereby RNA processing enzymes remove the intron sequences to produce an mRNA that can be translated into protein. The leader peptide sequence (L) is then removed by proteolytic enzymes (Fig. 6.3).

The V region of light chains is composed of V and J segments, and that of heavy chains is assembled from

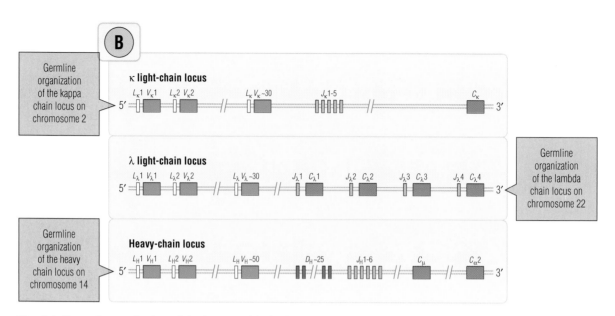

Fig. 6.1 Genomic organization of the immunoglobulin loci.

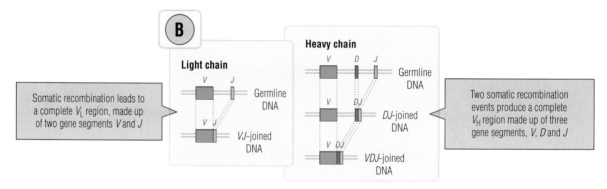

Fig. 6.2 Immunoglobulin variable regions are constructed from gene segments by recombination.

three segments: V, D and J (Fig. 6.2). In order for a complete V region to be transcribed, the V region gene segments (V and J, or V, D and J) have to be "cut out" and then joined together by enzymes responsible for DNA recombination. For example, one J segment from the array of J segments is combined with one V segment from the array of V segments to form a V_L region. Similarly, one V, one D and one J segment, are rearranged to make a V_H region. First the D and J segments are joined, then a V gene segment is joined to the DJ segment to create a complete V_H exon (Fig. 6.2). Since there are multiple V, D and J gene segments (Fig. 6.1), many different complete variable regions can be created. For example, V_1 combined with J_2 forms a different V_L region with a different specificity for antigen than that formed when V_6 combines with J_2.

The complex of enzymes involved in somatic recombination in lymphocytes is known as the V(D)J recom-

binase. These enzymes are responsible for the cleavage and rejoining of the DNA involved in rearrangement. Two of these enzymes, RAG-1 and RAG-2 (for *recombination activating genes*), are responsible for the first cleavage step involved in somatic recombination of immunoglobulin genes. RAG-1 and RAG-2 are only found in lymphocytes and defects in these enzymes lead to blockage of lymphocyte development (Box 7.1).

Gene organization and synthesis

Human light chain
As described in Chapter 4, there are two types of light chain, kappa (κ) and lambda (λ). The events leading to synthesis of a kappa light chain are shown in Figure 6.4 and described below. The process is essentially the same for lambda light chain synthesis.

Bone marrow   Thymus   Lymph node

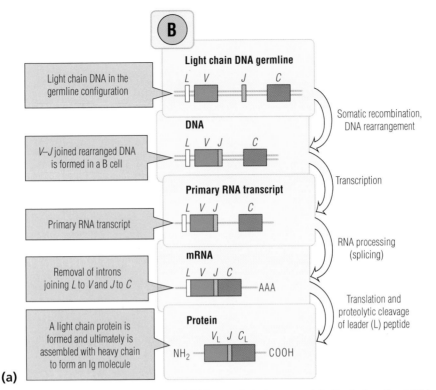

Fig. 6.3 Major steps in the synthesis of (a) light and (b) heavy chain immunoglobulin chains. *Fig. 6.3(b), see overleaf.*

In the germline of humans, there are approximately 30 different V_κ genes found in the kappa locus on chromosome 2. Each V_κ gene encodes the N-terminal 95 amino acid residues of a kappa variable region. Downstream (i.e., 3′) of the V_κ region there are five J_κ exons. Each J_κ segment encodes amino acids 96–108 of the kappa variable region. After a long intron, the kappa locus ends in the one C_κ exon encoding the constant region of the kappa light chain.

To synthesize a kappa light chain, a cell early in the B lymphocyte lineage (Ch. 14) selects a V_κ exon (e.g., $V_\kappa 3$), and after a process of DNA rearrangement involving the V(D)J recombinase, joins it to a J segment (e.g., $J_\kappa 2$). The intervening DNA, in this example from approximately the 3′ end of V_3 to the 5′ end of J_2, is deleted by looping it and cleaving it out for ultimate degradation. From this rearranged DNA, a primary RNA transcript is made (Fig. 6.4). This primary RNA transcript undergoes RNA splicing reactions to bring, for example, the $V_\kappa 3$, $J_\kappa 2$ and C_κ exons together as a mature mRNA. Splicing removes all the intervening sequences (e.g., J_3, J_4 and J_5), thereby allowing the RNA to be translated into a kappa polypeptide chain in the endoplasmic reticulum of the cell. The process is similar for lambda chain genes, except that lambda is found on chromosome 22 in humans, and there are about 30 V_λ and four J_λ genes. Each of the J_λ genes is associated with a different C_λ gene (see Fig. 6.5).

Consequently, there are four different subtypes of lambda light chain in humans.

Human heavy chain

In the human genome, there are approximately 50 V_H, 25 D_H and six J_H gene segments in the heavy chain locus on chromosome 14 (Fig. 6.1). The D, or diversity segment, like the J segment, encodes amino acids in the third **hypervariable** (hv3) or **complementarity determining** region (CDR3) of the heavy chain. The terms hypervariable region and complementarity determining region are used interchangeably but we will use hypervariable for discussions for both immunoglobulin and T cell receptor (Ch. 7).

The mechanism of heavy chain synthesis (Fig. 6.6) is very similar to that described for kappa light chains except that three segments, rather than two, are required for assembly of the V_H exon, and that multiple C_H exons are present in the heavy chain locus.

First the D and J segments are joined, then the V segment joins to the combined DJ segments to form the complete V_H exon. C region exons are spliced to the V_H exon during processing of the heavy chain RNA transcript.

As shown in Figure 6.6, there are multiple different C_H regions. Any given V_H region may be expressed with any of the C_H regions via a process of DNA rearrangement

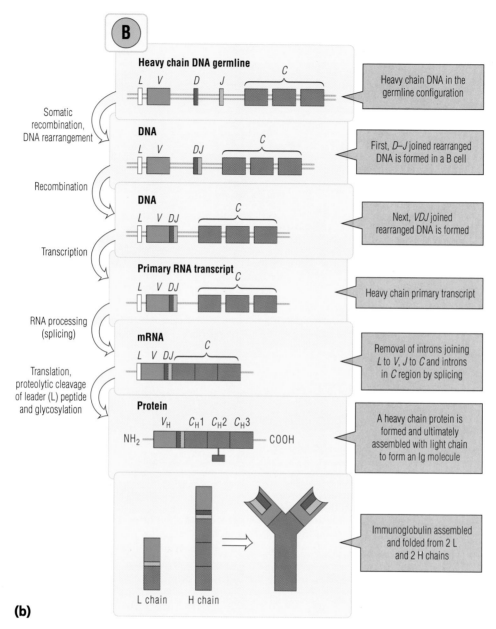

Fig. 6.3 *Continued*

referred to as isotype or **class switching**. The different C_H regions confer different biological (effector) functions. This allows yet more diversity because the same antigen specificity (V region) can be associated with C_H regions that confer different effector properties, e.g., ability to cross the placenta or to bind to different Fc receptors on different cell types (see Fig. 4.7).

Generation of antibody diversity

In order to generate the enormously diverse repertoire of antigen receptors that has been observed in humans, B cells use the genetic mechanisms summarized below.

1. V, D and J gene segments are present in multiple copies, e.g., there are approximately 30 V_κ gene segments. This is **germline diversity**.
2. VJ and VDJ gene segments can recombine in multiple combinations (**combinatorial diversity**), e.g., with 30 V_κ and five J_κ segments, there are $30 \times 5 = 150$ different human kappa light chains with different variable regions that can be formed.

 Bone marrow   Thymus   Lymph node

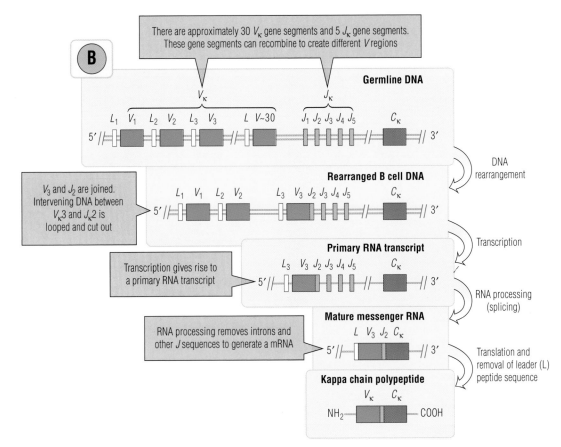

Fig. 6.4 Kappa light chain synthesis.

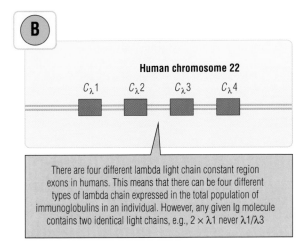

Fig. 6.5 Lambda light chain constant region genes.

3. The formation of the junction between gene segments, e.g., the joining of a *V* gene segment to a rearranged *DJ* gene segment, involves DNA cleavage, followed by the addition and subtraction of nucleotides to create a viable joint. The outcome of these events is that different coding sequences can be created at the joint in different B cells, e.g., through the random addition of nucleotides by the enzyme terminal deoxynucleotidyl transferase (TdT). Different sequences at the joint lead to greater antibody diversity, known as **junctional diversity**.

4. Multiple combinations of light and heavy chains. In principle, any heavy chain can associate with any light chain. Since both chains contribute to the antigen-binding site, this random assortment of light and heavy chains generates different antibody specificities. For example, 200 different light chains associating in random combination with 2000 different heavy chains potentially creates 4×10^5 different antibodies.

5. Somatic hypermutation after antigenic stimulation. After a functional antibody gene has been assembled and the B cell is responding to an antigen, there is another mechanism, **somatic hypermutation**, that generates additional diversity in the V region. This

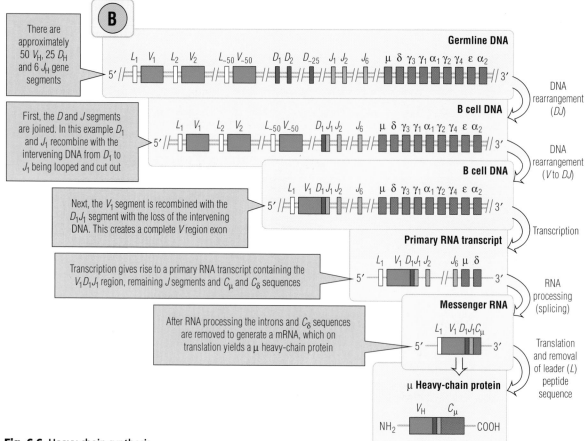

Fig. 6.6 Heavy chain synthesis.

mechanism operates to introduce point mutations at a very high rate into the V regions of heavy and light chains. Some of the mutations produce antibody molecules that are a better fit for antigen than the "original" antibody. These new antibodies tend to bind antigen with a higher affinity and B cells expressing them are preferentially selected for maturation into plasma cells (Ch. 14). This phenomenon is sometimes referred to as affinity maturation of the population of antibody molecules in an individual.

Fig. 6.7
Junctional diversity in joining V_H to a $D_H J_H$ segment (V_H ... A.GCG.CGA AAT.A ... $D_H J_H$)

	Initial gene segments	Nuclease deletion of one nucleotide	TdT addition of one nucleotide
Germline DNA sequence	V_H–A.GCG.CGA AAT.A–$D_H J_H$	V_H–A.GCG.CG☐ AAT.A–$D_H J_H$	V_H–A.GCG.CGA⬚G⬚ AAT.A–$D_H J_H$
	↓	↓	↓
VDJ joined DNA	V_H–A.GCG.CGA.AAT.A	V_H–A.GCG.CGA.ATA–	V_H–A.GCG.CGA.GAA.TA–
	↓	↓	↓
mRNA	–A.GCG.CGA.AAU.A–	–A.GCG.CGA.AUA–	–A.GCG.CGA.GAA.UA–
	↓	↓	↓
Protein	–Ala–Arg–Asn–	–Ala–Arg–Ile–	–Ala–Arg–Glu–

Bone marrow   Thymus   Lymph node

An example of the use of molecular genetic techniques for studies of the development of the immune response is shown in Box 6.1.

IMMUNOGLOBULIN CLASSES

Class switching

As described in Chapter 4, there are five classes of human immunoglobulin: IgM, IgD, IgG, IgE and IgA. There are also four subclasses of IgG: IgG1, IgG2, IgG3

and IgG4. There are C_H genes for each of these immunoglobulins (Fig. 6.6) and the same V_H exon can be rearranged to associate with a different C_H exon at different times in the course of an immune response. For example, early in the immune response to an antigen, a B cell will express IgM. Later, in the response to the same antigen the assembled V region may be expressed in an IgG antibody. This change involves DNA recombination between specific regions, called switch regions. Class switching is sometimes called **isotype switching** because the different classes of immunoglobulin are also called isotypes. Using a

BOX 6.1
Detection of immunoglobulin gene rearrangement

Immunoglobulin gene rearrangement can be detected using the technique of Southern blot analysis (see Fig. 6.8).

In this example, relatively intact, high molecular weight DNA was extracted from a non-B cell (e.g., skin fibroblast), a cloned B cell line (e.g., a B cell tumor line maintained in vitro) and polyclonal B cells purified from a normal (control) blood sample. Each of the DNA samples was then digested with the same

restriction enzymes that recognize randomly distributed base pair sequences throughout the genomic DNA. The fragments of DNA obtained after enzyme digestion (the so-called restriction fragments) are of different sizes. These DNA fragments are electrophoresed through a gel and separated according to size. The smaller fragments travel the farthest into the gel. The separated

continued

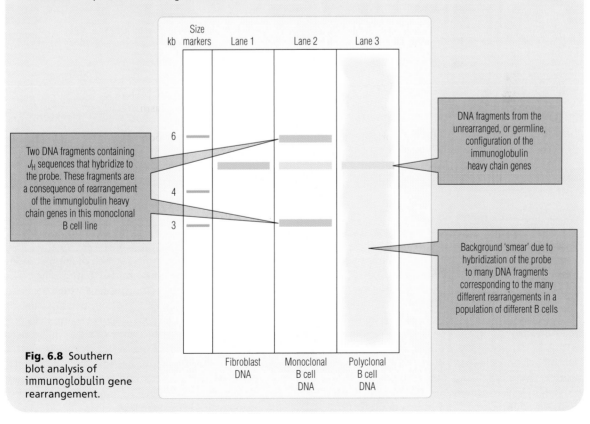

Two DNA fragments containing J_H sequences that hybridize to the probe. These fragments are a consequence of rearrangement of the immunglobulin heavy chain genes in this monoclonal B cell line

DNA fragments from the unrearranged, or germline, configuration of the immunoglobulin heavy chain genes

Background 'smear' due to hybridization of the probe to many DNA fragments corresponding to the many different rearrangements in a population of different B cells

Fig. 6.8 Southern blot analysis of immunoglobulin gene rearrangement.

> ### BOX 6.1
> ### Detection of immunoglobulin gene rearrangement (*contd.*)
>
> fragments are then "blotted" onto a piece of filter paper in a manner similar to that described for proteins in the Western blotting technique described in Chapter 5 (see Fig. 5.8). The DNA fragments remain fixed on the filter paper in their gel locations.
>
> A specific gene(s) can then be detected using a cloned piece of DNA as a probe. For example, if a cloned J_H segment from an immunoglobulin heavy chain gene is radiolabeled with radioactive phosphorus [^{32}P], this can be used to detect immunoglobulin heavy chain genes. The probe is denatured in a salt solution of high molarity into single-stranded DNA, and the filter is soaked in a salt solution containing the radioactive probe. The probe binds as a spot or band on the filter where there is sequence complementarity between the DNA fragments on the filter and the probe. The "hybridized probe" is detected when the filter is exposed to photographic film. Molecular weight markers are used to determine the size of the DNA fragment containing the immunoglobulin heavy chain gene that hybridizes to the J_H probe. This technique was first used to show that immunoglobulin gene rearrangements actually do take place, and it is still used to detect immunoglobulin gene rearrangements in certain lymphoid malignancies although it is largely being replaced by a more sensitive method involving the
>
> polymerase chain reaction (PCR).
>
> In Figure 6.8, a Southern blot analysis of immunoglobulin gene rearrangement is diagrammed. Lane 1 shows that in DNA from a fibroblast (non-B cell), the J_H probe detects one unrearranged, so-called, germline band of approximately 4.5 kb. The DNA from a cloned (i.e., monoclonal) B cell line (Lane 2), exhibits three bands that hybridize with the J_H DNA probe, i.e., the germline band and two other bands that result from the rearrangement of both alleles of the heavy chain gene in this B cell line. Lane 3 shows the results of hybridization of the J_H probe to DNA fragments from a polyclonal population of B cells. Since there are a very large number of B cells in a blood sample, and each exhibits a different immunoglobulin gene giving rise to DNA fragments of different sizes, there is a "smear" of DNA in the lane with no distinct bands other than the germline band.
>
> The techniques of molecular biology/molecular genetics, such as the Southern blot technique illustrated here, have been very useful for understanding the immune system and for the detection and monitoring of lymphoid malignancies (see Chs 14 and 34). Compare this diagram with Figure 4.4, which shows monoclonality and polyclonality of the protein product of these genes.

different constant region creates additional diversity, since different effector functions are associated with different C regions.

Expression of both IgM and IgD on B cells

IgD is frequently found on the surface of B cells co expressed with IgM. These two classes are co-expressed not by class switching but by alternative processing of a primary RNA transcript (Fig. 6.9). Transcription can proceed from a *VDJ* region through both the C_μ and C_δ exons to yield a long primary transcript RNA. This RNA can then be differentially processed by cleavage, polyadenylation and splicing. If processing utilizes the first polyadenylation site (pA1) then a μ heavy chain mRNA is derived. If processing utilizes the second polyadenylation site (pA2) then a δ heavy chain mRNA results. The mechanisms that regulate the choice of polyadenylation site are not fully understood. The significance of co-expression of IgM and IgD for B cell

function is also not clear but may be related to B cell memory (Ch. 17).

Membrane-bound and secreted immunoglobulin

B cells can produce immunoglobulins as membrane-bound or secreted forms. The membrane-bound form of immunoglobulin has an additional approximately 30 amino acid residues at the C-terminus of the heavy chain. These residues include a stretch of approximately 25 hydrophobic amino acids that anchor the immunoglobulin in the cell membrane where it can act as a receptor (see Ch. 11). The two different forms are encoded in different C_H exons, and alternative RNA processing (Fig. 6.10) is used to generate either the secreted or the membrane-bound form. Again, the mechanism of regulation of this alternative RNA processing or choice of polyadenylation sites is not fully understood. Presumably signals generated by antigen binding and/or interaction with T cells are involved (see Ch. 16).

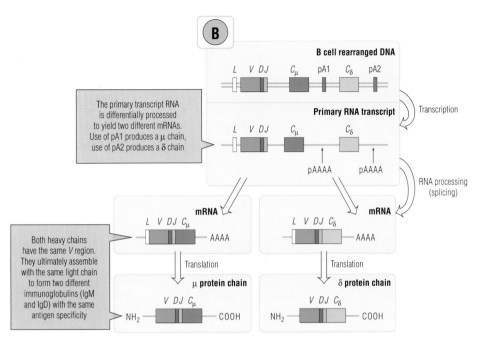

Fig. 6.9 Alternative RNA processing to allow co-expression of IgM and IgD. pA, polyadenylation site.

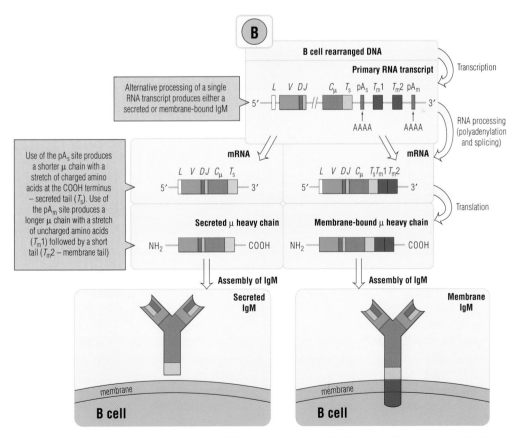

Fig. 6.10 Cell surface (transmembrane) and secreted forms of immunoglobulin. pA$_s$, polyadenylation site for the secreted form; pA$_m$, polyadenylation site for the membrane-bound form.

ALLELIC EXCLUSION

There are genetic polymorphisms (numerous different alleles at a single locus) of both heavy and light chain genes; these are known as **allotypes**. In heterozygous individuals who have, for example, inherited two alternative forms of the constant region gene for IgG1 (i.e., IgG1m(1) and IgG1m(2)), both forms will be found in the individual's total complement of immunoglobulins, but any one given B cell will express only immunoglobulins of one allotype. This phenomenon is known as **allelic exclusion**, and it indicates that only one of the two parental chromosomes expresses that gene in any given B cell (Fig. 6.11; see also Ch. 14).

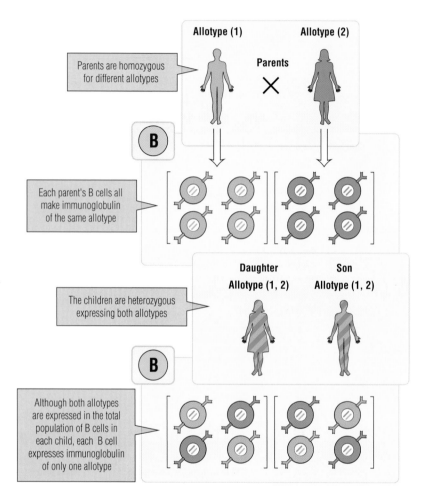

Fig. 6.11 Allelic exclusion.

LEARNING POINTS

Can you now:

- Explain how rearrangement of gene segments generates an antibody repertoire?
- Draw a diagram of immunoglobulin light chain gene organization and synthesis?
- Draw a diagram of immunoglobulin heavy chain gene organization and synthesis?
- Describe the various mechanisms that contribute to the generation of antibody diversity, e.g., rearranging multiple gene segments?
- Recall that there is allelic exclusion of immunoglobulin genes and explain why this is functionally significant?
- Draw a diagram of the process of class switching?
- Draw a diagram of the process used to generate membrane-bound and secreted forms of immunoglobulin?

 Bone marrow   Thymus   Lymph node

The T cell receptor

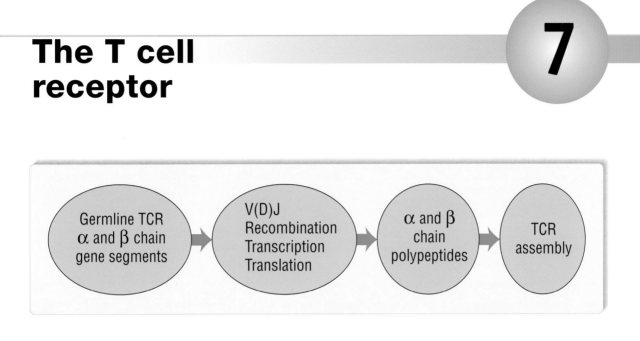

This chapter describes the antigen recognition molecule of T cells. As described in Chapter 2, T cell receptors (TCRs) recognize peptide antigens only when they are displayed by self-MHC molecules, i.e., they have a dual specificity. This is quite unlike the B cell antigen recognition molecule (antibody), which binds various kinds of peptide and non-peptide antigen directly. Despite the different mechanism of antigen recognition employed, the TCR is structurally similar to immunoglobulin (Fig. 7.1). The TCR, like the B cell antigen receptor, is clonally distributed. Every clone of T cells expresses a different antigen-receptor molecule.

BIOCHEMICAL CHARACTERIZATION AND RELATIONSHIP TO IMMUNOGLOBULIN

The TCR is a heterodimeric membrane protein. There are two types of receptor: receptors with $\alpha\beta$ (alpha/beta) chains are present on about 95% of human T lymphocytes; receptors with $\gamma\delta$ (gamma/delta) chains are found on about 5% of human T lymphocytes. Each of these chains has a molecular weight in the range 40 000–60 000. The extracellular portion of each chain is composed of two domains (Fig. 7.1). The overall structure is similar to that of a membrane-bound Fab fragment of immunoglobulin. The TCR domains farthest away from the membrane are similar to immunoglobulin variable (V) region domains, and the domains closest to the membrane are similar to immunoglobulin constant (C) region domains. Antigen binds to a site created by the V domains of the $\alpha\beta$- or $\gamma\delta$-chains. The

3D structure of the extracellular portion of the TCR has been determined (Fig. 7.2) and this also has a great deal of similarity with that of immunoglobulin.

Protein and nucleic acid sequence data have been obtained for many TCRs with different specificities. Analyses of these sequences suggest the existence of three **hypervariable** (hv) or complementarity determining regions (CDRs) in the variable region. We will use the term hypervariable since we used it for immunoglobulins in Chapter 6 and, in any event, the term hypervariable seems to communicate the concept more effectively. Determination of 3D structure shows that these hypervariable regions are arranged as a relatively flat surface (Fig. 7.2) that contacts amino acid residues of both the MHC molecule and the peptide antigen.

The $\alpha\beta$ T cell receptor

The $\alpha\beta$ TCR is the predominant (95%) human TCR found on MHC-restricted T cells. Most antigen-specific human T cells involved in host defense responses to intracellular microbes bear this form of the TCR. In general, when we refer to the TCR, we are referring to an $\alpha\beta$ TCR. The helper T cells that collaborate with B cells are $\alpha\beta$ T cells as are most of the cytotoxic T cells that kill virally infected cells. The $\alpha\beta$ TCR recognizes peptide antigens presented by MHC molecules (Chs 2, 3, 9 and 10).

The $\gamma\delta$ T cell receptor

The $\gamma\delta$ TCR is found on a few (5%) human T cells. These cells are derived in the thymus as a separate cell lineage from those cells expressing $\alpha\beta$ TCR molecules (Ch. 15). $\gamma\delta$ T cells have been found to be more

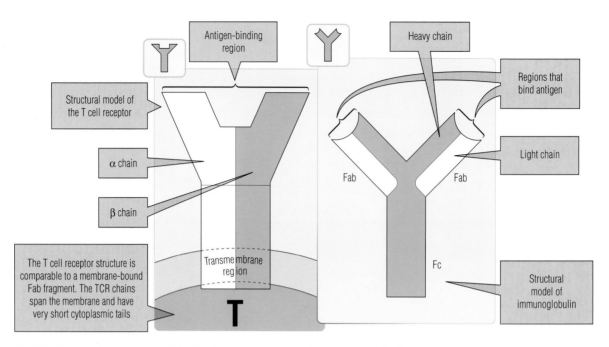

Fig. 7.1 Biochemical structure of the T cell receptor compared to immunoglobulin.

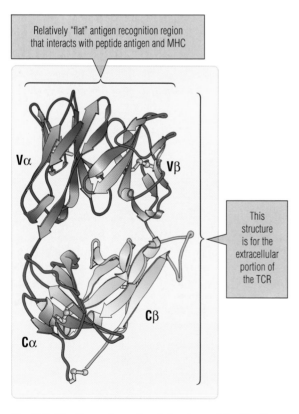

Fig. 7.2 The three-dimensional structure of the T cell receptor. (Adapted with permission from Garcia, K.C., Degano, M., Stanfield, R.L. et al. 1996. *Science*, 274:209.)

frequent in some epithelial tissues, which has led to the hypothesis that they are a "first line of defense" and may initiate responses to those microbes that are frequently encountered at epithelial boundaries such as the skin. At present, available data support the conclusion that human $\gamma\delta$ T cells do not recognize MHC-associated peptide antigens and are not MHC restricted. Some human $\gamma\delta$ T cells have been shown to recognize non-peptide phosphorylated compounds, including some carbohydrate moieties, presented by a molecule called CD1, which is similar to MHC class I molecules.

GENERATION OF DIVERSITY OF THE T CELL RECEPTOR GENES

The organization of the gene segments encoding the TCR chains is very like that for immunoglobulin heavy and light chain gene segments. As shown in Figure 7.3, genes for the α- and γ-chains are like the genes for immunoglobulin kappa and lambda light chains in that they use only V and J segments. The genes for the β- and δ-chains are like immunoglobulin heavy chain genes in that they utilize V, D and J gene segments. An unusual feature is that the TCR δ-chain gene segments are embedded in the TCR α-chain locus on chromosome 14. Another difference from the immunoglobulin genes is that there are fewer TCR C region genes. For example, there is only one C_α gene and although

Bone marrow   Thymus   Lymph node

there are two C_β genes, they appear to be functionally identical. This is in contrast to immunoglobulins where the C regions include the μ, δ, γ, ϵ and α classes, the γ1, γ2, γ3 and γ4 subclasses and the lambda subtypes (λ1–λ4), amongst others.

The mechanisms that generate diversity before antigenic stimulation of T cells are, in essence, the same as those already described for generation of diversity in B cells (Ch. 6). After stimulation by antigen, however, the pathway in T cells is quite different from that in B cells. Whereas immunoglobulin genes continue to diversify after antigenic stimulation (e.g., by somatic hypermutation and by class switching, attaching a V region to a different C region) the genes for the TCRs remain unchanged. TCR genes do rearrange in the thymus (Ch. 15). The basic molecular steps in synthesis of the TCR chains are very similar to those described for immunoglobulin light and heavy chains (Fig. 7.4). As for immunoglobulin genes in B lymphocytes, the V(D)J recombinase, including the RAG-1 and RAG-2 enzymes, is involved in TCR gene rearrangements (hence defects in these functions will affect B and T cells; Box 7.1). For the α-chain, a V gene segment (e.g., V_α2) and a J gene segment (e.g., J_α5) are recombined to form a V region exon (e.g., V_α2 J_α5). Transcription of the V region, along with the C_α exon, yields a primary RNA transcript. Splicing of this RNA yields an mRNA which on translation produces a TCR α-chain protein (Fig. 7.4) in a manner similar to that described for immunoglobulin light chains in Figures 6.3a and 6.4.

BOX 7.1
Severe combined immunodeficiency disease

Diseases that affect both T and B cells are called severe combined immunodeficiency diseases (SCIDs). Children with SCID are usually observed to have recurrent infections early in life that become life threatening because they cannot develop protective immunity. There are several defects that lead to SCID (Fig. 31.3). One defect is autosomal recessive and results in defective maturation of T and B cells. This rare defect results from a mutation in either of the recombinase-activating genes (*RAG-1* or *RAG-2*) causing a block in antigen receptor gene rearrangement. This form of SCID is expressed very early in the maturation of T and B lymphocytes (Chs 12, 14 and 15), and effectively terminates lymphocyte maturation, leading to problems in resisting viral and bacterial infections (see also Box 14.1).

Assembly of the β-chain is similar to assembly of the immunoglobulin heavy chain in that first a D and a J gene segment are combined, followed by combination of this DJ unit to a V gene segment, e.g., D_β1, J_β1 and V_β3 as shown in Figure 7.4. The complete V region exon is then transcribed along with C_β1 to form a primary RNA transcript. RNA splicing yields an mRNA which on translation yields the β-chain of the TCR (Fig. 7.4) in a manner similar to that described for immunoglobulin heavy chains in Figures 6.3b and 6.6. The α- and β-chains are translated in the rough endoplasmic reticulum and, like other membrane-bound glycoproteins, they are processed through the endoplasmic reticulum and Golgi compartments before expression at the cell surface membrane.

As with the immunoglobulins, TCR diversity is generated by (i) the existence of multiple V region genes, (ii) junctional diversity created by imprecise joining and addition of nucleotides by the TdT enzyme, and (iii) random combination of chains. Unlike immunoglobulin there is no somatic hypermutation in TCR genes. However, the total potential B and T cell antigen-receptor repertoires are similar in size because the lack of somatic hypermutation is offset by a greater potential for junctional diversity in TCR genes (see Ch. 9 for a summary). Theoretically, the T cell receptor repertoire may be as high as 10^{16}–10^{18}, with much of the repertoire contributed by junctional diversity. One illustration of the importance of junctional diversity to TCR diversity is that there are more than ten times as many J segments available for TCR α-chains as for the immunoglobulin kappa and lambda light chains.

Allelic exclusion

In allelic exclusion, only one of the two inherited parental alleles is expressed in any given cell although each one can be expressed. This occurs in B cells, where both alleles are expressed in the total population of immunoglobulins secreted by all the B cells in an individual but each individual B cell only expresses one allele (Ch. 6). Allelic exclusion is also observed in TCR β-chains but not in α-chains. In most T cells there is only one heterodimeric TCR expressed, but some mature human T cells can express two forms of the TCR, with two different α-chains associated with the same β-chain. How this influences the function of these T cells is unresolved.

RECOGNITION OF ANTIGEN

The TCRs only occur on the cell surface; T cells do not have the potential to express an alternative secreted form like the B cell antigen receptor. Figure 7.5 shows

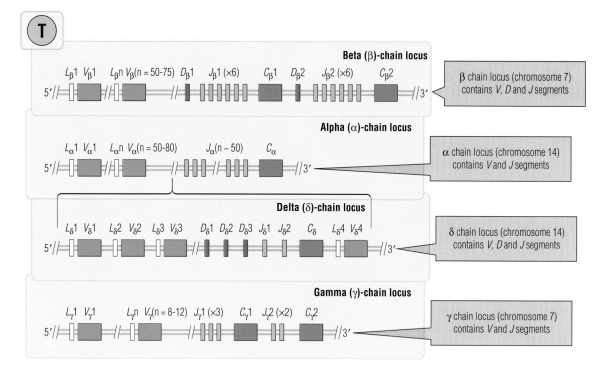

Fig. 7.3 Organization of human genes for T cell receptors.

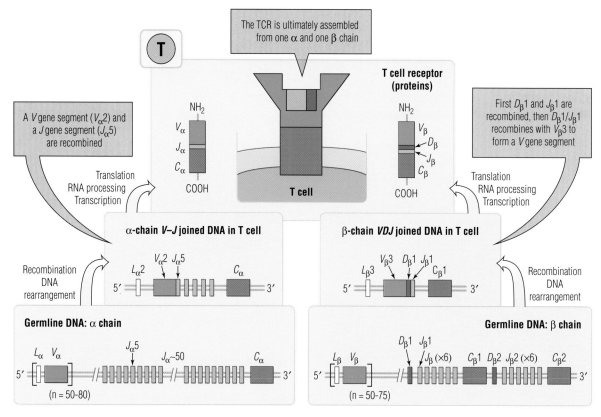

Fig. 7.4 Synthesis and expression of a human $\alpha\beta$ T cell receptor.

Bone marrow   Thymus   Lymph node

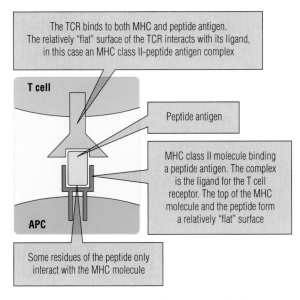

The TCR binds to both MHC and peptide antigen. The relatively "flat" surface of the TCR interacts with its ligand, in this case an MHC class II–peptide antigen complex

T cell

Peptide antigen

MHC class II molecule binding a peptide antigen. The complex is the ligand for the T cell receptor. The top of the MHC molecule and the peptide form a relatively "flat" surface

APC

Some residues of the peptide only interact with the MHC molecule

Fig. 7.5 Interaction of the T cell receptor with the peptide–MHC complex.

how the TCR interacts with peptide antigen presented by self-MHC molecules. Most peptide antigens after processing (Ch. 10) are displayed in the MHC groove (Chs 2, 3 and 8) for binding to the TCR. A few, known as superantigens, can activate T cells independent of antigen processing and presentation. These superantigens bind simultaneously to MHC class II molecules and to certain TCRs with particular β-chains. In doing so, they activate all T cells bearing this V_β region and give rise to a massive immune response (see Box 7.2).

A 3D structure analysis has been carried out on the trimolecular TCR–peptide–MHC complex and one example of this for MHC class I (HLA-A2), a viral peptide and a specific TCR is shown in Figure 7.7. This figure shows that the hypervariable sequences of this TCR V region create a "flat" surface that interacts with residues of the peptide antigen and with some of the polymorphic amino acid residues that are located in the α_1 and α_2 domains of the MHC molecule.

OTHER ACCESSORY MOLECULES INVOLVED IN T CELL FUNCTION

As shown in Figure 7.8, there are several molecules that contribute to T cell function; some are essential (e.g., the CD3 complex) while other accessory molecules assist in T cell function. This chapter has primarily focused on the TCR $\alpha\beta$- and $\gamma\delta$-chains, which bind antigen. The TCR cannot function as a receptor

BOX 7.2
Superantigens and toxic shock syndrome

Toxic shock syndrome kills several thousand people per year. Most of this mortality is caused by infection with virulent strains of staphylococcal or streptococcal bacteria that secrete peptide toxins. Some of these peptide toxins are superantigens that bind to certain TCR β-chains and directly activate T cells (Fig. 7.6). The activated T cells release cytokines. Since a large number (as much as 10%) of T cells are activated by superantigens, an extremely high level of certain cytokines appears in the blood and this induces the toxic shock phenomenon. Using knowledge about toxin binding to TCR β-chains, and extrapolating from principles of pharmacology, immunologists have designed synthetic peptide antagonists that block the activity of bacterial superantigens. This concept is further developed in Box 8.2. In animal model experiments, a peptide antagonist protected 100% of mice exposed to certain bacterial antigens. It is expected that such peptide antagonists will be used in clinical trials shortly.

Toxic shock syndrome can be brought on by infections spread in hospitals, from food poisoning, from complications of pneumonia, and from the use of tampons. This research is also of interest to those concerned about protecting military personnel and civilians who may be exposed to bacterial toxins as a result of bioterrorism.

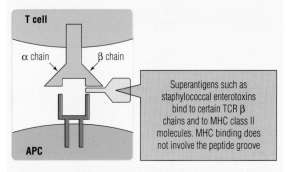

T cell

α chain β chain

Superantigens such as staphylococcal enterotoxins bind to certain TCR β chains and to MHC class II molecules. MHC binding does not involve the peptide groove

APC

Fig. 7.6 Superantigen binding to MHC class II and the T cell receptor.

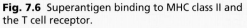

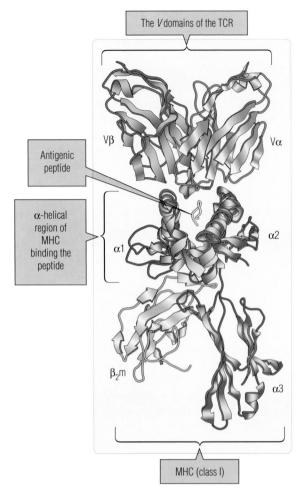

Fig. 7.7 The three-dimensional structure of the MHC-peptide-T cell receptor complex. (Adapted with permission from Bjorkman, P.J. 1997. *Cell*, 89:167.)

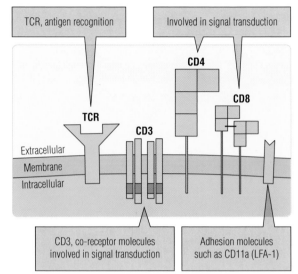

Fig. 7.8 Accessory molecules involved in T cell function.

without the CD3 complex comprising four different transmembrane protein chains: γ, δ, ϵ and ζ (zeta). CD3 molecules are necessary for a signal to be transduced to the cytoplasm after the TCR binds antigen (Ch. 11) thus allowing T cell activation. Several additional molecules (e.g., integrins such as CD11a; also known as leukocyte function-associated antigen 1

(LFA-1)) function in adhesion of the T cell to its target cell (Fig. 7.8), and yet others function both in adhesion and signal transduction. The most important of the latter are CD4 and CD8. (The surfaces of immune cells are covered with molecules that are vital to the functions of the cells. These molecules are detected using monoclonal antibodies and are given "CD" numbers, e.g., CD4, CD8.) CD4 and CD8 enhance the response of specific T cells both by stabilizing the TCR–peptide–MHC complex through binding to the class II or class I MHC molecules, respectively, and by bringing a tyrosine kinase (Lck, a member of the Src family), into the proximity of the cytoplasmic tails of the CD3 and zeta proteins, thereby facilitating signal transduction and cell activation. CD4 is the cellular receptor for HIV attachment to T cells. T cells carrying CD4 are known as T helper cells in that they promote the responsiveness of other cells. T cells carrying CD8 have killing functions, e.g., lysis of virally infected cells, and are also known as cytotoxic T lymphocytes (CTLs). The numbers of CD4+ T cells and CD8+ T cells are measured to assess disease progression in a number of infections including HIV.

LEARNING POINTS

Can you now:

- Draw the biochemical structure of the antigen recognition proteins of the TCR?
- Explain the roles of the various proteins in the TCR complex and list the major accessory molecules involved in T cell recognition?
- Recall the structural relationship between immunoglobulin and the TCR?
- Differentiate between the $\alpha\beta$ and $\gamma\delta$ TCRs and recall their different functional roles?
- Draw the TCR gene organization ($\alpha\beta$ and $\gamma\delta$)?
- Describe the genetic mechanisms involved in the generation of TCR diversity, e.g., junctional diversity?
- Compare and contrast the generation of diversity for immunoglobulin and the TCR?
- Compare and contrast the recognition of antigen and superantigen by the TCR?

Major histocompatibility complex

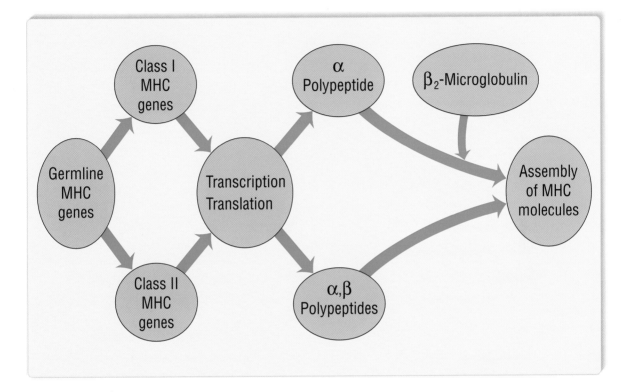

The major histocompatibility complex (MHC) is a region of DNA that encodes a group of molecules that recognize antigen. The molecules encoded by the MHC are referred to as MHC molecules and sometimes as transplantation antigens (Box 8.1). The MHCs of different organisms have specific names. For example, the human MHC, found on human chromosome 6, is known as human leukocyte antigen (HLA). The murine MHC, found on murine chromosome 17, is known as H-2. When we refer specifically to HLA we use the terms HLA genes or HLA molecules, e.g., *HLA-A* genes encode HLA-A molecules. As described in Chapter 3, HLA molecules are antigen-recognition molecules, just as antibodies and T cell receptors are antigen-recognition molecules. However, it was not until the three dimensional structure of an HLA molecule was obtained, that their role as antigen-recognition molecules became clear.

Genetic organization

Figure 8.1 shows the organization of the genes encoded in the human MHC. Only the major loci are shown. It should be noted that several hundred genes are encoded on this piece of human chromosome 6. Also note the breakdown of loci into three major classes: class I, class II and class III. As shown in Figure 8.2, there is extensive polymorphism (existence of a large number of allelic determinants) in the MHC. Indeed, this is the most polymorphic locus known. The alleles are also unusual in that they differ in approximately 10–20 amino acid residues rather than just one or a few residues. Figure 8.3 shows another unusual feature of this genetic region. Blocks of alleles (**haplotypes**) are inherited together and they are identical in families. This is largely because of a lack of genetic recombination in the MHC. Genetic recombination involves crossover and there are relatively few crossover events that take place involving the chromosomal segment that includes the MHC.

Regulation of gene expression

An important difference between the HLA class I (A, B and C) and II (DP, DQ, DR) gene products (Fig. 8.1), and the immunoglobulin and T cell receptor (TCR) gene products is that the MHC molecules are co-domi-

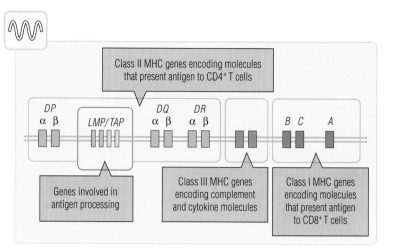

Fig. 8.1 Genetic organization of MHC. LMP, large multifunctional protease; TAP, transporter associated with antigen presentation.

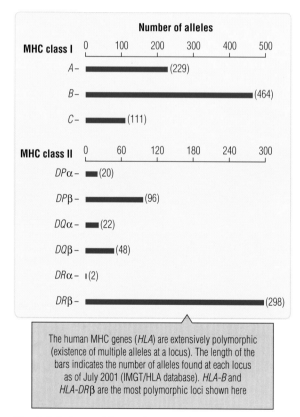

The human MHC genes (*HLA*) are extensively polymorphic (existence of multiple alleles at a locus). The length of the bars indicates the number of alleles found at each locus as of July 2001 (IMGT/HLA database). *HLA-B* and *HLA-DR*β are the most polymorphic loci shown here

Fig. 8.2 Polymorphism in the MHC. (Data courtesy of IMGT, The International Immunogenetics Database, http://imgt.cines.Fr:8104.)

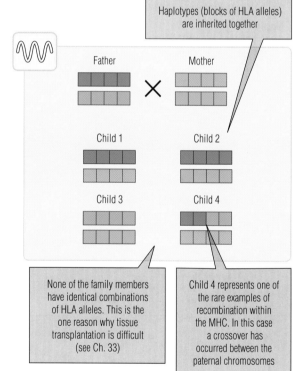

Haplotypes (blocks of HLA alleles) are inherited together

None of the family members have identical combinations of HLA alleles. This is the one reason why tissue transplantation is difficult (see Ch. 33)

Child 4 represents one of the rare examples of recombination within the MHC. In this case a crossover has occurred between the paternal chromosomes

Fig. 8.3 Haplotype inheritance.

nantly expressed. This means that both the maternally and the paternally derived allelic forms are expressed as cell surface proteins. By contrast immunoglobulin and TCR gene products have allelic exclusion (only one form is expressed on each cell; see Chs 6 and 7). This is illustrated in Figure 8.5 for a human family. Therefore except for the rare recombinant, children will express the haplotypes they inherit from their parents. Class I molecules are found on essentially every cell. This is in contrast to class II molecules, which are examples of differentiation antigens, and are found on only a few selected cells. Class II molecules are expressed on B cells, macrophages and dendritic cells; they can be induced on human T cells.

Bone marrow Thymus Lymph node

BOX 8.1
Transplantation antigens/graft rejection

The products of MHC-encoded genes were initially detected as transplantation antigens, i.e., antigens recognized as non-self when tissue was exchanged between individuals as a graft, e.g., kidney transplants. Transplantation antigens are the principal cause of graft rejection between non-identical individuals (Ch. 25). As shown in Figure 8.4, grafts between genetically identical individuals (syngeneic) succeed. All others eventually fail in the absence of other interventions, e.g., immunosuppressive drugs such as ciclosporin. This is the fundamental law of transplantation. Transplantation antigens (chiefly molecules encoded in the MHC) do not exist merely to frustrate the efforts of transplant surgeons. They are important antigen-recognition molecules that "display" antigen for "review" by T cells.

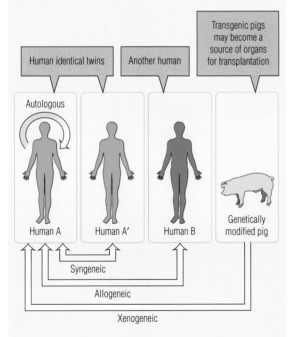

Fig. 8.4 Laws of transplantation.

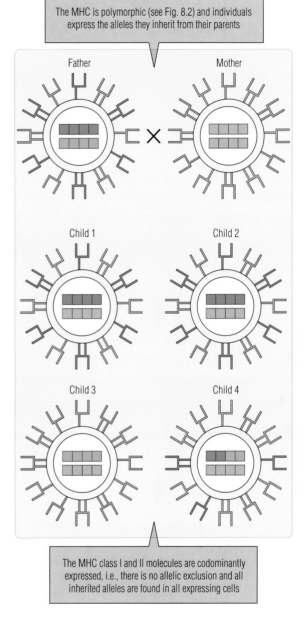

The MHC is polymorphic (see Fig. 8.2) and individuals express the alleles they inherit from their parents

The MHC class I and II molecules are codominantly expressed, i.e., there is no allelic exclusion and all inherited alleles are found in all expressing cells

Fig. 8.5 Co-dominant expression of MHC molecules.

Structure of the MHC gene products

Class I

Figure 8.6 shows the structure of the protein products of the class I genes. The class I molecules are non-covalently associated heterodimers of an approximately 45 000 molecular weight transmembrane glycoprotein (the α-chain, encoded in the MHC) with an approximately 12 000 molecular weight chain (β_2-microglobulin) encoded on a completely different chromosome (chromosome 15 in humans). Beta-2 microglobulin is a soluble protein that complexes with the α-chain during synthesis and assembly in the endoplasmic reticulum. It is essential for the peptide binding function of the MHC-encoded "heavy chain".

DNA and protein sequences obtained for a number of HLA molecules show that they are structurally

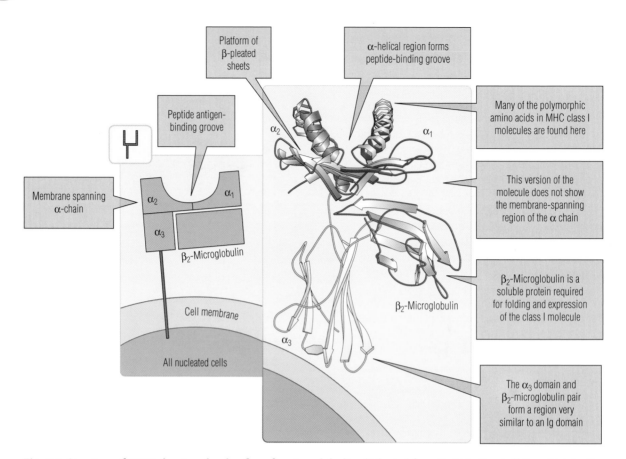

Fig. 8.6 Structure of MHC class I molecules. β_2m, β_2-microglobulin. (Adapted from Roitt I., Brostoff, J. and Male, D. 2001. *Immunology*, 6th edn. Mosby, London.)

homologous to one another, i.e., they have very similar sequences. HLA-A molecules have very similar sequences to HLA-B or HLA-C molecules. Alleles (alternative forms) of HLA-A, HLA-B or HLA-C are even more similar to one another. Thus two different HLA-A alleles might have about 90% sequence identity to each other.

The HLA class I genes have an exon/intron structure typical of genes encoding eukaryotic membrane proteins. There is no evidence for gene rearrangements, such as occur in immunoglobulin or TCR genes. Individuals inherit a set of HLA class I genes from their parents and they can express a maximum of six different class I molecules. However, the population as a whole is extensively polymorphic and large numbers of alleles, about 400 at *HLA-B* for example, exist in the human population.

Figure 8.6 also shows a ribbon-structure representation of the 3D structure of a HLA class I molecule. Once the structure was determined, it was clear that there was a binding groove in the molecule for peptide (antigen). This binding groove is formed entirely by the α-chain in class I molecules. The amino acid residues making up the groove are the chief sites of polymorphism, i.e., different *HLA-A* alleles produce different amino acids in the antigen-binding groove and they can, therefore, bind a different range of peptide antigens. The 3D structure also shows a β-pleated sheet platform structure (with homology to immunoglobulin) supporting the α-helical binding site. The peptide antigen has been said to fit into the groove like a "hotdog in a bun". Peptides of about 8–11 amino acid residues fit into the class I binding site. The precise sequence of the peptide is less important than the presence of certain amino acids (referred to as anchor residues) at particular positions.

Class II

The class II MHC molecules are non-covalently associated transmembrane heterodimers, where both chains are encoded in the MHC (Fig. 8.7). The molecular

Bone marrow   Thymus   Lymph node

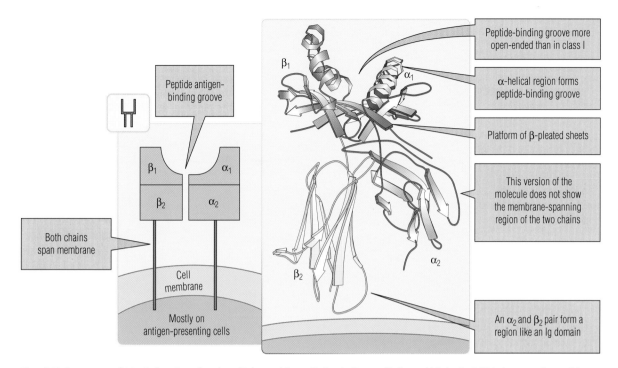

Fig. 8.7 Structure of MHC class II molecules. (Adapted from Roitt, I., Brostoff, J., and Male, D. 2001. *Immunology*, 6th edn. Mosby, London.)

weight of the α-chain is approximately 33 000 and that of the β-chain approximately 29 000 (Fig. 8.6). Both are polymorphic, transmembrane glycoproteins.

As for the class I genes, there is no evidence that gene recombination is used to generate diversity (polymorphism), and the class II genes have the typical exon/intron structure of membrane proteins. There are no variable and constant region gene clusters, as there are for immunoglobulin and TCR. When collections of gene and protein sequences for the many alleles at a class II locus are compared, however, there is evidence for regions of greater and lesser diversity. These regions of diversity are called "polymorphic" regions, and they come together in the folded molecule to form the antigen-binding groove. As shown in Figure 8.7, the 3D structure of a class II molecule has a β-pleated sheet platform structure, on top of which is an α-helical binding site for peptides. The binding groove in class II molecules is created by both the α- and β-chains.

The overall 3D structures of the class I and II molecules differ but there are similarities. The class II binding site for peptides is more "open" than the class I site, and longer peptides (30 amino acid residues or longer) can fit into the site and overlap at either end. Again, as is true for MHC class I molecules, the precise sequence of the peptide antigen is less important than that it contains particular residues at certain positions. Thus, any given MHC molecule can accommodate a wide range of peptides (one at a time). Hence the likelihood that any given complex antigen, such as a virus, would not contain a peptide antigen that could be efficiently recognized by, and bind to, at least one MHC molecule in an individual is very low. However, there is that possibility, and such an individual is said to be a non-responder or low responder to that antigen. Control of immune responsiveness is, therefore, also one of the genetic traits associated with the MHC because of the role that MHC molecules have of binding antigens and presenting them to TCRs prior to initiation of an immune response.

Restriction of antigen recognition

The discovery of an antigen-binding groove in MHC molecules helped to explain the concept of MHC restriction, which had been discovered earlier. It had been observed that T cells are specific for both MHC and antigen, and the MHC molecule must be self MHC. Whereas the B cell receptor can recognize antigen directly, the TCR only recognizes non-self antigen in association with self MHC, i.e., there is a dual recognition process. Figure 8.8 illustrates the observations that were made. Therefore, T cells must recognize foreign antigen *and* self MHC. The function of MHC is to be both a binding site (for non-self peptides) and a ligand (for the TCR). How the peptide antigens that are recog-

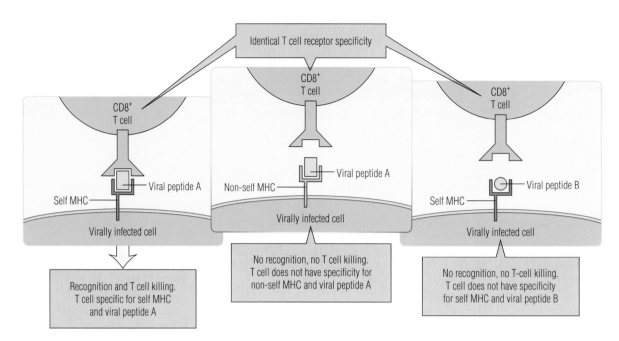

Fig. 8.8 T cell recognition of antigen is MHC-restricted.

nized by TCRs are derived from complex non-self antigens, such as viruses, and how they become associated with MHC molecules is the subject of Chapter 10—Antigen processing and presentation.

Models of the MHC–antigen–T cell receptor complex

Figure 8.9 shows a schematic model of the recognition complex involving an MHC class I molecule, a non-self peptide antigen and a TCR. The TCR contacts both amino acids from the MHC class I molecule and amino acids from the peptide antigen. Figure 8.9 also helps to illustrate how certain amino acids in the peptide antigen bind to amino acids of the MHC molecule in the peptide-binding groove, while other peptide antigen amino acids protrude out of the MHC groove and interact with the TCR.

The repertoire of TCRs that is selected during development in the thymus is dependent upon interaction with MHC molecules, i.e., T cells "learn" self MHC in the thymus during development and those that cannot bind appropriately to self MHC molecules are eliminated or made anergic (non-responsive; Ch. 15). This also helps to explain the phenomenon of MHC restriction, i.e., that the T cell receptors are specific for self MHC.

Further detailed molecular characterization of MHC–antigen–TCR interactions is relevant to various clinical situations, for example, designing peptide-

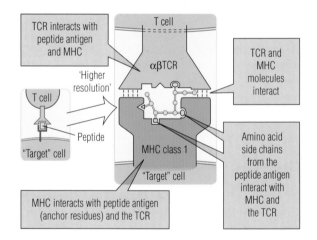

Fig. 8.9 Structure of MHC–antigen–T cell receptor (TCR) complex.

based vaccines. Investigations are underway to establish the usefulness of "altered peptide ligands", where the peptide antigen amino acids that would contact the TCR are altered to create a ligand that is an antagonist and there is no T cell activation. This is being investigated as a possible approach to therapy for autoimmune diseases that have a T cell involvement, e.g., multiple sclerosis (Box 8.2).

Bone marrow   Thymus   Lymph node

BOX 8.2
Specific immunotherapy with altered peptide ligands

The TCR contacts amino acids of both the peptide antigen and the presenting self MHC molecule in the trimolecular complex of TCR–peptide–MHC (Fig. 7.7). Amino acids at specific positions in the peptide antigen interact with the TCR, while others interact with the MHC molecule (Fig. 8.9). Borrowing a concept from pharmacology, and recognizing that the MHC–peptide complex is a *ligand* for the *receptor* on the T cell, some immunologists have reasoned that they could build altered peptide ligands (APLs) that are antagonists or partial agonists by substituting amino acids at certain positions in the peptide antigen. The approach has been shown to have validity in model systems and is now the subject of several clinical trials, e.g., for multiple sclerosis.

Multiple sclerosis is a demyelinating disease that can involve an autoimmune T cell response against myelin basic protein (MBP). A dominant T cell epitope in MBP is known to be peptide MBP_{83-99}. By substituting analogs for the amino acids at the positions in the peptide thought to contact the TCR, immunologists are hoping to "switch-off" the T cell response to MBP in patients with multiple sclerosis. Patients are given the APLs, which should bind to MHC molecules and be presented to the MBP-specific T cells. However, instead of activating the T cells, the APLs will either prevent signal transduction and cell activation (antagonist) or activate some functions but not all (partial agonist), hopefully deflecting some of the autoimmune T cells.

Population advantages of polymorphism in MHC

The existence of multiple different HLA class I and II genes means that there are numerous different peptide antigen-binding molecules available for the presentation of antigen to T cells. This is a selective advantage to the individual and to the population as a whole. A heterozygote can present more different pathogen-derived peptides than a homozygote (see Box 3.1). Each additional HLA gene in the individual or in the population makes it less likely that a pathogen will evolve that the immune system cannot recognize (see Box 3.1).

Disease correlations

There are many human diseases that appear to be linked to possession of certain HLA alleles. These diseases are often inflammatory or autoimmune in nature. Extensive HLA typing of families has revealed correlations of varying extents with possession of certain HLA alleles, e.g., a form of joint disease called ankylosing spondylitis is highly associated with the *HLA-B27* allele (Box 8.3). Another disease strongly correlated with HLA is insulin-dependent diabetes mellitus (IDDM). IDDM is associated with (linked to) *HLA-DQ2*. Approximately 50–75% of Caucasians with IDDM

BOX 8.3
Association between *HLA-B27* and the autoimmune disease ankylosing spondylitis

Both genetic and environmental factors contribute to autoimmune disease. Amongst the genes associated with autoimmune disease the strongest associations are with MHC genes (see Fig. 8.10). One of the strongest such associations is between *HLA-B27* and the presumed autoimmune disease ankylosing spondylitis. Patients with this disease develop inflammation of the vertebral joints. For example, a patient with ankylosing spondylitis may initially present with lower back pain and stiffness that leads to difficulty in walking. Eventually the spine may become bowed. Anti-inflammatory drugs will often alleviate the symptoms of the disease.

Individuals who possess *HLA-B27* are about 90 times more likely to develop the disease than other individuals in the population. Neither the mechanism of the disease nor the basis for its association with *HLA-B27* is known. However, environmental factors (perhaps infection) contribute at least as much to the likelihood of contracting the disease as does HLA type. For example, only a small proportion of the people who express *HLA-B27* ever develop ankylosing spondylitis (Ch. 27).

have *DQ2*. Some other high correlations are listed in Figure 8.10. These observations remain to be fully explained. They could be related to the role of MHC molecules in binding peptides to present to T cells, or they could be the result of another gene linked to HLA. In the example of systemic lupus erythematosus there is a linkage with complement genes (class III MHC)—see also Chapter 24.

Fig. 8.10
Correlations between some diseases and HLA alleles

Disease	HLA type
Ankylosing spondylitis	*B27*
Goodpasture's syndrome	*DR2*
Insulin-dependent diabetes mellitus	*DQ2*
Multiple sclerosis	*DR2*
Pemphigus vulgaris	*DR4*
Rheumatoid arthritis	*DR4*
Systemic lupus erythematosus	*DR3*

LEARNING POINTS

Can you now:

- Draw a diagram of the genetic organization of the human MHC, HLA?
- Describe the main structural features of the class I and class II MHC gene products?
- Recall that MHC gene products are co-dominantly expressed compared with the allelic exclusion demonstrated by immunoglobulin and TCR gene products?
- Explain the genetic basis of MHC polymorphism and its significance for the functioning of the immune system?
- Describe the concept of MHC restriction and draw a model of MHC–peptide–TCR interaction?
- Compare and contrast peptide antigen binding to class I and class II molecules?
- List some diseases associated with HLA alleles?

Bone marrow   Thymus   Lymph node

Review of antigen recognition

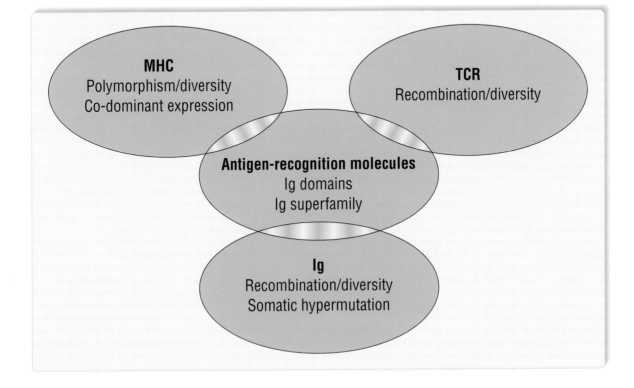

This section of the book has predominantly focused on the process of antigen recognition and the molecules involved in this process. This is key to understanding the immune system. The genes encoding the antigen-recognition molecules influence the functioning of just about the entire adaptive immune system. In the preceding chapters we have described the structure of various antigen-recognition molecules:

- antibodies (immunoglobulins)
- T cell antigen receptor (TCR)
- antigen-recognition molecules encoded in the major histocompatibility complex (MHC).

The genetic mechanisms involved in generating diversity in antibodies and TCRs were described. The generation of diversity in the genes for immunoglobulins and TCRs involves similar mechanisms, and chiefly involves somatic recombination of gene segments in each individual prior to exposure to antigen. MHC class I and II molecules are, by contrast, diverse through polymorphism. Many alternatives (alleles) exist in the human population as a whole, but the individual bears a restricted number, e.g., six different *HLA-A*, *B* and *C* (MHC class I) alleles. Chapters 3 to 8 should also have acquainted you with the various three-dimensional shapes of the antigen-recognition molecules and how they interact with antigen.

Important structural features

The immunoglobulin domain fold

As discussed in Chapter 4, the basic building block of the antibody molecule is a polypeptide chain of roughly 110 amino acid residues, folded to create an antiparallel β-pleated sheet structure and held in shape by intrachain disulfide bonds. This domain structure is shared by several other molecules and they are collectively referred to as the **immunoglobulin superfamily**. Most of the molecules in the superfamily are involved in recognition processes in the immune system, e.g., immunoglobulin, TCR, MHC class I and II molecules, CD4, CD8. Some representative examples of the members of this family of molecules are given in Figure 9.1.

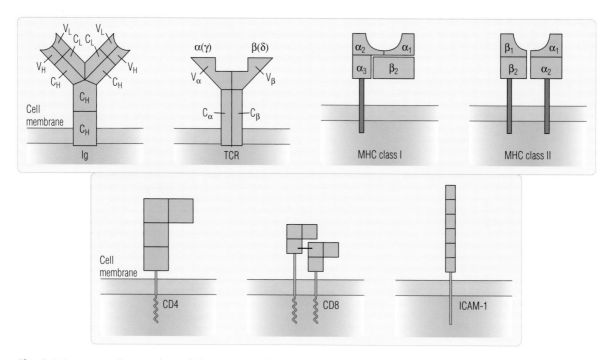

Fig. 9.1 Representative members of the immunoglobulin superfamily. B_2m, β_2-microglobulin; ICAM-1, intercellular adhesion molecule 1.

Some essential aspects of antibody and TCR structure are listed in Figures 9.2 and 9.3; Figure 9.4 highlights some important features of MHC molecules. These should help to focus your review of these molecules.

Antigen-recognition sites

As we have seen earlier (Chs 5, 6, 7 and 8), X-ray crystallographic analyses of several types of antigen-recognition molecule show that the antigen-binding site in antibodies can vary considerably in shape,

---

Fig. 9.2
Immunoglobulin and T cell receptor (TCR) proteins and gene segments

Immunoglobulin chains[a]	TCR chains[b]	V gene segments used
Heavy (γ1, μ, δ, etc.)	$\beta\delta$	V, D, J
Light (κ, λ)	$\alpha\gamma$	V, J

[a]May be both membrane bound and secreted.
[b]Membrane bound only.

Fig. 9.3
Immunoglobulin and T cell receptor (TCR) structure–function relationships

Structure	Recognition of antigen
Immunoglobulin	Directly: carbohydrate, protein, lipid, nucleic acid epitopes
TCR $\alpha\beta$	Dual recognition: self MHC + peptide antigen
TCR $\gamma\delta$	Directly: unusual phosphorylated non-peptide compounds including carbohydrates

Bone marrow   Thymus   Lymph node

Fig. 9.4
Selected features of MHC class I and II molecules

	MHC Class I	**MHC Class II**
Genes	*A, B, C*	*DP, DQ, DR*
Cellular expression	Essentially all nucleated cells	Chiefly, antigen-presenting cells
Structure	α-Chain plus β_2-microglobulin	α-Chain plus β-chain
Peptide binding	Peptides of 8–11 amino acid residues derived in the cytoplasm (endogenous antigen)	Peptides of 9–30 amino acid residues derived in intracellular vesicles (exogenous antigen)
Presentation to	CD8+ T cells	CD4+ T cells

while the TCR site for interaction with peptides presented by MHC molecules tends to be a flat surface area (Fig. 7.2) at least in the TCR variable regions that have been analyzed so far. The peptide-binding grooves of MHC class I and II molecules are similar in being formed from the α-helical regions of the polymorphic domains of the MHC molecules. The groove in class II molecules is open-ended, allowing longer peptides (approximately 9–30 amino acid residues) to "hang over" the groove, whereas the class I peptide groove is closed, only allowing binding of peptides of a fixed size (approximately 8–11 residues). Knowledge being built up about how immune molecules recognize antigens is being exploited medically in immunotherapy (see Box 9.1).

Molecular analyses of the antigen-recognition molecules highlight the fundamental difference between recognition by B cell receptors and by TCRs: immunoglobulin binds antigen directly whereas the TCR interacts with peptide antigens presented by MHC molecules. The ligand for the B cell receptor is antigen alone, but the ligand for the TCR is a peptide antigen–MHC molecule complex (Fig. 7.7).

Generation of diversity

Several mechanisms have evolved to generate a wide range of antigen-recognition molecules (repertoire) capable of interacting with antigen. With respect to MHC, the MHC molecules are polygenic and polymorphic, i.e., there are multiple copies of similar genes. For example, the MHC class I locus is represented by the *HLA-A*, *HLA-B* and *HLA-C* loci in the human. In the human population, there are also a large number of

---

BOX 9.1
Molecular genetic engineering: immunotherapy for B cell lymphoma

Anti-CD20 is a mouse monoclonal antibody developed against a molecule found on most or all B cells. CD20 may be a calcium channel protein involved in B cell activation. Antibody to CD20 has been found to be useful in treating human lymphoma. Unfortunately, the mouse antibodies are eventually recognized by the patient and human anti-mouse antibodies are produced, which interfere with the action of anti-CD20 after about 2 weeks of therapy. Knowledge of the structure of antibodies led to development of a chimeric "humanized" anti-CD20. This involved linking the gene segments for the variable region of the mouse antibody with the gene segments encoding a human Fc region. The antibody produced retained the anti-tumor specificity and it had fewer mouse epitopes to stimulate a human immune response.

Intact immunoglobulin is a large molecule, which is not always efficient at penetrating a tumor mass. It was reasoned that improved penetration could be achieved with a "single-chain antibody". This was achieved by "genetic engineering" which attached a single variable region from the mouse anti-CD20 to a single constant region from a human immunoglobulin. The single-chain antibody molecule still bound complement and the CD20 protein on B cells and was useful in anti-tumor therapy.

Several humanized monoclonal antibodies are in clinical trials for specific anti-tumor therapy and this would not have been possible without the detailed molecular knowledge we have obtained about immunoglobulins.

alleles at these loci. This is polymorphism—existence of multiple alleles at a locus in the population. Much of the diversity in MHC (polymorphism) was created by gene conversion mechanisms, not by the somatic recombination mechanisms used by immunoglobulin and TCR genes. Gene conversion does not occur widely in the immune system and it will not be explained further here.

The immunoglobulin and TCR genes are extremely diverse. Again, like MHC alleles, which pre-exist exposure to antigen, the repertoire of immunoglobulin and TCR genes largely precedes contact with antigen. The same enzymes, i.e., the V(D)J recombinase including RAG-1/RAG-2, are involved in gene segment recombination in B and T cells. These enzymes do not appear to function in other cells. Most immunoglobulin and TCR diversity is a result of junctional diversity created during the recombination of V region gene segments, e.g., D to J, V to DJ, V to J. The various genetic mechanisms contributing to diversity in immunoglobulin and TCR genes are listed in Figure 9.5. Clearly junctional diversity, created by imprecise joining and by insertion and addition of nucleotides by the enzyme terminal deoxynucleotidyl transferase as gene segments are recombined, is a major contributor to this diversity (Fig. 9.6). Another point that should be highlighted is that although there is extensive "improvement" of the immunoglobulin binding site for antigen after exposure to antigen, the TCR repertoire does not continue to change after antigenic exposure (Fig. 9.5).

Fig. 9.5
Mechanisms used to generate diversity in immunoglobulin and T cell receptors

	Immunoglobulin	T cell receptor
Prior to exposure to antigen		
Multiple V region gene segments	✓	✓
Somatic recombination of gene segments	✓	✓
Junctional variability	✓	✓
Multiple combinations of chains, e.g., light/heavy or α/β	✓	✓
After exposure to antigen		
Somatic hypermutation	✓	–
Class switching	✓	–

Fig. 9.6
Generation of diversity: contribution of different mechanisms

Mechanisms	Immunoglobulin	T cell receptor	
		$\alpha\beta$	$\gamma\delta$
V segment recombination (V, D, J)	~2.5×10^5	~2×10^3	~10^2
Estimated total repertoire	~10^{11}	~10^{16}	~10^{18}

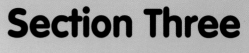

Section Three
Physiology

Antigen processing and presentation

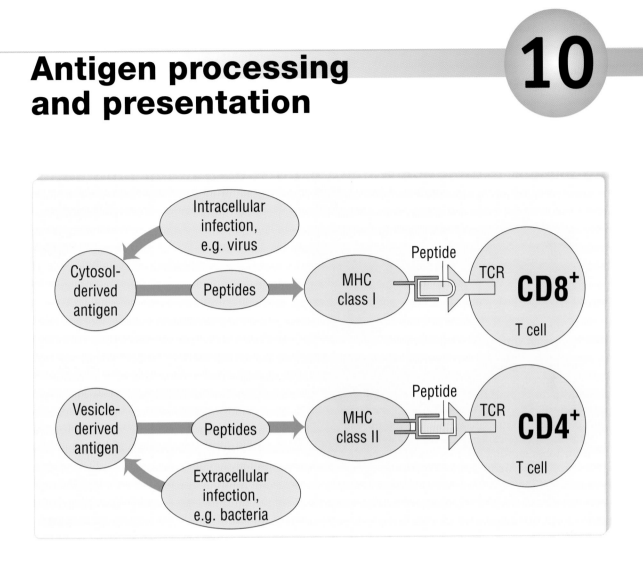

The topic for this chapter is the formation of the MHC–foreign antigen complexes, which are the ligands for the T cell receptor (TCR).

As we have seen earlier, the body has developed "barriers" that are very effective in preventing foreign "antigens", such as bacteria or viruses, from gaining entry and inducing disease. If a foreign organism or antigen (such as a toxin) gains entry, the protective systems of the innate immune system (e.g., phagocytic cells) may destroy the antigen before it is encountered by B or T cells and induces an adaptive immune response. Very little foreign antigen typically survives the innate immune system's various host defense systems intact, but if it does then fortunately it only requires a very small number of B or T cell antigen receptors to be engaged to initiate a protective adaptive immune response.

B cell antigen receptors may interact directly with an invading microbe but TCRs only recognize "processed" antigenic peptides. In addition, the TCR recognizes foreign antigen only when the antigen is attached to the surface of other cells (antigen-presenting cells (APCs) or target cells; Fig. 10.1). Examples of APCs are macrophages, B cells and the various dendritic cells (see Chs 2 and 20). Dendritic cells, as discussed later, are APCs "par excellence" (see Box 10.1 and Chs 12 and 20). These accessory cells, in addition to presenting antigen, usually provide co-stimulator activities that complete the immune activation process. Antigen is presented by APCs in association with MHC molecules (see also Ch. 8). Antigen recognition by T lymphocytes is thus said to be **MHC restricted**. The major subsets of T lymphocytes, the helper T cells (CD4+)and the cytotoxic T cells (CD8+) have different "MHC restrictions", thus the CD4+ T cell–APC interaction is MHC class II restricted and the CD8+ T cell–target cell interaction is MHC class I restricted (Chs 7, 8 and 15). The process whereby antigen becomes associated with self-MHC molecules for presentation to T cells is termed antigen processing.

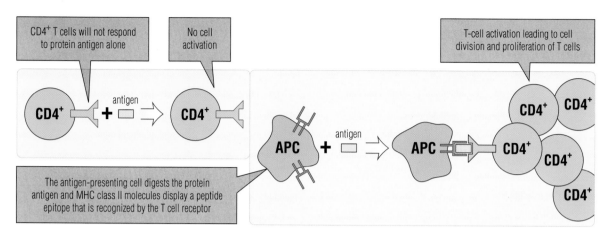

Fig. 10.1 Antigen presentation to T cells by antigen-presenting cells (APCs).

Pathways of antigen processing

Peptide antigens generated in the cytosolic compartment of the cell (e.g., from viruses and bacteria that replicate in the cytosol) bind to class I MHC molecules for presentation to CD8+ T cells (Ch. 7). Peptide antigens generated in intracellular vesicles from the endocytic uptake of extracellular antigens, such as toxins, or from microbes growing in intracellular vesicles (e.g., after the phagocytic uptake of certain bacteria by macrophages) bind to class II MHC molecules for presentation to CD4+ T cells. This means that CD8+ T cells can monitor the intracellular environment, and CD4+ T cells can monitor the extracellular environment for pathogens.

The intracellular pathway traversed by an antigen is the primary factor in determining if an antigen will be presented on class I or class II MHC molecules, not anything particular about the antigen itself. If a protein that is normally extracellular, and would therefore be processed to create an MHC class II peptide antigen complex, is instead transfected directly into the cytoplasm in a gene expression system, then the peptides

Box 10.1
Dendritic cells—antigen-presenting cells par excellence

The dendritic cells (DCs) make up a system of cells critical to the immune response, especially T-cell mediated immunity. These cells were originally detected by their atypical cell shape (see Fig. 2.7). They have extensive "dendritic" processes that continually form and retract. Dendritic cells are found in several places in the body and are motile, migrating in the blood and lymph from peripheral organs to the lymphoid organs, particularly to T-cell areas of organs such as the lymph nodes. In essence, DCs function to capture antigens at sites of contact with the external enviroment, e.g., the skin and mucosal epithelia, and they then transport the antigen until they encounter a T cell with specificity for that MHC–antigen complex.

Dendritic cells in different organs have been given different names (see Ch. 13). For example, in lymphoid organs DCs are known as interdigitating cells (IDCs) and they are prevalent in T cell areas. In the skin they are known as epidermal Langerhans cells (LCs) and in other organs, e.g., the heart, as interstitial dendritic cells. Finally, DCs found in the blood and lymph are known as veiled cells. All of these dendritic cells are antigen-presenting cells, although they may have a slightly different morphology or role. Amongst the characteristics of DCs that contribute to their ability to present antigen effectively are: (1) they express high levels of MHC class II molecules; (2) they express high levels of co-stimulatory molecules, e.g., CD80 (B7); and (3) they retain MHC–peptide antigen complexes on their surface for long periods of time, thereby enhancing the likelihood of T-cell binding and subsequent activation. DCs initiate both CD4+ and CD8+ T-cell responses (see Ch. 15). Their importance as antigen-presenting cells is leading to clinical research to investigate their use in new approaches to vaccination against tumor antigens and certain viruses.

 Bone marrow   Thymus   Lymph node

that are now generated in the cytoplasm after proteolytic breakdown of the transfected protein will be presented on class I MHC molecules.

Protein antigens need to be processed by APCs to produce the antigenic peptides recognized by T cells. This processing requires time (minutes to hours) and metabolism and so will not occur in killed APCs, although killed cells may present pre-formed peptide antigens to T lymphocytes (e.g., vaccines or peptides from extracellular pathogens).

Mechanisms of antigen processing

Extracellular (or exogenous) antigens

Extracellular (or exogenous) antigens are either extracellular proteins (e.g., a protein vaccine) or a protein derived from a pathogen in a cytoplasmic vesicle after uptake. These antigens are processed for eventual presentation on MHC class II molecules to CD4$^+$ T lymphocytes (Fig. 10.2a). First, however, they must be internalized by the APC. Mostly this involves fluid phase endocytosis, but if antigen is bound by the immunoglobulin receptor, for example, then internalization is via the much faster route of receptor-mediated endocytosis. Other antigens in this processing pathway are those derived from microbes that grow in intracellular vesicles after uptake by phagocytosis in cells such as macrophages. In any event, the antigen is first found inside the cell in an acidic membrane-bound compartment that can enter the endosomal pathway of the cell. The endosomal pathway is critical to both biosynthetic and degradative events in the cell. Much is known about the multiple stages that proteins in the endosomal processing pathway go through. Figure 10.2 illustrates only the most important stages of degradative processing, and the principal stages in the biosynthesis of integral membrane glycoproteins, such as the MHC class II α- and β-chain molecules.

The antigen derived in the intracellular vesicle moves through various acidic endosomal/lysosomal compartments where it is degraded by cellular proteases, first to peptides of different sizes then ultimately to amino acids. During this process, peptides are generated in the size range that can bind to class II MHC molecules (9 to 30+ amino acid residues). The APC also synthesizes new class II MHC molecules in the endoplasmic reticulum. These molecules move out through the Golgi apparatus, where they are glycosylated, eventually becoming part of a vesicle that buds off the Golgi and may fuse with an endosomal vesicle containing peptides from an extracellular or vesicle-derived antigen. In the pathway from the endoplasmic reticulum through the Golgi and so on, the empty binding site of class II MHC is "protected" from binding other peptides (e.g., self peptides) by a molecule known as the **invariant chain** (Ii). In the acidic environment of the endosome

this protection is removed by proteolytic action, and the class II binding site is available for occupancy by any appropriate peptide available in the endosome. "Occupied" MHC class II molecules are then expressed at the cell surface when the endosomal vesicle fuses with the cell surface membrane. In this way, a foreign antigen can be presented to the repertoire of TCRs and can induce the appropriate T cell to proliferate (Fig. 10.2a).

Intracellular (or endogenous) antigens

Endogenous (intracellular) antigens such as viral proteins are processed by "target cells" for eventual presentation on class I MHC molecules to CD8$^+$ T cells (cytotoxic T lymphocytes (Fig. 10.2b)). In this case, peptides that are foreign antigens are generated in the cytoplasmic compartment. These may be derived by breakdown, via the normal cellular machinery, of viral proteins that are being synthesized and assembled in the cytoplasm of a virally infected cell (e.g., a fibroblast). In Figure 10.2b, a viral protein is being synthesized in the cytosol. The cellular degradative machinery, most importantly a complex of proteases known as the **proteasome**, may enzymatically cleave some of the viral protein molecules through various polypeptide and peptide intermediate steps until peptides of 8–11 residues are formed; these can bind to class I MHC molecules. Many of the peptides will undergo further degradation, making them irrelevant to the immune system. However, some will enter the endoplasmic reticulum carried by a two-chain molecule known as TAP (transporter associated with antigen presentation; see Box 10.2). TAP permits the peptides to traverse the membrane bilayer of the endoplasmic reticulum and bind in the empty peptide-binding groove of nascent MHC class I molecules being synthesized in the endoplasmic reticulum. Binding of these small peptide antigens is critical for the final stages of assembly of MHC class I molecules. In the absence of peptide, class I molecules are unable to fold correctly and are not found at the cell surface. MHC class I molecules complete their biosynthesis in the Golgi and move out to the surface membrane via the exocytic pathway. After fusion of an exocytic vesicle with the surface membrane, foreign antigenic peptides associated with MHC class I molecules may interact with T lymphocytes bearing receptors capable of binding this MHC–antigen complex (CD8$^+$ or cytotoxic T cells).

Class I or II association

It is important to underline that, as illustrated in Figure 10.2, the likelihood of an antigen becoming associated with class I or class II MHC is determined solely by the route of trafficking through the cell, not by some special property of the antigen. The process-

(a)

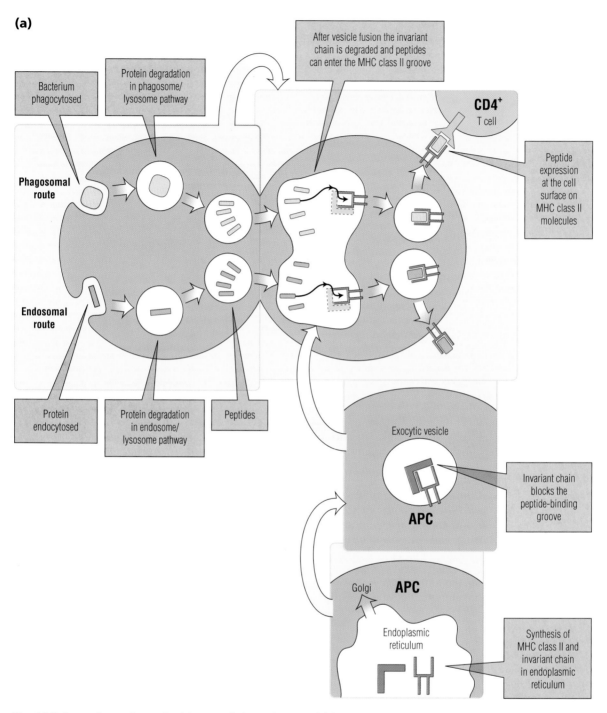

Fig. 10.2 Processing pathways for (a) extracellular antigens and (b) intracellular antigens. TAP, transporter associated with antigen presentation; TCR, T cell receptor. (*Fig. 10.2(b), see opposite*)

ing of antigens in this way also explains why polysaccharides, lipids and nucleic acids are not recognized by $\alpha\beta$ T cells—they are not processed to fit into the binding groove of the MHC molecules.

Processing of cytosol- and vesicle-derived antigens to result in association with MHC class I or class II molecules respectively, results in the activation of different subsets of T cells (Figs 10.3 and 10.4).

Bone marrow   Thymus   Lymph node

(b)

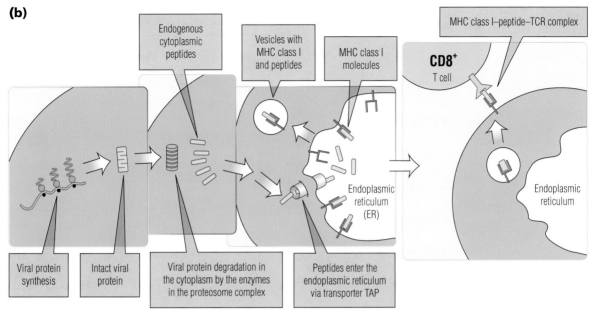

Endogenous cytoplasmic peptides

Vesicles with MHC class I and peptides

MHC class I molecules

MHC class I–peptide–TCR complex

CD8⁺ T cell

Endoplasmic reticulum (ER)

Endoplasmic reticulum

| Viral protein synthesis | Intact viral protein | Viral protein degradation in the cytoplasm by the enzymes in the proteosome complex | Peptides enter the endoplasmic reticulum via transporter TAP |

Fig. 10.2 *Continued*

BOX 10.2
TAP deficiency

The peptide transporter (TAP) found in the endoplasmic reticulum membrane is encoded by two genes, *TAP-1* and *TAP-2*, located in the class II region of the MHC. The transporter is a heterodimer of the two proteins TAP-1 and TAP-2. Rare mutations exist in *TAP-1* or *TAP-2* that alter the function of TAP and prevent the efficient entry of peptides into the lumen of the endoplasmic reticulum. In the absence of peptide antigen, the MHC class I molecules are unstable and only a small fraction are transported through the exocytic pathway to the cell surface.

This reduced expression of class I MHC molecules interferes with the development of cytotoxic T lymphocytes (CTL).

In humans with TAP mutations, chronic upper respiratory infections are observed. Humoral immunity is intact in these patients and some aspects of cellular immunity are also normal, e.g., the patients' CD4⁺ T cells can respond to antigen. However, the lack of expression of class I MHC molecules results in reduced numbers of CTL and in difficulties responding appropriately to some respiratory viruses.

ACTIVATION OF T CELLS INDEPENDENT OF PROCESSING

There are some antigens, termed **superantigens**, that can activate T cells without requiring antigen processing (Ch. 7). These superantigens are typically bacterial exotoxins such as Staphylococcal enterotoxin B or some retroviral antigens. The superantigen binds simultaneously to the external surface of MHC class II molecules on the APC and to an external site on V_β chains of the TCR (Figs 7.5 and 7.6). They are not a part of the typical MHC–antigen binding site complex. As a result of this binding, they activate and expand T cells bearing this V_β molecule, explaining why comparatively large percentages of T cells are activated by these superantigens, leading to severe systemic complications, e.g., toxic shock syndrome and even death in some cases (see Box 7.2). Figures 7.5 and 7.6 contrast T cell activation by the normal antigen-processing mechanism with that occurring with a superantigen.

(a)

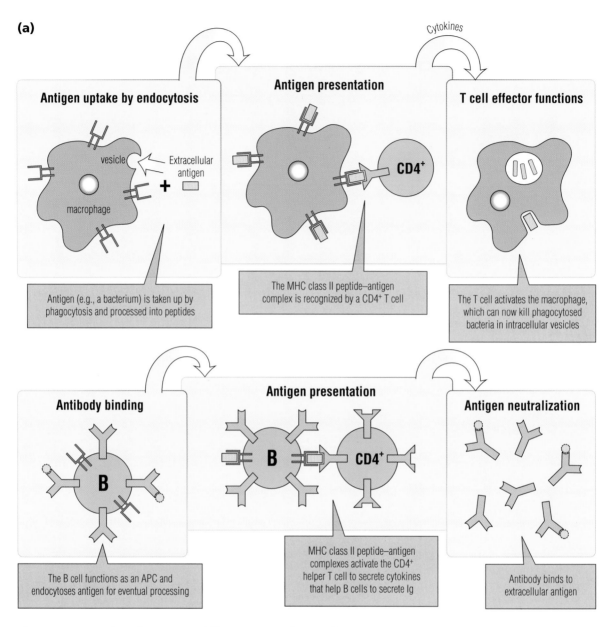

Fig. 10.3 Presentation of antigens to different subsets of T cells. (a) Class II MHC-associated extracellular antigen is presented to T helper cells (CD4⁺ T cells) either by macrophages or by B cells. (b) Class I MHC-associated cytosolic antigen is presented to cytotoxic T cells (CD8⁺ T cells). (*Fig. 10.3(b), see opposite*)

EVASION OF PROCESSING PATHWAYS BY PATHOGENS

If pathogens can avoid having their peptide antigens displayed by MHC molecules then they can avoid detection by the adaptive immune system. Consequently, numerous pathogens have developed strategies to interfere with antigen processing. For example, bacteria such as *Mycobacterium tuberculosis* have acquired the capacity to inhibit phagosome–lysome fusion. This inhibits their exposure to lysosomal proteases and reduces the likelihood that mycobacterial peptides will be generated that will bind to MHC molecules and be expressed at the cell surface. Amongst the viruses, several have found ways to interfere with the processing steps leading up to binding to MHC class I molecules. For example, a protein of herpes simplex virus (HSV) binds to TAP and inhibits

 Bone marrow   Thymus   Lymph node

(b)

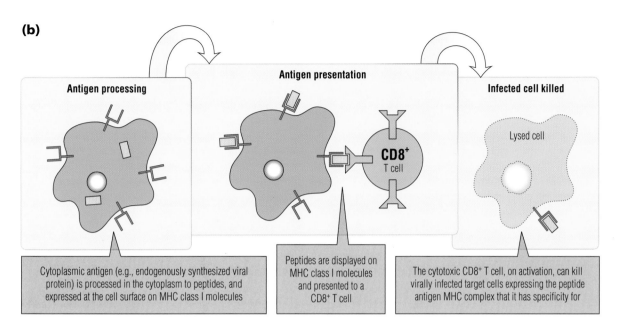

Antigen processing | Antigen presentation | Infected cell killed

CD8⁺ T cell

Lysed cell

Cytoplasmic antigen (e.g., endogenously synthesized viral protein) is processed in the cytoplasm to peptides, and expressed at the cell surface on MHC class I molecules

Peptides are displayed on MHC class I molecules and presented to a CD8⁺ T cell

The cytotoxic CD8⁺ T cell, on activation, can kill virally infected target cells expressing the peptide antigen MHC complex that it has specificity for

Fig. 10.3 *Continued*

Fig. 10.4
Pathways of antigen processing

	Cell compartment		
	Cytosol	**Phagocytic vesicles**	**Endocytic vesicles**
Source of antigen	Viruses and some bacteria	Bacteria taken up by phagocytosis, some of which are able to grow in cellular vesicles (phagosomes), e.g., the mycobacteria that cause tuberculosis	Extracellular proteins (vaccines, toxins, etc.), which are taken into the cell by endocytosis and processed in cellular vesicles (endosomes)
Molecule binding antigenic peptides	Class I MHC	Class II MHC	Class II MHC
Type of cell reacting with MHC–peptide complex	CD8⁺ T cells, which kill infected cells	CD4⁺ T cells* which activate macrophages. The activated macrophages can then destroy the intravesicular bacteria	CD4⁺ T cells* which activate B cells to make antibody

* The roles of different subsets of CD4⁺ T cells are explained further in Chapter 15.

peptide transport into the endoplasmic reticulum. A consequence of this is that there are fewer HSV peptides available to bind to class I MHC. Certain strains of adenovirus express a protein that inhibits the transcription of class I MHC molecules, thereby reducing the number of class I MHC molecules available to display adenoviral peptides to CD8⁺ lymphocytes (see also Ch. 24).

Some of the ways pathogens have found to avoid detection by the host defense systems by interfering with several steps in antigen processing is a reflection of the dynamic interchange between host and microbe as both try to survive and propagate. Equally medical research is using knowledge of the process of antigen presentation to devise new and better therapies (Box 10.3).

BOX 10.3
DNA vaccination

Alternatives to standard vaccination techniques are being developed. One of these involves vaccines composed of bacterial plasmids containing complementary DNA (cDNA) sequences encoding protein antigens (e.g., a viral protein) against which a protective immune response is desired. Following inoculation, the bacterial plasmid transfects APCs, where the cDNA is transcribed, translated and some of the protein molecules are eventually broken down into peptide antigens. Some of the peptides enter the endoplasmic reticulum and bind to MHC class I molecules. Following transport to the cell surface, they are detected on the surface of the APC by T cells. Early results indicate that this approach leads to a strong and long-lived immune response to certain antigens. Furthermore, because the cDNA-encoded proteins are synthesized in the cytosol, this can provide a way to introduce antigen into the intracellular processing pathway, leading to presentation on class I MHC molecules and the elicitation of a cytotoxic T cell response. Standard vaccine approaches (e.g., protein vaccine injected intramuscularly) would result in the protein being introduced to the endocytic/class II pathway, with eventual presentation to CD4+ T cells and the likelihood of stimulating an antibody response.

The relative ease of creating plasmids that include cDNAs encoding other immune system-enhancing proteins, e.g., cytokines, in conjunction with the "vaccine" protein, makes this a very attractive approach to consider adopting widely for vaccines in the future. A cDNA vaccine prepared with plasmids encoding melanoma tumor antigens is presently in clinical trials and others will undoubtedly follow.

LEARNING POINTS

Can you now:

- List at least three examples of antigen-presenting cells (APCs; e.g., macrophages) and describe their role in antigen processing and presentation?
- Describe how T lymphocytes recognize antigens on the *surface* of other cells associated with MHC molecules?
- Explain why linear protein antigenic determinants are recognized by T cells and conformational determinants are recognized by B cells?
- Draw diagrams of the different pathways of processing of an extracellular (exogenous) and an intracellular (endogenous) protein antigen (indicating the role of intracellular proteolytic compartments)?
- Describe with a diagram the molecular interactions involved in MHC-restricted antigen presentation to CD4+ and CD8+ T cells?

Bone marrow   Thymus   Lymph node

Lymphocyte activation

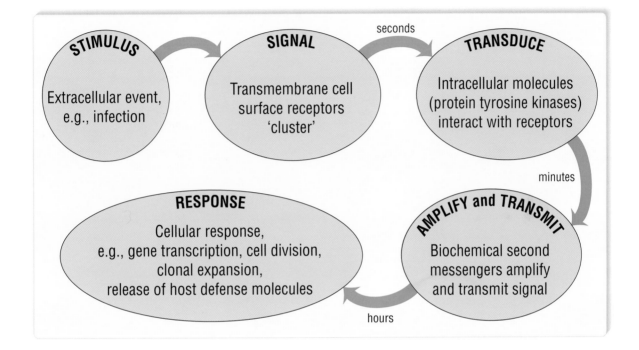

Events, such as an infection, produce a stimulus, in the form of antigens, to the immune system. As discussed earlier in Chapters 1 and 2, antigen-recognition molecules exist as cell surface receptors on B and T lymphocytes and are able to recognize these foreign molecules. Binding to the receptors initiates a protective response. The topic for this chapter is the mechanisms involved in B and T lymphocyte activation to produce the host defense response.

Firstly, antigen must be recognized, then notice (a signal) of this recognition must be transmitted to the cellular interior and a response generated. The process of translating the molecular events of antigen recognition into a cellular response is known as **signal transduction**. Intracellular molecules are very important in signal transduction. They cause biochemical "second messengers" to be induced and biochemical pathways to be activated that amplify the signal throughout the cell. At the end of the biochemical pathways are transcription factors, which upon activation initiate the new gene transcription that leads to cell functional changes including proliferation, division and differentiation.

In this overview of the activation of B and T lymphocytes we will also explain the action of some immuno-

suppressive drugs and indicate how enhanced knowledge of lymphocyte activation mechanisms is leading to the design of new immunomodulatory agents.

ANTIGEN RECEPTORS

The B and T cell antigen receptors (BCR and TCR) are multimolecular protein complexes at the cell surface (TCRs are described in Ch. 7 and BCRs in Chs 4 and 5). Although both membrane-bound immunoglobulin and the $\alpha\beta$ (or $\gamma\delta$) TCR have protein chains that span the cell surface membrane and extend into the cytoplasm, they have very short cytoplasmic sequences. These short cytoplasmic "tails" are ineffective at interfacing with the intracellular molecules that activate lymphocytes. Consequently, other proteins must interact with the "receptor" proteins before there can be effective signal transduction. Both the BCR and the TCR are multimolecular protein complexes in which these proteins are non-covalently linked together with the antigen-receptor proteins in the cell surface membrane. The major protein components of the BCR and the TCR are illustrated in Figures 11.1 and 11.2.

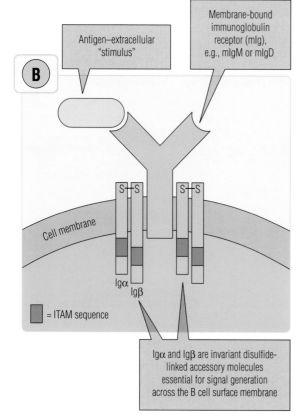

Fig. 11.1 The structure of the B cell receptor multimolecular complex. ITAM, immunoreceptor tyrosine-based activation motif.

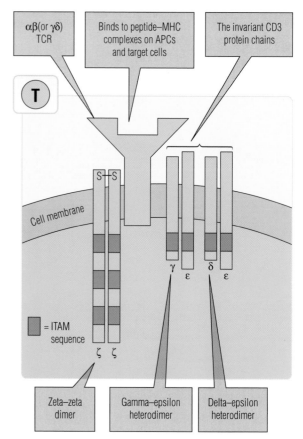

Fig. 11.2 The structure of the T cell receptor multimolecular complex. APC, antigen-presenting cell; ITAM, immunoreceptor tyrosine-based activation motif.

The B cell receptor

Functionally, the BCR is a complex of membrane-bound immunoglobulin (mIg) and the invariant protein chains, Igα and Igβ. As shown in Figure 11.1, Igα and Igβ are associated with mIg as a disulfide-linked heterodimeric complex. It is not known how many Igα–Igβ heterodimers are a part of the complex—only two are shown in Figure 11.1. The Igα–Igβ heterodimer is required for expression of mIg at the cell surface and for signal transduction. The intracellular regions of Igα–Igβ are large enough to interact with cellular signaling proteins. Igα and Igβ each contains sequences found in several receptor molecules, including proteins of the TCR complex, called the immunoreceptor tyrosine-based activation motif (**ITAM**). ITAMs are essential for signal transduction in B and T cells.

The T cell receptor

Functionally, the TCR complex comprises the TCR αβ (or γδ) chains and six other protein chains involved in signal transduction. The TCR αβ (or γδ) chains bind the MHC–antigen complex on an antigen-presenting cell but alone cannot effectively signal to the T cell that antigen is bound. This is achieved in cooperation with the accessory protein chains: CD3 and ξ. CD3 is made of four chains, one each of γ and δ and two ε-chains. There are two ξ-chains in the TCR complex (see Fig. 11.2). Both CD3 and ξ-chains have substantial intracellular regions that contain ITAMs. These sequences contain tyrosine, which becomes phosphorylated. The phosphorylated ITAMs interact with cytoplasmic signaling proteins.

Initiation of B and T cell activation

There are several requirements for B and T cell activation. For the primary signal, the receptor complexes must be clustered. For B cells this can occur by crosslinking of receptor molecules by multimeric antigens. This rarely occurs with soluble protein antigens and other surface molecules become involved to enhance signaling (see below). Both B and T cells require a second signal for activation. The nature of the second signals, referred to as a co-stimulatory signals, will be described in Chapter 16 along with further details of the interaction of B and T cells. Other cell surface molecules, referred to as co-receptor molecules, do contribute to the primary signal. The role of co-receptors in B cell and T cell activation will be explained below.

Clustering of TCRs involves binding of the TCR to MHC–peptide antigen complexes on the antigen-presenting cell (APC). Immunotherapy using "altered peptide ligands" (APLs) is intended to act by modulating T cell activation at this stage (see Box 11.1 and Box 8.2). It appears that occupancy of as little as a few hundred TCRs is sufficient to initiate a primary activation signal. Again, T cell activation requires a second co-stimulatory signal provided by the APC. As in B cells, co-receptor molecules contribute to the activation of T cells. CD4 and CD8 act as co-receptor molecules on T cells. Their role is also discussed further below. Finally, so-called accessory molecules facilitate T cell–APC contact and TCR–MHC–peptide binding. These accessory molecules are mostly adhesion molecules such as CD11a or leukocyte function associated antigen 1 (LFA-1) on T cells, which binds to CD54 or intercellular adhesion molecule 1 (ICAM-1) on APCs. These adhesion molecules are discussed further in Chapter 12.

Co-receptor molecules in B cell activation

As described above, the antigen-specific receptors on B and T cells are unable to transduce signals without the help of invariant proteins such as Igα/Igβ and CD3, respectively. However, optimal signaling requires yet more cell surface molecules, known as co-receptor molecules. The B cell co-receptor (Fig. 11.3) can co-cluster with the BCR and increase the efficiency of signaling by several thousandfold. As shown in Figure 11.3, the B cell co-receptor comprises three proteins: CD21 (also known as complement receptor 2 (CR2)), CD19 and CD81. Protein antigens bound to complement component C3d (see Ch. 19) can bind simultaneously to both CD21 and the BCR. This enables the CD21/CD19/CD81 co-receptor complex to cluster and crosslink with the BCR, and induce phosphorylation reactions on the intracellular tail of CD19. This phosphorylation allows kinases belonging to a family of similar enzymes (the Src family) to bind to the cytoplasmic tail of CD19 and to increase the concentration of signaling molecules around the BCR, thereby enhancing the efficiency of signaling.

BOX 11.1
Altered peptide ligands and lymphocyte activation

Altered peptide ligands (APLs) are designed to be antagonists or partial agonists of the TCR for use in specific immunotherapy for certain diseases. Box 8.2 describes the trial of APLs in multiple sclerosis. Now that we have reviewed lymphocyte activation, we can discuss the actions of APLs on T lymphocytes in more detail. APLs that are partial agonists partially activate the cell, e.g., causing secretion of some cytokines but not cell division. T cell recognition of APLs that are partial agonists appears to result in altered phosphorylation of receptor complex molecules, e.g., CD3 ε- and the ζ-chains. This partial phosphorylation reduces the ability of the receptor complex to concentrate protein tyrosine kinases (e.g., ZAP-70) on the cytoplasmic tails of the receptor proteins (Figs 11.6 and 11.8), and impairs signal transduction. This has the ultimate effect of partially inhibiting T lymphocyte responses.

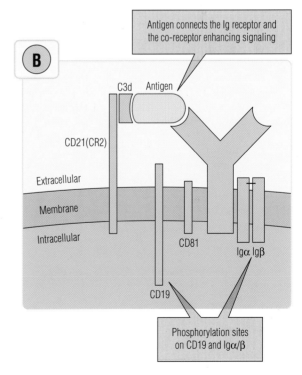

Fig. 11.3 The B cell receptor/co-receptor complex.

Co-receptor molecules in T cell activation

Optimal signaling through the TCR only occurs when co-receptor molecules are involved. The TCR co-receptor molecules are CD4 or CD8. As discussed in Chapters 7 and 10, CD4 binds to MHC class II molecules and CD8 binds to MHC class I molecules. When, for example, the TCR binds to an MHC class II–peptide complex on an APC, CD4 on the T cell binds to the MHC class II molecule (Fig. 11.6). The tyrosine kinase Lck (a Src kinase) is associated with the cytoplasmic domain of CD4 (and CD8). Consequently Lck is localized with the TCR complex when CD4 binds to MHC class II–peptide complexes.

Lck is integral in the signaling cascade in T cells and again co-receptor molecule involvement increases the concentration of these signaling molecules in the vicinity of the TCR. The presence of the CD4 or CD8 co-receptors has been estimated to reduce the number of MHC–peptide complexes required to trigger a T cell response by about 100-fold.

SIGNALING EVENTS

Intracellular molecules, chiefly protein tyrosine kinases (PTKs) and protein tyrosine phosphatases (PTPs), form the link between receptor activation and activation of biochemical pathways that amplify and transmit the signal. Within seconds of cross-linking the BCR, PTK enzymes of the Src family (Box 11.2) phosphorylate ITAMs in the receptor protein cytoplasmic tails (Fig. 11.5). Phosphorylation of the receptor tails attracts other signaling molecules to the cytoplasmic side of the receptor. In B cells, the critical molecule is another PTK known as Syk. Syk is found at high levels in B cells but is also found in other cells, including some T cells. Syk binds to the phosphorylated ITAM sequences in Igα and Igβ and is then itself activated by phosphorylation. Syk may be phosphorylated by the Src family kinases associated with the BCR, as shown in Figure 11.5, or it may be phosphorylated by another Syk molecule bound to an adjacent BCR chain.

BOX 11.2
Intracellular signaling: the role of protein tyrosine kinases and protein tyrosine phosphatases

Phosphorylation is a common biochemical mechanism by which cells regulate the activity of proteins. Protein kinases affect protein function by adding phosphate groups to proteins. These phosphate groups are added to tyrosine residues by tyrosine kinases, e.g., ZAP-70, and to serine or threonine residues by serine/threonine kinases, e.g., protein kinase C. The phosphate groups can be removed by protein phosphatases. In general phosphorylation activates enzymes, and dephosphorylation inactivates enzymes.

Several protein kinases are essential in signal transduction in lymphocytes and it is important that you recognize some of the most important. For example, activation of the receptor-associated tyrosine kinases of the Src (pronounced as "Sark") family informs the interior of B and T lymphocytes that the antigen receptor is occupied. Two of the major Src family kinases in lymphocytes are known as Lyn and Lck. Another family of tyrosine kinases particularly important in lymphocytes is the Syk family. There are two members of this family: Syk and ZAP-70.

Tyrosine kinases, such as Lyn and Lck, tend to be activated early in signaling pathways, whereas serine/threonine kinases, such as protein kinase C and calcineurin, tend to be important in later stages of signaling.

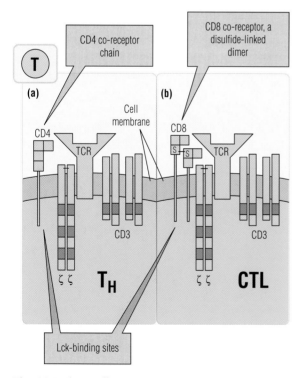

Fig. 11.4 The T cell receptor/co-receptor complex.

Bone marrow   Thymus   Lymph node

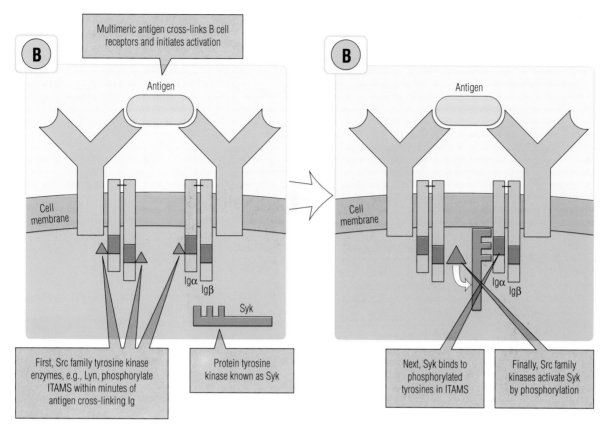

Fig. 11.5 Earliest events in activation of B cells.

A related series of steps occurs in T cells. Clustering of the TCR, CD3 and CD4/CD8 proteins on recognition of peptides displayed by MHC molecules on APCs brings the PTK known as Lck into the receptor complex (Fig. 11.6). Lck phosphorylates the ITAMs in the cytoplasmic sequences of CD3 and ξ-chain. This attracts the PTK ZAP-70, which is unique to T cells and natural killer cells. ZAP-70 is part of the same PTK family as Syk. ZAP-70 binds to the ITAMs of the ξ-chains. More than one ZAP-70 molecule may bind to a ξ-chain because of the multiple ITAMs per ξ-chain (Fig. 11.6). ZAP-70 is then phosphorylated by Lck. Phosphorylation activates the PTK activity of ZAP-70.

Once a critical number of Syk or ZAP-70 kinases are activated in B or T cells respectively, then the signal is transmitted onwards from the membrane, and amplified by activation of several pathways. The important role of PTKs in lymphocyte function is indicated by the occurrence of immunodeficiency in the presence of mutations affecting PTK function (see Box 11.3).

AMPLIFICATION THROUGH SIGNALING PATHWAYS

In order for the signal to be propagated from the membrane to the nucleus, where it can have a major impact on a cellular response, several biochemical pathways are utilized that are similar in B and T cells and which amplify the signal while propagating it.

In both B and T cells three main signaling pathways are used. The first involves phosphorylation and activation of the enzyme phospholipase Cγ (PLC-γ). This is triggered by Syk or ZAP-70 (Figs 11.7 and 11.8). Activated PLC-γ then stimulates two pathways involving (i) diacylglycerol and protein kinase C and (ii) inositol 1,4,5-trisphosphate (IP$_3$) and the serine/threonine-specific protein phosphatase calcineurin. The third main pathway involves activation by Syk or ZAP-70 of adapter proteins that then activate single-chain guanosine trisphosphate (GTP)-binding proteins (e.g., Ras). The Ras family of proteins then activates

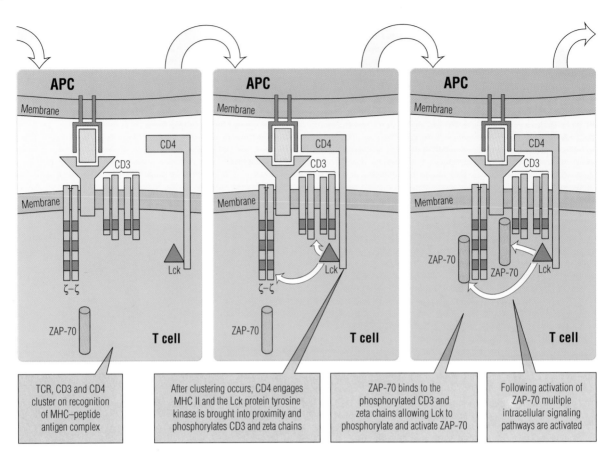

TCR, CD3 and CD4 cluster on recognition of MHC–peptide antigen complex	After clustering occurs, CD4 engages MHC II and the Lck protein tyrosine kinase is brought into proximity and phosphorylates CD3 and zeta chains	ZAP-70 binds to the phosphorylated CD3 and zeta chains allowing Lck to phosphorylate and activate ZAP-70	Following activation of ZAP-70 multiple intracellular signaling pathways are activated

Fig. 11.6 Earliest events in activation of T cells.

BOX 11.3
Immunodeficiency diseases and protein tyrosine kinases

The important role of PTKs in lymphocyte function is underlined by the effects of mutations in the genes encoding two of these enzymes, i.e., ZAP-70 and Bruton's tyrosine kinase (Btk).

Defects in ZAP-70 lead to a severe combined immunodeficiency (SCID) syndrome in humans. In these patients, there are abnormalities in T cell development and only mature CD4+ T cells are found. In addition, these CD4+ T cells have defective TCR signal transduction, leading to altered T cell function and severe immunodeficiency disease (see also Ch. 31).

Defective Btk leads to agammaglobulinemia. In this X-linked agammaglobulinemia, serum immunoglobulin is absent. Btk is involved in phosphoinositide hydrolysis during BCR signaling and defects in Btk result in impaired B cell development and prevent antibody production. The complications these patients experience in resisting bacterial infection are reduced by regular injections of pooled gammaglobulin preparations containing antibodies against commonly encountered pathogens (passive immunotherapy—see also Chs 2 and 31 and Box 4.2).

signaling pathways leading through the mitogen-activated protein kinases (MAP kinases) directly to activation of transcription factors (Figs 11.7 and 11.8).

Phosphorylation of PLC-γ by Syk in B cells (Fig. 11.7) and phosphorylation of PLC-γ by ZAP-70 in T cells (Fig. 11.8) leads to migration of PLC-γ to the cell

Bone marrow   Thymus   Lymph node

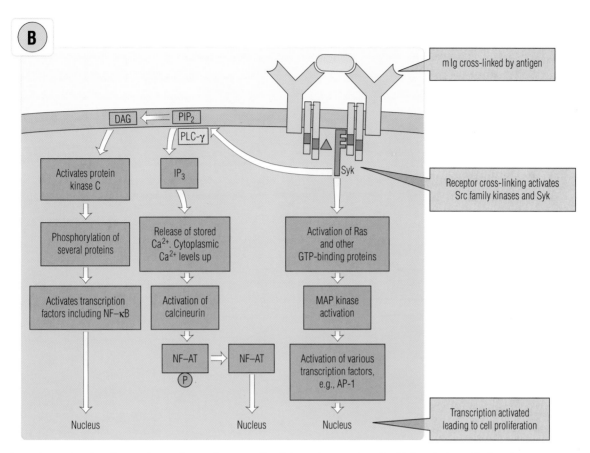

Fig. 11.7 Major signaling pathways in B cells. DAG, diacylglycerol; PIP$_2$, phosphatidylinositol 4,5-bisphosphate; IP$_3$, inositol 1,4,5-trisphosphate; PLC-γ, phospholipase Cγ; MAP kinase, mitogen-activated protein kinase; NF-AT, nuclear factor of activated T cells; NF-κB, nuclear factor kappa B; AP-1, activation protein 1.

membrane where it catalyses the cleavage of phosphatidylinositol 4,5-bisphosphate to produce diacylglycerol and inositol 1,4,5-trisphosphate. The latter causes cytoplasmic calcium ion levels to increase, which, among other events, activates several calcium-dependent enzymes including a serine/threonine-specific protein phosphatase called **calcineurin**. Calcineurin is responsible for dephosphorylating the NF-AT (nuclear factor of activated T cells) family of transcription factors. NF-AT is required for expression of genes for cytokines in T cells (e.g., interleukin 2) but is also found in other cell types and is activated by BCR stimulation in B cells.

The serine/threonine kinase protein kinase C is activated by interaction with diacylglycerol and phosphorylates several cellular proteins, leading eventually to the activation of transcription factors, including NF-κB. The third signaling pathway involves activation of the

small GTP-binding proteins of the Ras family. These signaling molecules operate through activation of the MAP kinase family of enzymes. The MAP kinases activate several transcription factors including one called activation protein 1 (AP-1).

RESPONSE

The various transcription factors including NF-AT, NF-κB and AP-1 act on several lymphocyte genes to enhance their transcription. This prepares B cells for proliferation and differentiation and in T cells leads to enhanced expression of cytokines such as interleukin 2, which is an essential component of an effective T cell response, being responsible for clonal expansion etc. Immunosuppressive drugs can modulate this response (Box 11.4).

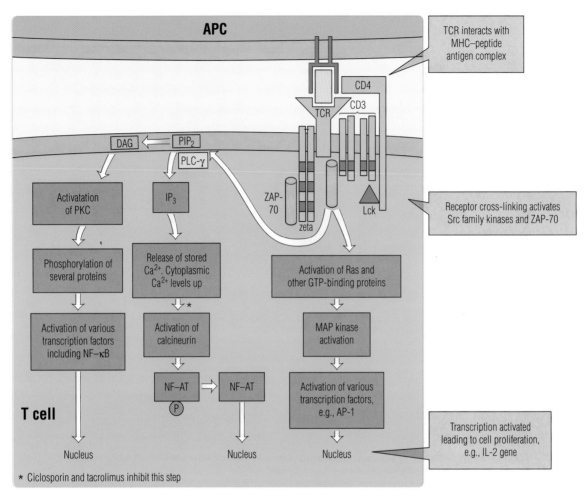

Fig. 11.8 Major signaling pathways in T cells. DAG, diacylglycerol; PIP$_2$, phosphatidylinositol 4,5-bisphosphate; IP$_3$, inositol 1,4,5-trisphosphate; PLC-γ, phospholipase Cγ; MAP kinase, mitogen-activated protein kinase; NF-AT, nuclear factor of activated T cells; NF-κB, nuclear factor kappa B; AP-1, activation protein 1.

BOX 11.4
Immunosuppressive drugs: mechanism of action

There are several immunosuppressive drugs in use to prevent allograft rejection (see Ch. 33). Two of the most useful are ciclosporin and tacrolimus. These are remarkable drugs that have revolutionized the field of transplantation surgery. Their availability has saved thousands of lives and made organ transplantation "do-able" even when there is no perfect HLA match available. Studies of the mechanism of action of these drugs have also helped to elucidate some of the signaling pathways in T cells.

Both ciclosporin and tacrolimus function by preventing T cell cytokine gene transcription

mediated by NF-AT. They accomplish this by forming a complex with cytoplasmic proteins called immunophilins. The drug–immunophilin complex inhibits the action of calcineurin (Fig. 11.8). Without the dephosphorylation reaction mediated by calcineurin, NF-AT is unable to enter the nucleus and promote gene transcription, e.g., of the gene for interleukin 2 (IL-2). In the absence of this cytokine, lymphocyte proliferation is inhibited, and the immune response is suppressed. This prevents graft rejection but has the disadvantage of leaving the patient open to infectious disease because the immune response is inhibited.

 Bone marrow   Thymus   Lymph node

LEARNING POINTS

Can you now:

- Draw the B and T cell receptor complexes and list the molecules involved?
- Recall that B and T cell activation is more optimal with the aid of co-receptor complexes?
- Describe with a diagram the earliest biochemical events in B and T cell activation?
- List the major signaling pathways triggered in B and T cells by antigen recognition?
- Recall the mechanism of inhibition of T cell activation by immunosuppressive drugs such as ciclosporin and tacrolimus?

Hematopoiesis

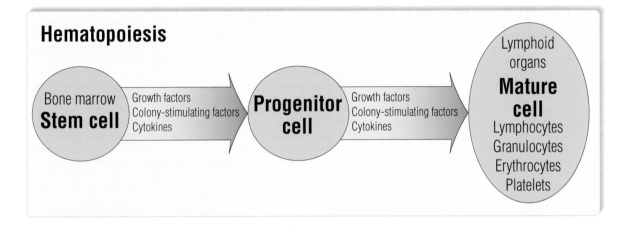

Hematopoiesis

Bone marrow **Stem cell** — Growth factors / Colony-stimulating factors / Cytokines → **Progenitor cell** — Growth factors / Colony-stimulating factors / Cytokines → Lymphoid organs **Mature cell** Lymphocytes Granulocytes Erythrocytes Platelets

Hematopoiesis is the process whereby all blood cells are formed; in humans the bone marrow is the major site for hematopoiesis and all of the differentiated blood cell types from lymphocytes to granulocytes to red blood cells are continuously generated in the adult human bone marrow. Several hundred million white blood cells (leukocytes) are generated every hour in the human adult bone marrow along with about ten billion red blood cells.

The leukocytes, both lymphoid and myeloid cells, have been briefly described already in Chapter 2, and this chapter will explain their development from progenitor cells, and provide some additional characterization. In addition, Chapter 13 will describe the structure and function of the lymphoid organs where lymphocytes are generated and/or mature. The process by which lymphocytes move from the organs of lymphoid generation (chiefly the bone marrow and thymus in humans) to the spleen, lymph nodes, skin, mucosa, etc., where they encounter antigen, is known as lymphocyte recirculation (or trafficking) and homing. Chapter 13 will also describe how lymphocytes recirculate and home to different tissues, and it will explain the important role of cell adhesion molecules in these processes.

The three major stages of hematopoiesis

Hematopoiesis can be divided into three major parts. Each part involves very different types of cells: stem cell, progenitor cell, mature cell (Fig. 12.1). **Hematopoietic stem cells** (HSCs) are pluripotential,

and self-renewing. They give rise to all the blood cell types (lineages). HSCs do not express cell lineage specific marker proteins (such as CD3 on T cells or CD19 on B cells) but they do express a protein designated as CD34, which has allowed them to be enriched, by fluorescence-activated cell sorting (FACS) techniques (see Ch. 5), for further study and for use in autologous stem cell transplantation (Box 12.1).

HSCs migrate during embryonic development to the fetal liver and bone marrow. There they are induced to differentiate further by the large number of growth factors found in these tissues. Included amongst these growth factors are the **colony-stimulating-factors** (CSFs). Specific CSFs induce differentiation of particular cell lineages as discussed below.

In the presence of these various growth factors, including the CSFs, the HSCs become **progenitor cells** (Fig. 12.1). Progenitor cells are less primitive than HSCs and they have some commitment to develop along a particular cell lineage. Two separate immune system progenitor cells develop, i.e., the lymphoid and myeloid progenitor cells, under the influence of growth factors. These cells give rise to **mature cells**, which have fully differentiated, such as T cells (Fig. 12.1).

Lymphoid cells

Development
Figure 12.2 illustrates the major overall stages in the development of B and T cells from the lymphoid progenitor. The initial stages of T lymphocyte precursor (thymocyte) development, but not human pre-B cell

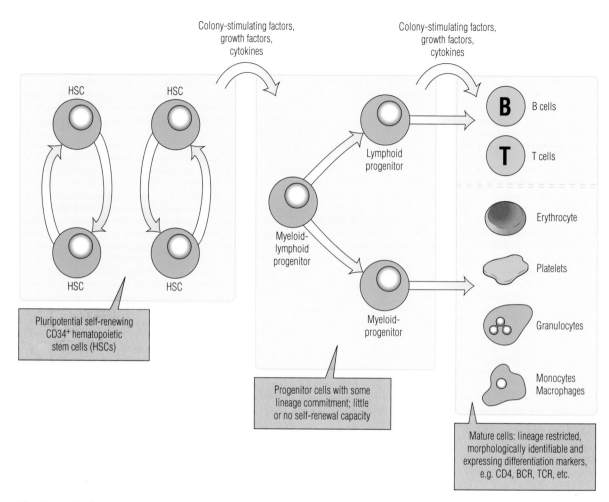

Fig. 12.1 The three major stages of hematopoiesis. HSC, hematopoietic stem cell; BCR, B cell receptor; TCR, T cell receptor.

BOX 12.1
Autologous hematopoietic stem cell transplantation

For several weeks following chemotherapy/ radiotherapy treatments for cancer, patients have severely depressed blood and immune systems. They are substantially at risk from infections. In certain circumstances, the patient's own bone marrow, which contains stem cells, is obtained prior to cancer therapy for use in treatment. This bone marrow is stored at very low temperatures in a medium that preserves the cells from destruction. It is returned to the patient (autologous bone marrow transplant) after chemotherapy/radiotherapy to help quickly to reconstitute the immune and blood cells. Since this is the patient's own marrow there are no complications with regard to transplant rejection. However, the process of obtaining the bone marrow

usually involves a relatively painful surgical procedure to aspirate cells from the pelvic bones under general anesthetic.

Large numbers of hematopoietic stem cells (HSCs) can be mobilized into the blood by giving patients granulocyte colony-stimulating factor (G-CSF). The HSCs are then identified by their expression of the CD34 molecule and harvested from the blood. Peripheral blood harvesting has been found to generate more stem cells than does bone marrow aspiration. It is also less painful for the patient, and it is becoming the approach of choice in preference to autologous bone marrow transplants in the treatment of certain patients. The general topic of transplantation is discussed in greater detail in Chapter 33.

Bone marrow   Thymus   Lymph node

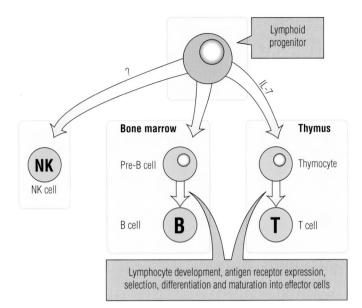

Fig. 12.2 Overview of the development of the lymphoid cell lineage.

development, are under the influence of the cytokine interleukin 7 (IL-7). IL-7 is produced and released from non-lymphoid stromal cells in the bone marrow. The bone marrow stromal cells include macrophages and adipocytes, and these are discussed further in Chapter 13. IL-7 is one of several cytokines affected by X-linked SCID (Box 12.3). Much of B lymphocyte development takes place in the bone marrow (see Chs 13 and 14). Most T lymphocytes develop in the thymus from thy-

mocyte precursors derived in the bone marrow (see Chs 13 and 15). The developmental pathway for natural killer (NK) cells is not yet well defined. NK cells are part of the innate immune system and their role in viral and tumor immunity is further described in Chapters 21 and 34.

X-linked severe combined immunodeficiency disease, in which both B and T cells are absent, is discussed in Box 12.2.

Box 12.2
X-linked severe combined immunodeficiency disease (XL-SCID)

Boys affected by XL-SCID are born with absent T and B cells and, if untreated, will rapidly die from infection. Bone marrow transplant is an effective treatment for these boys, but, tragically, in many cases an HLA-matched donor is unavailable.

In the 1990s, the mutation on the X chromosome responsible for XL-SCID was identified. The mutation is in the gene for a subunit of several T cell cytokine (growth factor) receptors, including the receptors for IL-2, IL-7 and IL-4. The cytokine receptor subunit is referred to as the γ chain.

Once the gene for the γ chain had been cloned, it became possible to repair the defect in the affected boys by **gene therapy**. Recombinant viruses are used to insert the corrected γ chain gene into precursor cells removed from the affected boys, in a process called transfection. The precursor cells are then

returned to the patient.

Up to the present, several children with XL-SCID have been treated with this gene therapy, which has been an overwhelming success. Although attempts at treating some other diseases caused by mutations have failed, gene therapy for XL-SCID has been successful because:

- The transfected cells are able to respond to the cytokines (growth factors) and hence start proliferating rapidly. They soon replace the cells containing the mutated gene.
- In other diseases, the protein product of the corrected gene is recognized as a "foreign" protein and elicits a destructive immune response. This cannot happen in immunodeficient children with XL-SCID.

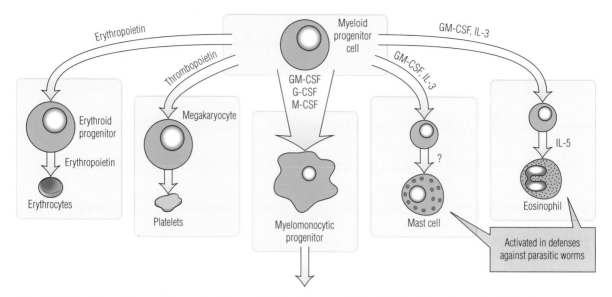

Fig. 12.3 Overview of the development of the myeloid cell lineage. IL, interleukin; CSF, colony-stimulating factors; GM, glanulocyte–macrophage; G, granulocyte; M, macrophage.

Lymphoid cell types

B cells (Fig. 2.6). These are the cells that produce antibody. They express immunoglobulin as an antigen-specific receptor along with several other important molecules such as MHC class II molecules and the co-receptor molecule CD19. Morphologically, they have a large nucleus surrounded by a small rim of cytoplasm. In addition to producing antibody to combat extracellular infections they can also function as antigen-presenting cells. They may be stimulated by antigen to form a larger blast cell with more cytoplasm, extensive endoplasmic reticulum, and secretory capacity for antibody.

T cells (Fig. 2.6). Morphologically T cells resemble unstimulated B cells, i.e., small lymphocytes with a large nucleus and small cytoplasm. They can be stimulated by antigen to become lymphoblasts with more cytoplasm and organelles. T cells consist of two subsets: CD4+ helper cells and CD8+ cytotoxic cells (Ch. 15). They also express an antigen-specific T cell receptor and they are the major source of antigen-specific protection against viral infection and other intracellular infections.

Natural killer cells (Fig. 2.6). NK cells are lymphocytes that do not have clonally distributed antigen-specific receptors. They are part of the innate immune system and lyse certain virally infected cells and some tumor cells (see Ch. 21).

Myeloid cells

Development

Figure 12.3 depicts the main stages in development of the other major white blood cells—the granulocyte and monocyte/macrophage lineages. These cells derive from the same myeloid progenitor that gives rise to erythrocytes and platelets. The various differentiation pathways are stimulated by the actions of different growth factor combinations, e.g., erythropoietin stimulates development of erythrocytes, and the CSFs (granulocyte–macrophage CSF (GM-CSF), granulocyte-CSF (G-CSF) and monocyte/macrophage-CSF (M-CSF)) stimulate development of the myelomonocytic progenitor cell and, ultimately, neutrophils, monocytes, macrophages and dendritic cells (DCs) (Fig. 12.4).

Various specific CSF/cytokine combinations are necessary for the differentiation of each myeloid cell type (Figs 12.3, 12.4 and 12.5).

Myeloid cell types

Neutrophils (Fig. 2.6). Neutrophils exhibit phagocytic and cytotoxic activities and they migrate to sites of inflammation and infection in response to chemotactic factors. They are short lived with a half-life of about 6 hours. About 10^{11} neutrophils are estimated to be generated every day in the adult human. They contain both primary granules, loaded with lysosomal enzymes including myeloperoxidase and elastase, and secondary granules containing lysozyme, collagenase, etc. These cells are often referred to as polymorphonuclear neutrophils (PMNs) because they have nuclei with two to five lobes. Their role as a first line of defense in the innate response to bacterial infections is discussed further in Chapter 24. Their development under the influence of G-CSF is discussed in Box 12.3.

Mast cells (Fig. 2.6). Mature mast cells have large granules which can be stained purple with dyes. These

Bone marrow   Thymus   Lymph node

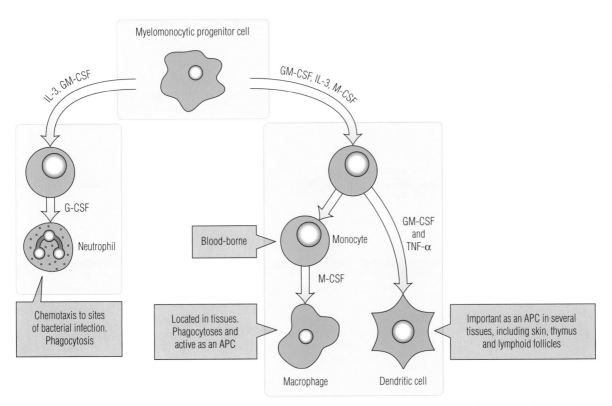

Fig. 12.4 Overview of the development of the monocyte/macrophage lineage. TNF, tumor necrosis factor; IL, interleukin; CSF, colony-stimulating factors; GM, glanulocyte–macrophage; G, granulocyte; M, macrophage.

granules contain heparin and histamine but do not contain hydrolytic enzymes. Mast cells express specific receptors on their surface for the Fc region of certain immunoglobulins, i.e., FcR_γ and FcR_ϵ. These cells have important roles in allergic responses (Ch. 26). They are activated through their receptors for IgE to release the above substances.

Eosinophils (Fig. 2.6). Eosinophils are characterized by a nucleus with two or three lobes. They have large specific granules, which contain heparin, as well as peroxidase and other hydrolytic enzymes. These cells have

phagocytic and cytotoxic activity and express Fc receptors, specifically FcR_γ and FcR_ϵ. These cells also function to combat certain parasitic infections—particularly worms (Ch. 21).

Monocytes/macrophages (Figs 2.6 and 2.7). Monocytes are the largest blood cells. They contain many granules and have a lobular shaped nucleus. Monocytes phagocytose, have bacteriocidal activity and can carry out antibody-dependent cell-mediated cytotoxicity (ADCC; see Ch. 21). Monocytes migrate out of the blood into the tissues and become tissue macrophages, e.g., the Kupffer

---

BOX 12.3
Administration of granulocyte colony-stimulating factor for neutropenia

Granulocyte colony-stimulating factor (G-CSF), because of its important role in hematopoiesis, has become a well-characterized protein. The G-CSF gene has been cloned, and a recombinant form of G-CSF has been produced for use in treatment. G-CSF causes an increase in neutrophil production in the bone marrow. Apart from its role in autologous stem cell transplantation, in vivo administration of G-CSF

has been approved for the treatment of neutropenias caused by several conditions including cancer chemotherapy and acute leukemia. The enhanced neutrophil levels produced by G-CSF treatment have been shown to protect these otherwise immunosuppressed patients from life-threatening bacterial infections (Box 20.1).

cells of the liver. They express the monocyte/ macrophage marker protein designated CD14. Macrophages have a central role at the dividing line between the innate and specific immune response because of their role in antigen processing and presentation.

Dendritic cells (Fig. 2.7). DCs are irregularly shaped cells with many branch-like membrane processes. Mature DCs are non-adherent and non-phagocytic. They express large amounts of MHC class II molecules and consequently they are excellent antigen-presenting cells (see Box 10.3). There are several different types of DC in different tissues. The type found in the skin is referred to as an epidermal Langerhans cell. DCs have a critical role in several aspects of lymphocyte development, and, because of their role in antigen presentation, they are also important in lymphocyte activation.

Fig. 12.5
Colony stimulating factors and cytokines important for hematopoiesis

Molecule	Major cellular sources	Major biological activity
Colony-stimulating factors		
Granulocyte	Monocytes, macrophages, fibroblasts, endothelial cells	Stimulates neutrophil formation
Granulocyte–macrophage	T cells, monocytes, macrophages, fibroblasts, endothelial cells	Stimulates proliferation and differentiation of myeloid progenitors
Monocyte/macrophage	Monocytes, macrophages, fibroblasts, endothelial cells	Stimulates proliferation and differentiation of monocytes and macrophages
Interleukins		
3	T cells	Stimulates multiple hematopoietic cells
4	T cells, natural killer cells, basophils, mast cells	Stimulates B cell proliferation
5	T cells	Stimulates differentiation of eosinophils
7	Stromal cells in the bone marrow	Stimulates T cell progenitor proliferation and differentiation

LEARNING POINTS

Can you now:

- Draw the developmental pathway from stem cell through progenitor cell to mature lymphoid and myeloid cells?
- Describe the role of colony-stimulating factors and other growth factors in the developmental pathways to lymphoid and myeloid cells?

- List several important morphological features and functional activities of B and T lymphocytes, natural killer cells, neutrophils, mast cells, eosinophils, monocytes, macrophages and dendritic cells?

Bone marrow   Thymus   Lymph node

The organs and tissues of the immune system

13

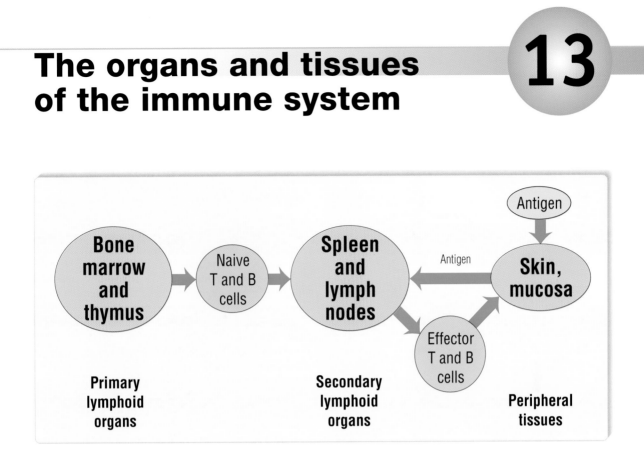

Up until this point in the book we have primarily discussed the genes, molecules and cells that function in the immune response. However, host defense responses take place in a whole organism, not in isolated cells or amongst subcellular components! It is now necessary to consider the immune response in the context of a physiological system.

PRIMARY AND SECONDARY LYMPHOID ORGANS

The immune system is made up of distinct compartments, the organs and tissues, that are interconnected by the blood and lymphatic systems. This chapter will describe several important features of the lymphoid organs and tissues and will introduce a systems view of the immune response. In the last few years, it has become obvious that although we know much about the genes, molecules and cells that are the basis of an immune response there is still much more to learn about how the immune response is coordinated at a systems level, and how the complex series of physiological events in vivo can influence the outcome of an immune response. Further discussion of how the immune system is integrated with other physiological systems, including the neural and endocrine systems, that can also influence immune response outcomes is provided in Chapter 35.

The immune system is thought of as being composed of those organs and tissues in which lymphocytes are produced—the **primary lymphoid organs**—and those where they come into contact with foreign antigen, are clonally expanded and mature into effector cells—the **secondary lymphoid organs**.

In the embryonic human (Fig. 13.1), the primary lymphoid organs (i.e., where lymphocytes are generated) are initially the yolk sac, then the fetal liver and spleen, and finally the bone marrow and thymus. In adult humans (Fig. 13.2), the primary lymphoid organs are the bone marrow and thymus. By puberty, most lymphopoiesis is B lymphocyte production in the marrow of the flat bones, e.g., the sternum, vertebrae and ribs.

The human secondary lymphoid organs are generally considered to be the spleen, lymph nodes and mucosa-associated lymphoid tissue (MALT) lining the respiratory, gastrointestinal and reproductive tracts. Some consider the skin (cutaneous immune system) in this category also. These organs are distributed as shown in Figure 13.2. Lymphocytes lodge in the secondary lymphoid organs and they expand clonally on contact with the antigen appropriate for their specific antigen receptors. They also recirculate between these organs via the blood and lymphatic systems. This lymphocyte recirculation or *trafficking* connects the various lymphoid compartments, creating one system (see below).

Lymphocytes are dispersed to almost all tissue sites and so almost all the tissues in the human body could be

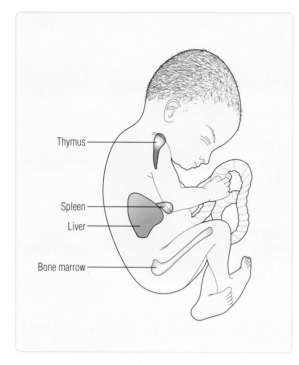

Fig. 13.1 Organs of lymphocyte production in the developing human.

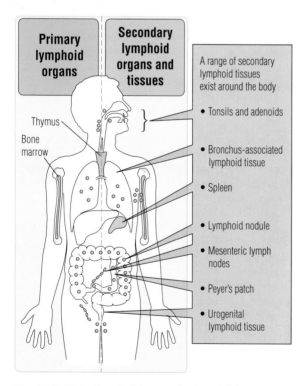

Fig. 13.2 Major lymphoid organs in the adult human. (Adapted from Roitt, I., Brostoff, J. and Male, D. 2001. *Immunology*, 6th edn. Mosby, London.)

thought of as "lymphoid tissues". However, some sites, e.g., eye, testis and brain, do not have lymphoid cells and these are said to be **immunologically privileged**. The most important sites of lymphocyte dispersal are the spleen, lymph nodes, MALT and skin. Each of these will be described briefly in this chapter to create a context for understanding the physiology of the immune response.

Bone marrow

As described in Chapter 12, the bone marrow is the major hematopoietic organ in humans. It is a richly cellular organ system. All of the blood cell types except mature T lymphocytes are found in the extensive cavities in the bone marrow. The extensive internal cavity structures in this organ can be seen on electron micrographs (Fig. 13.3). B cell generation takes place in these internal cavities; development from B cell progenitors to immature B cells occurs in a radial direction toward the center of the bone. This process will be described in more detail in Chapter 14.

Hematopoiesis is facilitated in the bone marrow by a mixture of cells and extracellular matrix components. This environment not only provides mechanical support but is also a source of the growth factors and cytokines essential for the development of the various blood cell types. The bone marrow reticular stroma, a mixture of extracellular matrix molecules, macrophages and adipocytes, is particularly important in B lymphocyte development, supplying cytokines and other molecules critical to the development of mature B cells.

Thymus

The thymus is a bilobed organ, found in the anterior mediastinum. The base of the thymus rests on the surface of the heart and because of this location the thymus is usually removed during some pediatric cardiothoracic surgical procedures, for example, surgery to repair a heart defect shortly after birth (Box 15.1). It is notable that removing the thymus after birth seems to have little effect on the ability of these children to mount an effective T cell-mediated immune response.

The thymus forms from two types of epithelial cell (endoderm and ectoderm) derived from the third pharyngeal pouch, the corresponding branchial clefts and the pharyngeal arch. The thymus grows until puberty; it then undergoes progressive involution, and it is largely adipose tissue, with only a small amount of lymphoid tissue remaining, by late adulthood.

Each of the lobes of the thymus is divided further into lobules by connective tissue septae called trabeculae. Figure 13.4a shows a stained section of a thymus. There are three main areas:

- the **subcapsular zone** containing the earliest progenitor cells

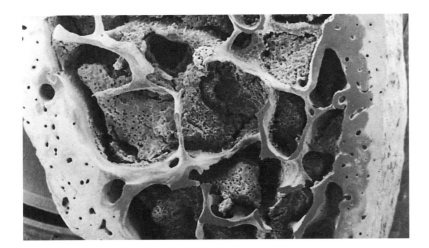

Fig. 13.3 Bone marrow as seen in a low-power scanning electron micrograph. (Reproduced with permission from Stevens, A and Lowe, J. 1999. *Human histology*, 2nd edn. Mosby, London.)

- the **cortex**, which is densely packed with developing T cells that are undergoing selection
- the **medulla** containing fewer, but more mature, T lymphocytes; these have survived the selection processes and are about to be released to the periphery (see Ch. 15).

The thymus is the primary site of T cell development. The vast majority of T cell progenitors (more than 95%) die in the thymus, through the process of apoptosis. There is an extensive network of epithelial cells and antigen-presenting cells that are involved in the selection process leading to the development of an appropriate T cell receptor repertoire. An outline of some of the important cell–cell interactions in T cell development is found in Figure 13.4b, and this topic is developed in more detail in Chapter 15.

Spleen

The spleen, a secondary lymphoid organ about the size of a clenched fist, is found in the left upper quadrant of the abdomen and cannot usually be palpated. It is a major "filter" for the blood, removing opsonized microbes and dead red blood cells. It is also the main site for responses to blood-borne antigens, and the source of B cells that respond in the absence of T cell help to bacterial cell wall polysaccharide antigens. Figure 13.5a shows a stained section of a spleen. There are two main areas: the **red pulp**, containing chiefly red blood cells in the process of disposal, and the **white pulp**, containing dense lymphoid tissue. The spleen has been estimated to lodge about 25% of the total lymphocytes in the body. The white pulp is segregated into B and T lymphocyte areas. The T cells are chiefly found in the **periarteriolar lymphoid sheaths** (PALS; Fig. 13.5b). The PALS are concentric cuffs of lymphocytes associated with central arterioles. Lymphoid follicles (Fig. 13.5c), some with germinal centers (GC; Fig. 13.5b and 13.5c), appear within the PALS. Most B cells are found in follicles. Follicles with germinal centers containing chiefly activated B cells are generally referred to as secondary follicles (Fig. 13.5c) to distinguish them from primary follicles (no germinal center), which contain chiefly resting B cells. The marginal zones (Fig. 13.5c) contain marginal zone B cells, macrophages and some T cells. The marginal zone B cells are particularly important in making responses to polysaccharide antigens (so-called T cell-independent antigens or TI-antigens; Ch. 14 and Box 13.1).

Lymph nodes

A lymph node is a bean-shaped structure (see Fig. 13.6b), usually found clustered in groups at sites where numerous blood and lymph vessels converge. For example, a large collection of nodes is found in the armpit (axillary nodes). Lymph nodes function to concentrate lymph-borne antigens for presentation to T cells. Lymph is absorbed extracellular fluid, and the lymph nodes filter (or survey) its contents for antigens before it drains into the blood stream.

A lymph node is organized into several areas (Fig. 13.6). The cortex is predominantly the site of B cells. As for the spleen, B cells are generally found in primary or secondary follicles (Fig. 13.6a), depending on their state of activation. The lymph node paracortex is predominantly a CD4+ T cell area. The medulla of the node contains a mixture of B cells, T cells and macrophages.

Circulating lymphocytes enter the node via specialized high endothelial venules (HEVs) in the paracortex.

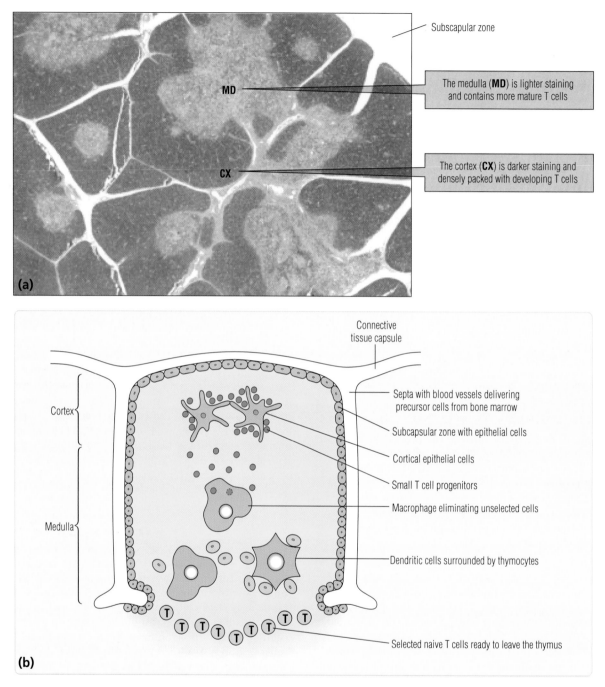

Subscapular zone

MD

The medulla (**MD**) is lighter staining and contains more mature T cells

CX

The cortex (**CX**) is darker staining and densely packed with developing T cells

(a)

Connective tissue capsule

Cortex

Medulla

Septa with blood vessels delivering precursor cells from bone marrow

Subcapsular zone with epithelial cells

Cortical epithelial cells

Small T cell progenitors

Macrophage eliminating unselected cells

Dendritic cells surrounded by thymocytes

Selected naive T cells ready to leave the thymus

(b)

Fig. 13.4 Thymus. (a) A stained section of the thymus. (Reproduced with permission from Kerr, J.B. 2000. *Atlas of functional histology*. Mosby, London. (b) A simplified schematic showing the cellular organization of the thymus.

Fig. 13.5 Spleen. (a) Stained section of the spleen. (b) Stained section of the spleen showing detail of PALS and GC. ((a) and (b) reproduced with permission from Kerr, J.B. 2000. *Atlas of funtional histology*. Mosby, London.) (c) A Simplified schematic showing the organization of the spleen.

Bone marrow   Thymus   Lymph node

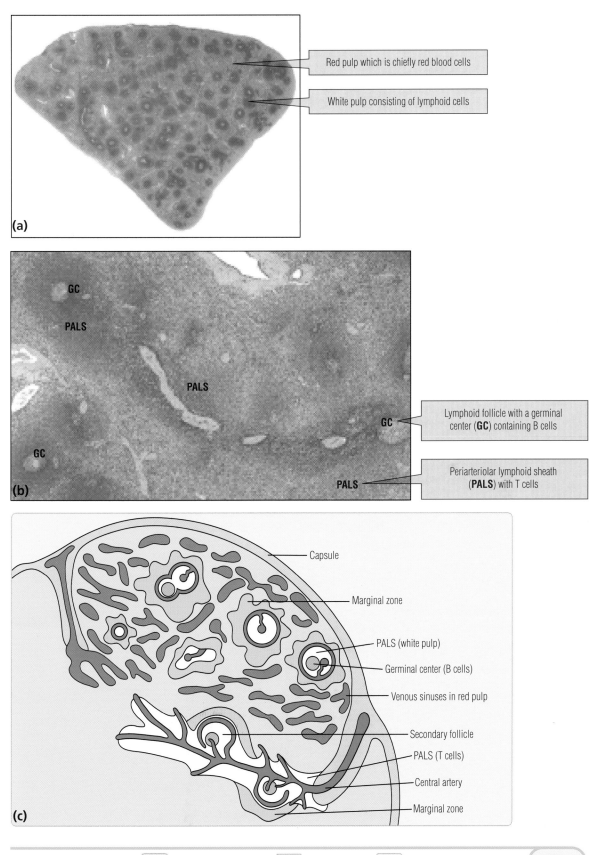

(a)

Red pulp which is chiefly red blood cells

White pulp consisting of lymphoid cells

(b)

GC

PALS

PALS

GC

GC

PALS

Lymphoid follicle with a germinal center (**GC**) containing B cells

Periarteriolar lymphoid sheath (**PALS**) with T cells

(c)

Capsule

Marginal zone

PALS (white pulp)

Germinal center (B cells)

Venous sinuses in red pulp

Secondary follicle

PALS (T cells)

Central artery

Marginal zone

Blood vessel   Gut   Peripheral tissue

BOX 13.1
Risks of splenectomy

The spleen is a soft, "spongy" organ that bleeds easily following trauma. In certain situations, for example lap-belt-mediated trauma sustained to the mid-section in a car accident, the spleen can be ruptured and it has to be surgically removed.

Splenectomized patients are more susceptible to infection by encapsulated bacteria, e.g., pneumococci, that are usually cleared by opsonization with antibody followed by phagocytosis by splenic macrophages. These patients are also less able to make antibody responses to polysaccharide antigens (T-independent

(TI) responses; Ch. 14). The marginal zone B cells in the spleen are particularly important in responses to the polysaccharide antigens found on bacterial cell walls, and splenectomy predisposes these patients to certain infections that require a TI-antibody response for protection.

Splenectomized patients are immunocompromised and they are significantly at risk of infectious disease. They are usually maintained on life-long prophylactic antibiotics.

(a)

(b)

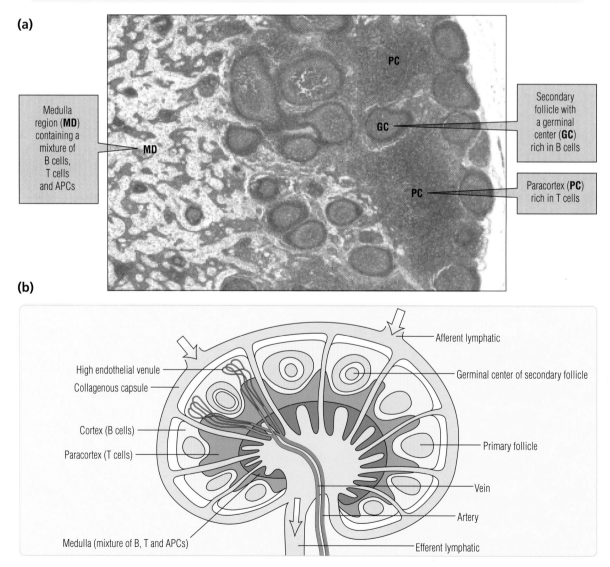

Fig. 13.6 Lymph nodes. (a) Stained section of a node. (Reproduced with permission from Kerr, J.B. 2000. *Atlas of functional histology.* Mosby, London.) (b) A simplified schematic showing the organization of a node. APC, antigen-presenting cell.

The important role of HEVs in lymphocyte trafficking is discussed below.

During a response to an infection, B and T cells in the node are activated. Fluid and cells are accumulated in the node during lymphocyte activation, leading to lymph node enlargement (the "swollen gland" typical of response to infection). After the immune system clears the infectious agent, the node returns to its normal size and it can no longer be palpated. The location of the swollen lymph nodes reflects the site of infection. For example, an infected finger leads to swollen axillary nodes. More generalized swollen nodes (lymphadenopathy) reflect a generalized infection or tumor.

Mucosa-associated lymphoid tissue

The mucosal immune system is principally composed, in humans, of lymphoid tissue in the respiratory and gastrointestinal tracts, known as nasopharyngeal-associated lymphoid tisue (NALT; e.g., tonsils and adenoids) and gut-associated lymphoid tissue (GALT; e.g., Peyer's patches), respectively. These tissues contain a specialized epithelial cell type—M cells—that takes up antigens that are inhaled or ingested. Antigens are taken up by M cells by the process of **pinocytosis**. Pinocytosis is the cellular intake of small vacuoles containing fluid and/or molecules. It is not clear if M cells also process and present antigens. The mucosal immune system handles antigen at a contact point between the host and the environment, and it is an important first line of defense. The mucosal tissues are enriched in IgA-producing plasma cells and they also contain T cells and macrophages.

Intraepithelial lymphocytes

The mucosal epithelium of the gastrointestinal, respiratory and reproductive tracts contains large numbers of lymphocytes. These lymphocytes are mostly T cells (~90%) and about half of these T cells are CD8+ $\gamma\delta$ T cells (Fig. 13.7d).

Intraepithelial lymphocytes are thought to develop locally without the influence of the thymus, although this is controversial. They appear to have T cell receptors of limited diversity and to recognize antigen directly, i.e., not as peptide–MHC complexes. The antigens recognized by intraepithelial lymphocytes tend to be expressed as a consequence of infection, e.g, heat-shock proteins. In general, intraepithelial lymphocytes act to protect the host against viral and bacterial pathogens encountered in the gut. In addition to their role as effector T cells, the intraepithelial T cells secrete cytokines that have a role in regulating immune responses in the mucosa. This regulatory role may, for example, prevent excessive responses to food antigens. Regulatory intraepithelial lymphocytes may maintain IgA responses during regimens designed to induce oral tolerance (Box 13.2).

Peyer's patches are closely associated with the lumen of the gut and form part of the GALT. Figure 13.7a shows a stained section of a Peyer's patch. The M cells transport antigens by a process called transcytosis into the subepithelial tissues where they encounter lymphocytes. Figure 13.7d shows a section of mucosa in which

BOX 13.2
Oral tolerance

Tolerance is defined as a state of immunological unresponsiveness to an antigen that can be induced by prior exposure to that antigen (see also Chs 14 and 15). Oral administration of a protein antigen in large doses has been found in many cases to lead to tolerance, i.e., a suppressed response on subsequent immunization with the antigen.

Since mucosal tissues are rich in lymphocytes and accessory cells, we might expect a significant immune response to a dose of oral protein antigen. Oral immunization with some antigens, e.g., oral poliovirus vaccine, is known to produce an effective long-lived protective immune response. However, several protein antigens, particularly if taken in large oral doses, have been found to induce immune tolerance. It is not known why oral tolerance is such a prevalent phenomenon. However, it has been suggested that it is a mechanism to protect against unwelcome and even life-threatening immune responses to food proteins. The possibility that oral tolerance could be used to inhibit the immune response against proteins implicated in various human autoimmune diseases has been considered for some time. Some success has been obtained with this approach in animal model systems. In addition, some preliminary clinical trials of oral tolerance have also been reported. However, much remains to be done before inducing tolerance orally becomes an accepted approach to therapy for human disease.

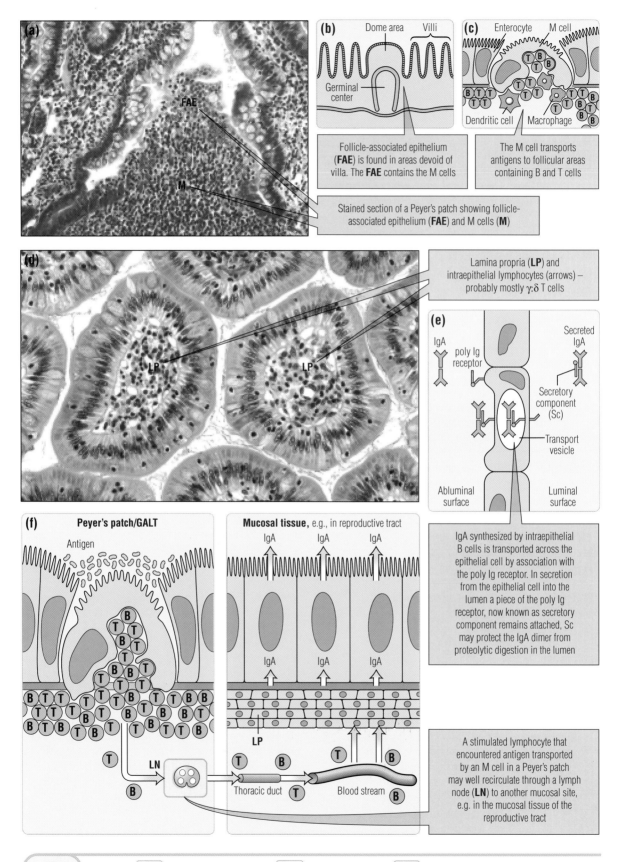

(a) FAE, M

(b) Dome area — Villi — Germinal center

(c) Enterocyte — M cell — Dendritic cell — Macrophage

Follicle-associated epithelium (**FAE**) is found in areas devoid of villa. The **FAE** contains the M cells

The M cell transports antigens to follicular areas containing B and T cells

Stained section of a Peyer's patch showing follicle-associated epithelium (**FAE**) and M cells (**M**)

(d) LP, LP

Lamina propria (**LP**) and intraepithelial lymphocytes (arrows) – probably mostly γ:δ T cells

(e) IgA — poly Ig receptor — Secreted IgA — Secretory component (Sc) — Transport vesicle — Abluminal surface — Luminal surface

IgA synthesized by intraepithelial B cells is transported across the epithelial cell by association with the poly Ig receptor. In secretion from the epithelial cell into the lumen a piece of the poly Ig receptor, now known as secretory component remains attached, Sc may protect the IgA dimer from proteolytic digestion in the lumen

(f) Peyer's patch/GALT — Antigen

Mucosal tissue, e.g., in reproductive tract — IgA IgA IgA — IgA IgA IgA — LP

LN — Thoracic duct — Blood stream

A stimulated lymphocyte that encountered antigen transported by an M cell in a Peyer's patch may well recirculate through a lymph node (**LN**) to another mucosal site, e.g. in the mucosal tissue of the reproductive tract

Bone marrow   Thymus   Lymph node

Fig. 13.7 Mucosa-associated lymphoid tissue (MALT). (a) A stained section of a Peyer's patch (gut MALT: GALT). (b) The organization of GALT in Peyer's patches. (c) An M cell in the intestinal follicle-associated epithelium (FAE). (d) A section of mucosa showing T and B cells in the lamina propria (LP). (e) Transport of IgA across epithelium. (f) Trafficking of lymphocytes from MALT. ((a) and (d) Reproduced with permission from Kerr, J.B. 2000. *Atlas of functional histology*. Mosby, London.)

the lamina propria contains T and B lymphocytes. Typically, the B cells are in follicles surrounded by a T cell zone. The B cells secrete IgA across the epithelium (Fig. 13.7e). IgA is initially bound to the poly-Ig receptor (Fig. 13.7e) and, after transport across the epithelial cell membrane, it retains a piece of this receptor (now known as secretory component), which may help protect it from degradation in the lumen.

After exposure to antigen in the MALT, lymphocytes may leave and home to other mucosal tissues. Figure 13.7f shows this migration (recirculation or trafficking) from Peyer's patches in the gut to other mucosal surfaces, e.g., the reproductive tract. This trafficking provides a potential target for vaccination, using mucosal vaccines for the initial stimulation (Box 13.3). Mucosal immune responses also occur in the lamina propria of secretory glands such as mammary and salivary glands.

Skin (cutaneous immune system)

The skin is the major physical barrier to pathogen entry, and it is a very important interface between the immune cells and the external environment. The skin has many lymphoid accessory cells, e.g., dendritic cells, that have critically important roles in handling environmental antigens that penetrate the skin. Many immune responses are initiated in the skin and, consequently, some view the skin as another peripheral organ of the immune system—the cutaneous immune tissue.

Figure 13.8a shows a photograph of inflamed skin during a delayed type hypersensitivity (DTH) response. This type of response is described in more detail in Chapter 30. The lymphoid cells involved in immune reactions in the skin are shown in Figure 13.8b. The epidermal layer of the skin has numerous dendritic cells called Langerhans cells, which are very important in antigen processing and presentation (see also Ch. 10) in the skin. The T cells found in the epidermal layer (intraepidermal T cells) in association with the Langerhans cells are chiefly CD8$^+$ cells. Frequently, these CD8$^+$ T cells carry $\gamma\delta$ T cell receptors (Ch. 7), similar to the situation described earlier for the intraepithelial T cells of the MALT. The underlying dermis is rich in macrophages and T cells (Fig. 13.8b).

BOX 13.3
Mucosal vaccines

Many pathogens, both bacterial and viral, invade the host via mucosal tissue. For example, HIV, which is primarily sexually transmitted, influenza, which invades through the respiratory mucosa, or *Shigella* and *Escherichia coli*, which cause enteric infections and diarrhea. For this reason, it would be very desirable to be able to vaccinate and induce a mucosal immune response that would prevent entry of such pathogens.

Attempts to produce effective mucosal vaccines have been frustrated by the phenomenon of oral tolerance described in Box 13.2. Other routes of administration to other mucosal sites include intranasal and intravaginal. Recent advances in mucosal vaccines have come from the use of mucosal adjuvants to prevent the induction of tolerance. Subunit proteins of certain bacterial

enterotoxins, including the B subunit of the heat-labile toxin (LT-B) of *E. coli*, have been shown to be mucosal adjuvants when co-administered with other vaccine proteins. Vaccination at one mucosal site can confer immunity at other mucosal sites because of lymphocyte migration to other mucosal tissues (Fig. 13.7f).

For example, a recent clinical trial has shown that intranasal immunization with an influenza vaccine together with LT-B stimulated effective anti-influenza immunity in human subjects. It is likely that our rapidly developing understanding of the mucosal immune system will lead to effective mucosal vaccines that will confer long-term protection against pathogens such as HIV, influenza, rotaviruses and the enteropathogenic bacteria. The impact worldwide of such mucosal vaccines would be enormous.

 Blood vessel   Gut   Peripheral tissue

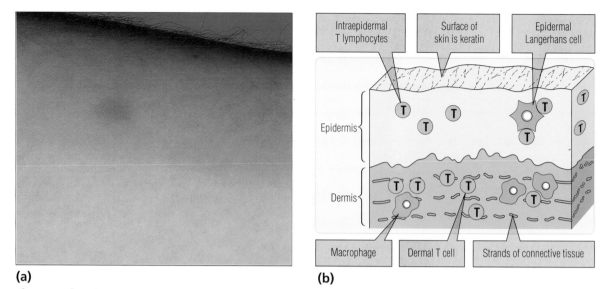

Fig. 13.8 Skin: the cutaneous immune system. (a) A photograph of inflamed skin during a DTH test. (b) A simplified schematic of skin showing antigen-presenting cells (APCs) and Langerhans cells.

LYMPHOCYTE RECIRCULATION (TRAFFICKING) AND HOMING

At this point we will confine our discussion of trafficking to lymphocytes. Trafficking of other white blood cells is discussed in Chapter 20. Most mature lymphocytes are in constant circulation via the bloodstream and lymphatics (Fig. 13.9). They move constantly from one lymphoid tissue to another, and from lymphoid tissue to peripheral tissue. It has been estimated that a lymphocyte makes a circuit of the human body, from the blood, to the tissues, to the lymphatic system and returns to the blood, once or twice a day. This circulation is important to ensure that the small number of lymphocytes specific for any given antigen have the best chance to find that antigen in any possible body site. Most of the circulating lymphocytes are T lymphocytes. B lymphocytes, since they secrete a soluble effector molecule (antibody) that interacts directly with antigen, have less requirement to recirculate, and so they spend longer time periods than T cells in the lymphoid organs.

Naive T lymphocytes, i.e., T lymphocytes that have not yet encountered the antigen they have specificity for (see Ch. 15), constantly circulate among the secondary lymphoid organs until they encounter antigen or die. This circulation through the lymphoid organs maximizes the chance to encounter antigen displayed on a professional antigen-presenting cell: a requirement to activate a naive T cell (see also Ch. 15). Effector (or memory, i.e., long-lived cells that retain "memory" of contact with antigen and respond faster;

see Ch. 17) T lymphocytes, by comparison, migrate to and lodge in selected tissue sites, where they may remain for some time. This process is referred to as **lymphocyte homing**. Posting T cells that have already been primed by contact with antigen in peripheral sites where they can screen for antigen enhances the likelihood of effective protection via a secondary immune response (Ch. 17).

Lymphocyte recirculation and homing is regulated by receptor–ligand interactions between members of the different families of cell adhesion molecules (CAMs; Fig. 13.10). There are several extensive families of CAMs. The major ones are the selectins, addressins, integrins and the CAMs that are a part of the immunoglobulin superfamily. These molecules have a variety of important roles in the immune response. Figure 13.10 illustrates some of the molecules that are most important in leukocyte recirculation and homing. The same molecules, and others in these families, have roles in several physiological processes that involve cell migration, including development, tissue repair and the adaptive and innate immune responses.

The most important of these adhesion protein interactions is between proteins on the lymphocyte surface (mostly the naive T lymphocyte surface) and proteins on the surface of the endothelial cells lining postcapillary venules, particularly HEVs. The HEVs have thicker than usual endothelial cell linings and are found in lymph nodes and MALT (e.g., Peyer's patches). They facilitate lymphocyte transport out of the bloodstream into the tissues, a process known as lymphocyte extravasation.

Bone marrow   Thymus   Lymph node

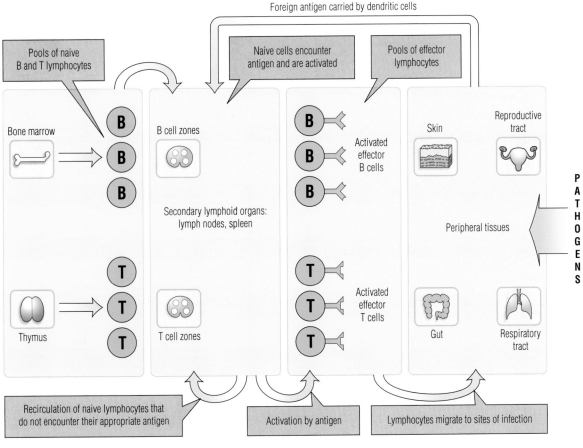

Fig. 13.9 Recirculation of lymphocytes.

Fig. 13.10
Cell adhesion molecules that are important in lymphocyte recirculation

Receptor	Function and tissue distribution	Ligand	Function and tissue distribution
L-Selectin (CD62L) (selectin family)	Leukocyte homing receptor, binds carbohydrates	GlyCAM-1 (addressin family)	Endothelial cell adhesion molecule found on the high endothelial venules of lymph nodes
		MAdCAM-1 (addressin family)	Endothelial cell adhesion molecule found on the high endothelial venules of mucosal lymphoid tissue
Leukocyte function associated antigen (LFA-1; CD11a/CD18) (integrin family)	Secondary adhesion molecule found on T cells, monocytes, polymorphonuclear cells, etc.	Intercellular adhesion molecules (immunoglobulin superfamily)	Found on endothelial cells; function in secondary adhesion and transmigration
Very late antigen 4 (VLA-4; CD49d/CD29) (integrin family)	Role in primary adhesion of effector lymphocytes that are homing to sites of infection	Vascular cell adhesion molecule (CD106) (immunoglobulin superfamily)	Found on endothelial cells that have been activated by an inflammatory response

Blood vessel   Gut   Peripheral tissue

Lymphocyte extravasation

Figure 13.11 is a simplified representation of the four steps in lymphocyte extravasation. The four steps are:

1. primary adhesion to endothelium
2. lymphocyte activation
3. secondary adhesion (arrest)
4. transmigration/chemotaxis.

Lymphocytes normally flow freely through the blood vessels. Analyses by videomicroscopy show that they can roll along endothelial cells, slowed down by low-affinity interactions between receptor molecules on the lymphocyte cell surface, known as homing receptors, and ligands known as addressins on the vascular endothelial cell surface (Fig. 13.10). If the lymphocyte detects signals that there is an infection in the tissue, e.g., by detecting inflammatory mediators such as chemokines (see Ch. 20), then the lymphocyte may be

triggered, or activated, to express other adhesive molecules that can mediate strong, high-affinity, adhesive interactions. This primary adhesion, triggering and expression of new adhesion molecules takes place in a few seconds, and lymphocyte movement is stopped even in the presence of considerable sheer forces from the ongoing blood flow.

The secondary adhesion phase is mediated by high-affinity interactions between different families of CAMs found both on the lymphocyte surface and on the endothelial cells in the tissues. Expression of different addressin molecules in different tissues allows lymphocytes to home to various tissue sites based on selective homing receptor–addressin expression and interaction (Fig. 13.10).

Lymphocyte arrest is followed by passage (**diapedesis** or transmigration) through the tight junction between adjacent endothelial cells into the tissues (Fig. 13.11). Once recruited into tissues, lymphocytes

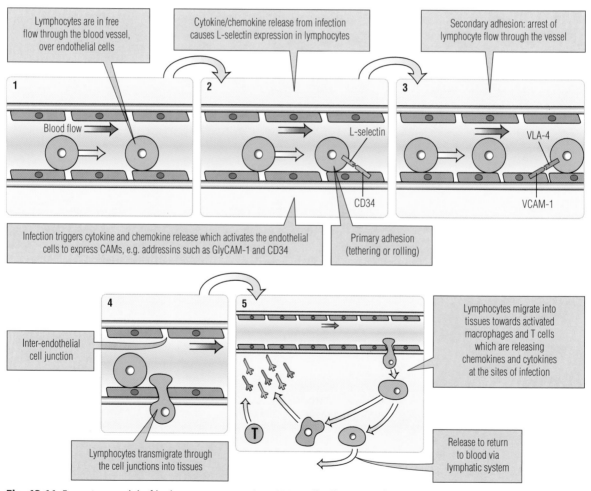

Fig. 13.11 Four-step model of leukocyte extravasation. CAM, cell adhesion molecule; VLA, very late antigen; VCAM, vascular cell adhesion molecule.

Bone marrow   Thymus   Lymph node

then disperse into specialized areas, e.g., B lymphocytes to primary B cell follicles, T cells to PALS, etc.

It is important to point out that the specificity of the recirculation/homing process is entirely a function of homing receptor–addressin interactions and is independent of antigen. In fact, most lymphocytes recruited to an infected tissue are not specific for the antigen causing the infection. However, an ongoing immune response does influence the retention of lymphocytes at a tissue site, and it causes release of various factors that stimulate expression of adhesion proteins.

LEARNING POINTS

Can you now:

- Describe the immune response in terms of a systemic physiological response?
- Describe the role of the bone marrow in lymphocyte generation and B cell maturation?
- Draw the cellular organization of the thymus and describe the role of the thymus in T lymphocyte generation and maturation?
- Draw the structure of the spleen and describe its role:
  - as a major site of responses to blood-borne antigens
  - as a "filter" for the blood
  - as a site of T-independent antibody synthesis?
- Draw the structure of a lymph node and describe its role as a "filter" for the lymph and as a major site for responses to lymph-borne antigens?
- Describe the role of the various mucosa-associated lymphoid tissues (GALT, NALT, etc.) as a first line of defense, trapping environmental pathogens and presenting them to lymphocytes?
- Describe the important role of the skin as a part of the immune system?
- Draw the major recirculation pathways of lymphocytes around the organs and tissues of the immune system?
- Draw the four-step model of lymphocyte extravasation?

B cell development

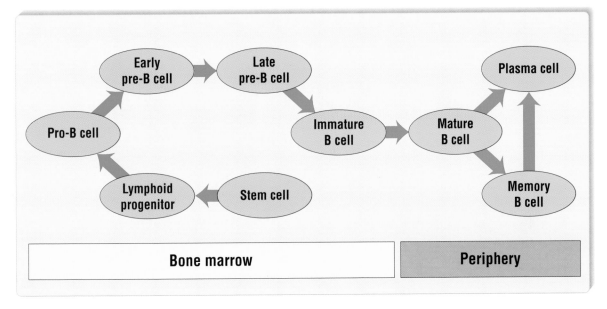

As discussed in Chapters 6 and 11, membrane-bound antibody molecules on the surface of B cells comprise a key part of the B cell receptor (BCR) that is responsible for recognizing antigen. A series of developmental stages (defined largely by the receptor gene rearrangements that occur during these stages) results in expression of the antigen-specific BCR. B lymphocytes expressing a diverse repertoire of BCRs, as yet unselected, are generated continually in the bone marrow. Before reaching maturity, the developing B cells undergo a selection process (referred to as **negative selection**) in an attempt to ensure that their antigen receptor does not display self-reactivity. Anti-self reactivity may result in autoimmunity (Ch. 27). Those B cells surviving negative selection disperse to the peripheral lymphoid organs (Ch. 13) where they may encounter the foreign antigen they have specificity for, become activated and, ultimately, terminally differentiate into antibody-producing cells. Those cells that do not encounter the appropriate antigen die in a matter of days or at most a few weeks. In this chapter, the developmental stages of the B cell, from hematopoietic stem cell to mature B cell will be discussed; the stages include:

- pro-B cells
- pre-B cells
- immature B cells
- mature B cells
- plasma or memory cells.

Early B lymphocyte development

Stem cell to immature B cell

The B cell lineage is derived from lymphoid progenitor cells that differentiate from hematopoietic stem cells (Ch. 12). B cells are produced throughout life, with differentiation first occurring in the fetal liver and then shifting to the bone marrow soon after birth (Chs 12 and 13). In the adult bone marrow, B cell development can be seen to follow a radially organized maturation pathway, with the least developed cells close to the endosteal (inner) surface of the bone and the more mature cells concentrated in the central marrow space (Fig. 14.1). Immature B cells exit the bone marrow via the sinusoids and migrate to the periphery. Their development in the bone marrow depends on a variety of growth factors contributed by bone marrow stromal cells (Ch. 12).

From the earliest cell progenitor, the hematopoietic stem cell, the B cell differentiation pathway can be subdivided into several developmental stages. These stages are defined by the rearrangement status of the

Material in this chapter contributed by Dr Patrick Swanson, Department of Medical Microbiology and Immunology, Creighton University School of Medicine, Omaha, Nebraska, USA.

 Blood vessel Gut ▨ Peripheral tissue

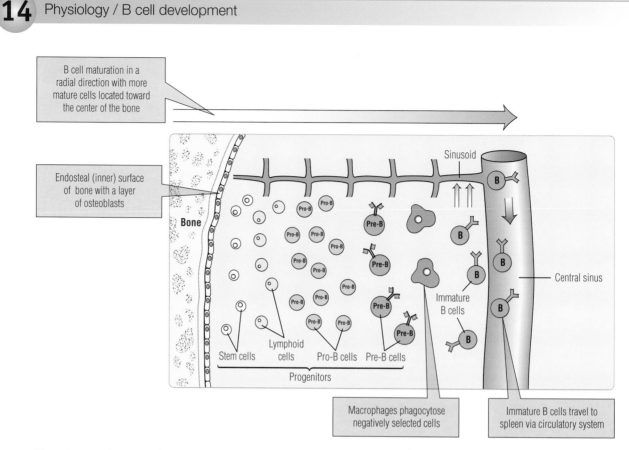

Fig. 14.1 Development of B cells in bone marrow.

Fig. 14.2

Steps in B cell development pathway. Other molecules not shown in this figure have been used to define B cell maturation. For simplicity, other stages of differentiation have also been omitted

	Stem cell	Pro-B cell	Early pre-B cell	Late pre-B cell	Immature B cell
Surface markers					
CD34	+	+	–	–	–
CD19	–	+	+	+	+
Expression of *RAG* genes	–	++↑	+↓	++↑	+↓
Status of immunoglobulin genes					
H	Germline	D_H to J_H and V_H to $D_H J_H$ rearrangement	$V_H D_H J_H$ rearrangement	$V_H D_H J_H C_\mu$	$V_H D_H J_H C_\mu$
L	Germline	Germline	Germline	V_L to J_L rearrangement	$V_L J_L C_L$
Expression of pre-BCR or BCR proteins					
ψL	–	+	+	–	–
μ	–	–	+	+	+
Pre-BCR	–	–	+	–	–
BCR	–	–	–	–	+

Bone marrow   Thymus   Lymph node

immunoglobulin heavy and light chain genes and the expression of differentiation-specific molecules (markers) on the cell surface (Fig. 14.2). The earliest committed B lineage cell is called the **pro-B** cell. This cell is recognized by the appearance of surface markers characterizing the B lineage (e.g., CD19, a part of the co-receptor complex; Ch. 11). The rearrangement of immunoglobulin heavy chain diversity (D_H) and joining (J_H) gene segments, i.e., the joining of D_H to J_H occurs during this developmental stage. Next, attempts are made to rearrange immunoglobulin heavy chain variable region (V_H) gene segments to be adjacent to the rearranged $D_H J_H$ segments. Productive V_H to $D_H J_H$ recombination generates a contiguous variable region gene segment from which a μ heavy chain is eventually expressed (see also Ch. 6). At the **early pre-B stage**, two invariant polypeptides associated non-covalently with one another to form a light chain-like structure, called the surrogate light chain (ψL), pair with the μ_H chain. The resulting complex is expressed on the cell surface in association with immunoglobulin α- and β-chains (Ch. 11) to form a receptor complex termed the **pre-B cell receptor** (pre-BCR). The pre-BCR plays an important role in tranducing signals leading to proliferative expansion of the pre-B cells and thereby facilitating their further development. Proliferation promotes further development and progression towards the next main stage—the **late pre-B cell**.

Acquisition of the pre-BCR coincides with rapid cellular proliferation and downregulation of the *V(D)J* recombinase machinery: *RAG-1*, *RAG-2* (recombination activating genes 1 and 2) and terminal deoxynucleotidyl transferase (TdT) (Ch. 6). These events have the dual effect of selecting B cells with functionally rearranged receptor genes and also preventing further V_H to $D_H J_H$ rearrangements, thereby limiting the possibility that two different antigen-binding regions are expressed on the same B cell. The recombination activating genes are essential for the immune response to function and defects can lead to deficiency diseases (Box 14.1).

Later in the **pre-B cell stage**, the *V(D)J* recombinase machinery is upregulated and light chain gene rearrangement is initiated. The appearance of paired light and heavy chain polypeptides on the cell surface as a complete IgM molecule, the BCR, constitutes the transition to an **immature B cell**.

It is worth pointing out that until the BCR is present on the cell surface, the antigenic specificity of the receptor cannot be tested. Consequently, the recombinational processes involved in B cell development that give rise to extensive receptor diversity necessarily generate some antigen receptors that possess self-reactivity. The next phase of B cell development involves screening this as-yet unselected receptor repertoire against self-antigen, a process that occurs during the transition from the immature to mature B cell, as discussed in greater detail below.

Ordered immunoglobulin gene segment rearrangement and allelic exclusion

As discussed in Chapter 6, the developing B cell has an extensive array of possible *V*, *D* and *J* gene segments from which to assemble functional immunoglobulin

---

BOX 14.1
Autosomal recessive SCID due to defects in the recombination activating gene (RAG-1, RAG-2) products

The RAG enzymes initiate immunoglobulin gene rearrangements in B cells. They are also essential in T cells for TCR gene rearrangements (see Chs 7 and 15). Further evidence of their importance comes from the fact that deficiencies in *RAG-1* or *RAG-2* lead to autosomal recessive severe combined immunodeficiency disease (SCID). The form of autosomal recessive SCID that results from *RAG-1/RAG-2* mutations is different from other forms of the disease in that there is a complete absence of both T and B cells. There are, however, NK cells found in the circulation. Hence, this form of the disease is known as T–B–SCID.

T–B–SCID is a rare syndrome that without bone marrow transplantation (BMT) from an HLA-compatible donor is invariably fatal by two years of age. The disease presents in infants during the first few weeks of life as lymphopenia with recurrent infections. Only a very small thymus can be detected. These babies have recurrent episodes of pneumonia, otitis and skin infections. They have persistent infections with opportunistic organisms such as *Candida albicans* and *Pneumocystis carinii*. For the parents and the pediatrician this is an extreme emergency situation. These children are at great risk. However, if BMT is performed early enough, over 80% of children survive. SCID as a syndrome is rare and T–B–SCID even rarer. However, there are several hundred individuals who are alive today after BMT to correct the various forms of SCID that they suffered from. BMT is further discussed in Chapter 34.

---

heavy and light chain genes. Moreover, each cell has two different light chain loci (κ and λ), either of which could undergo rearrangement to generate a light chain to pair with a given heavy chain. Finally, each cell possesses two copies of each immunoglobulin locus (one donated from each set of parental chromosomes), and both are capable of being rearranged. Yet, only a single parental chromosome is used to synthesize a given heavy or light chain, resulting in the expression of a single heavy and light chain combination (a **monospecific** BCR), a phenomenon termed **allelic exclusion** (Ch. 6 and Fig. 6.11). This outcome is critical because it prevents different antibodies with distinct antigenic specificities from being secreted from the same cell, a situation that is wasteful and potentially dangerous to the organism. So how is allelic exclusion achieved?

The developmentally ordered process of heavy and light chain gene rearrangement plays an important role in ensuring that only a single type of receptor locus is rearranged at a time; i.e., first the heavy chain, then the light chain (Figs 14.3 and 14.4). But why is it that a given locus is only rearranged on one allele at a time? The answer to this question is related to how heavy and light chain gene rearrangements are developmentally regulated. Specifically, the general molecular processes responsible for rendering a given

immunoglobulin heavy or light chain locus physically accessible to the *V(D)J* recombination machinery are also involved in keeping one allele inaccessible to the recombination machinery while the other allele undergoes *V(D)J* rearrangement. The mechanistic details underlying these processes have not been completely elucidated, but it appears that actively rearranging loci assume a less compact chromosomal organization than their quiescent counterparts. How the rearrangement status of a given allele is communicated to the other allele is also not yet clear.

The transition from immature to mature B cell

Once the B cell completes the early maturation stages in the bone marrow, it begins to migrate to peripheral lymphoid organs to complete its development. As immature B cells mature, they pass through a transitional stage. During this stage the *V(D)J* recombination machinery (RAG-1 and RAG-2) is downregulated, surface expression of IgM is increased, and membrane-bound IgD, arising after alternative splicing of heavy-chain transcripts (Ch. 6), begins to appear on the B cell surface (Fig. 14.5). Once B cells progress through this stage, they become

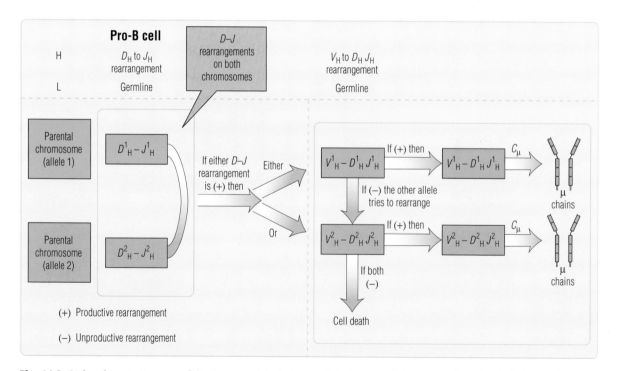

Fig. 14.3 Ordered rearrangement of the immunoglobulin heavy chain locus, enabling expression of a single heavy chain.

Bone marrow   Thymus   Lymph node

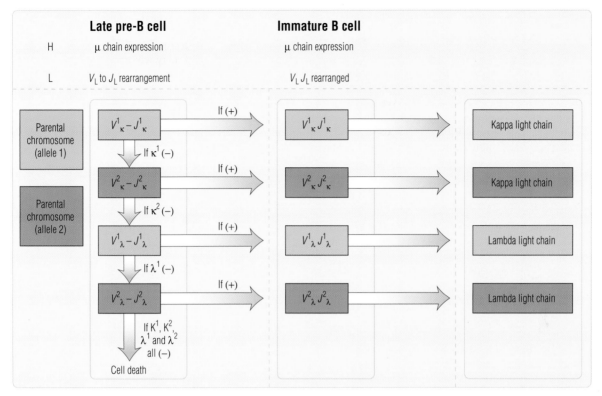

Fig. 14.4 Ordered rearrangement of the immunoglobulin light chain locus, enabling expression of a single light chain.

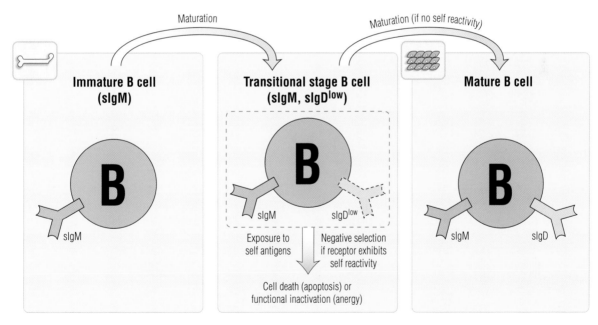

Fig. 14.5 Transition from immature to mature B cell; migration from bone marrow to periphery.

mature B cells, expressing both surface IgM and IgD. B cells that have fully rearranged immunoglobulin genes but have not yet encountered non-self antigen are often known as **naive** or **virgin B cells**. The rearrangement of immunoglobulin genes can be followed using Southern blotting (Box 14.2).

 Blood vessel · Gut · Peripheral tissue

BOX 14.2
Molecular genetic analysis of B cell tumors

As described in Chapter 6, the techniques of molecular genetics, e.g., Southern blotting, can be used to follow immunoglobulin gene rearrangement. Immunglobulin genes rearrange in normal and neoplastic human B lymphocytes, and Southern blotting, for example, is useful in the clinical diagnosis and monitoring of lymphoma. As described in Chapter 6, Box 6.1, Southern blot analysis with a J_H probe of a normal, polyclonal population of B cells purified from blood does not detect specific DNA fragments from rearranged immunoglobulin genes (see Fig. 14.6, Lane 1). However, if there is malignant expansion of a clone of B cells in a patient then rearranged immunoglobulin genes can be detected. As the "monoclonal B cell population" increases in the blood, the one or two rearranged immunoglobulin genes in this population of B cells will appear as one or two distinct bands that hybridize to the J_H probe (see Fig. 14.6, Lanes 2 and 3). The intensity of the bands from the neoplastic B cells increases as the tumor grows (see Lanes 2 and 3), and decreases after tumor therapy, e.g., chemotherapy or immunotherapy with anti-CD20 (see Box 9.1 and Ch. 34), as shown in Lane 4. Thus, Southern blotting and other molecular genetic techniques can be very useful to the hematopathologist in monitoring lymphoid malignancies. These molecular techniques enhance the morphological interpretations of the pathologist, and provide the physician with "molecular markers" that can guide diagnosis and the selection of new therapies.

Fig. 14.6 Analysis of follicular lymphoma by Southern blotting with J_H probe.

Induction of tolerance

During the transitional phase, an important event occurs that helps to shape the final BCR repertoire. As immature B cells begin to encounter self antigens, those cells with antigen receptors that display self-reactivity are deleted or functionally inactivated, a process termed **negative selection**. This selection process results in a pool of immature B cells that do *not* become activated when challenged with self antigen, a condition called **tolerance**. The process of selection leading to the induction of tolerance to self is important in reducing potential self-destructive responses. One of the downsides of generating an enormous repertoire of receptors is the potential for anti-self receptors with potentially negative effects. Removing or inactivating the cells bearing these anti-self receptors is critical to avoiding pathology, i.e., autoimmune disease. By the process of negative selection the immune system fine-tunes the B cell repertoire and avoids contributing to disease states.

While self antigens comprise the bulk of the antigens with potential to induce tolerance that an immature B cell will encounter, it is important to note that foreign antigens can also induce tolerance when presented to immature B cells, thereby tricking the immune system into believing that the foreign antigen is part of the "self" milieu.

If the immature B cell does not recognize any antigens present in the bone marrow, it will continue to develop into a mature B cell. However, antigen binding by the immature BCR triggers a series of events designed to induce tolerance toward the antigen. How tolerance is rendered depends on both the relative ability to crosslink the BCR and the dose of the antigen (Fig. 14.7). Let us first consider the fate of cells recognizing antigens that are abundant on the cell surface and that can extensively crosslink immature BCRs (multivalent antigens). Extensive crosslinking of the immature BCR by a multivalent antigen induces a state of maturational arrest. During this period, the *V(D)J* recombination machinery is upregulated to try to alter receptor specificity away from (perceived) autoreactivity by reinitiating *V(D)J* rearrangement, a process known as **receptor editing** (Fig. 14.8). Typically, additional light chain gene rearrangements are attempted in order to replace the existing light chain with one that does not display self-reactivity when paired with the heavy chain. If new, productive, gene rearrangements cannot be obtained that alter receptor specificity so that it is no longer self-reactive, the cell will die by apoptosis, an outcome called **clonal deletion**. Because multivalent antigens (e.g., abundant cell surface molecules) are capable of crosslinking multiple BCRs on a single cell, the dose required to achieve tolerance to these antigens is quite low.

Immature B cells respond somewhat differently to univalent antigens: small, soluble proteins that cannot effectively crosslink the immature BCR. Since these antigens can support less-extensive BCR crosslinking than do multivalent antigens, they display more dose dependence. When immature B cells are exposed to high doses of such a soluble antigen, responding B cells downregulate expression of IgM and are rendered incapable of becoming activated upon subsequent antigenic challenge, a condition called **anergy** (Fig. 14.7).

When there is an established peripheral B cell population (e.g., in the adult) only about 20% of new cells will survive the migration to the peripheral lymphoid organs and subsequently enter a long-lived pool of recirculating follicular B cells. The remaining 80% die within about 1 week. This observation suggests that maturing B cells must compete for limited anatomic sites in the periphery (most likely the follicles of the lymphoid organs) that provide suitable environments for supporting their continued survival and development (see also Ch. 17).

The mature B cell

Additional tolerance induction

Since not all self antigens are present in the bone marrow, mechanisms have evolved to ensure that the

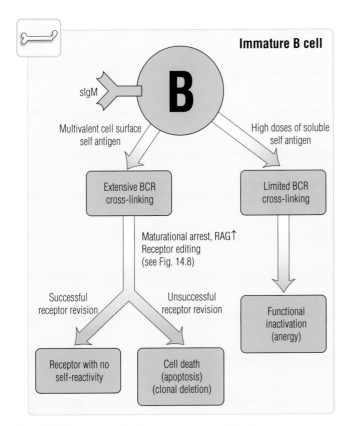

Fig. 14.7 Receptor selection: generating self-tolerance.

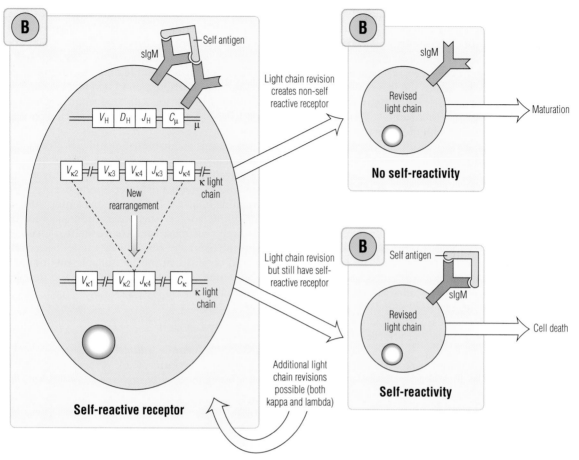

Fig. 14.8 B cell receptor editing.

mature B cell pool is rendered tolerant to self antigens encountered in the periphery. As has been introduced in Chapters 10 and 11, and will be discussed below and in more detail in Chapter 16, specific T cell help is generally required for the mature B cell to produce antibody. If the mature B cell engages an antigen and no T cell specific for the antigen responds to provide the necessary signals (Chs 11 and 16) for the B cell to become fully activated, the cell will undergo clonal deletion or become anergic. As with immature B cells, the outcome of receptor engagement depends on the antigen encountered. Multivalent antigens generally cause clonal deletion, and univalent antigens induce anergy (Fig. 14.7). An important difference, however, is that the *V(D)J* recombination machinery, present through most stages of B cell development, appears to be permanently shut off when B cells acquire mature levels of surface IgM and IgD. Therefore, the option to undergo additional receptor editing in fully mature B cells is lost.

Activation and antibody production

Specialized anatomical structures in the secondary lymphoid organs (Ch. 13) provide an environment where

antigen is concentrated and displayed on antigen-presenting cells (e.g., follicular dendritic cells) to incoming naive B cells, which in turn interact with localized T cells that support B cell activation and differentiation. Each type of secondary lymphoid tissue traps antigen from different sources: the spleen collects blood-borne antigens, antigens present in the afferent lymphatic system are trapped in lymph nodes, and mucosa-associated lymphoid tissues (MALT, e.g., Peyer's patches in gut and tonsils/adenoids in nasopharynx) acquire antigen from the surrounding mucosal epithelia.

The activation of a naive B cell and its subsequent differentiation into an antibody-secreting **plasma cell** is a multistep process that usually begins when the B cell exits the bloodstream and enters a secondary lymphoid organ (Fig. 14.9). Upon entry, the B cell migrates into a region rich in T cells (called the paracortex in lymph nodes, and the periarteriolar lymphoid sheath in spleen; Ch. 13). In the absence of its target antigen, the B cell traverses this region and eventually re-enters the circulation. If the B cell encounters its target antigen, antigen engagement by the BCR triggers the B cell to internalize the BCR–antigen complex. Then the antigen

Bone marrow   Thymus   Lymph node

is degraded and, in the case of protein antigens, processed into peptide–MHC class II complexes, which are subsequently displayed on the cell surface (Ch. 10).

As a general rule, naive B cells cannot be activated by antigen alone. A second accessory signal is required to initiate full activation of the B cell (Ch. 16). In the case of protein antigens, the second signal is delivered by an activated T cell with an antigen receptor (TCR) that recognizes the peptide–MHC class II complex displayed by the B cell or by antigen presented by a neighboring antigen-presenting cell. Antigens that require this form of B cell–T cell collaboration to initiate an immune response are termed **thymus-dependent** (TD) antigens,

because athymic animals that lack T cells are unable to mount an immune response to these antigens.

Continued selection of B cells in lymphoid follicles

Signals derived from the antigen–BCR complex and the TCR–MHC class II complex cause the B cell to become activated and begin proliferating (Chs 11 and 16), forming a primary focus of B blast cells at the boundary of the T cell zone and follicle (Fig. 14.9). Some of the progeny differentiate into plasma cells secreting IgM. Others migrate into the lymphoid follicles to establish a germinal center (Ch. 13), where they undergo a period of rapid proliferation (dividing about once every 6 hours). During this period, somatic mutations are introduced into the antigen-receptor genes (Ch. 6) resulting in the expression of BCRs that vary in their affinity toward the antigen that initiated the immune response.

B cells positively selected by interaction with antigen encountered in the network of follicular dendritic cells and germinal center T cells may undergo an additional round of proliferation and somatic mutation. Alternatively they may leave the germinal center and terminally differentiate into a plasma cell, or they may become a recirculating **memory B cell** (Ch. 17). The memory cells do not secrete antibody but can be rapidly reactivated upon subsequent antigenic challenge. As the process of somatic mutation is repeated several times, populations of B cells bearing receptors with increasing affinity toward dwindling levels of antigen are selected. This process is referred to as **affinity maturation** and occurs in BCRs (Ch. 6) but not TCRs (Ch. 7). The presence of T cells in the germinal center also supports immunoglobulin class switching (Chs 6 and 16), which provides an important means of altering the effector function of the antibodies produced by the B cells.

Upon terminally differentiating, the plasma cell homes to the bone marrow or intestinal lamina propria (Ch. 13), where it secretes large amounts of antibody for a period of at least several weeks. Expression of surface immunoglobulin is downregulated on these B cells and, hence, they no longer respond to antigen. By comparison, the recirculating memory B cells (Ch. 17) readily respond to subsequent antigenic challenge as they express a functional (and affinity-matured) BCR. Once reactivated, memory cells can terminally differentiate into plasma cells.

Thymus-independent antigens

As was briefly described earlier, B cells responding to polypeptide antigens require two signals to become fully activated: one derived from crosslinking the BCR, and one obtained from TCR recognition of peptide–MHC complexes displayed on the B cell surface

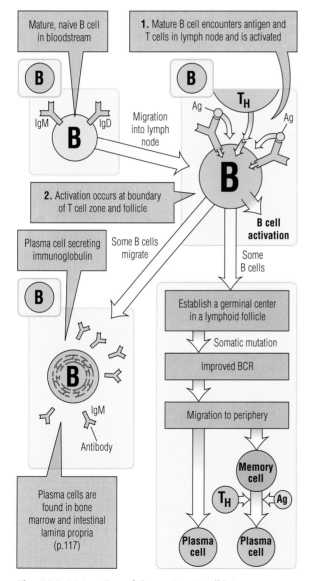

Fig. 14.9 Maturation of the mature B cell into an effector B cell (plasma cell).

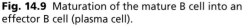

(Ch. 16). However, some antigens are able to activate B cells directly in the absence of T cell help; hence, they are called **thymus-independent** (TI) antigens. In this case, the second signal is derived from the antigen itself.

Figure 14.10 illustrates how TI antigens activate B cells. TI antigens include repeating polymers, such as dextran and bacterial polysaccharides, and certain bacterial cell wall components, such as lipopolysaccharides.

It is important to consider the protective mechanism that responses to TI antigens play in host defense. As these antigens are often of bacterial origin, TI responses provide a means to generate an early and specific antibody response against bacterial pathogens that can proliferate quickly and overwhelm the immune system. However, since T cells are not usually mobilized, the antibody repertoire generated during TI responses is limited because T cell-dependent events that promote affinity maturation and class switching are not induced.

The B cell repertoire and human development

In adults, most peripheral B cells belong to a pool of long-lived, recirculating follicular B lymphocytes collectively termed conventional (or B-2) B cells. However, other B cell populations also emerge from the precursors of conventional B cells. An important subset is referred to as B-1 cells. B-1 cells appear to develop from immature B cell precursors, but they are phenotypically distinct from conventional B cells and they express different cell surface markers (Fig. 14.11). For example, many, but

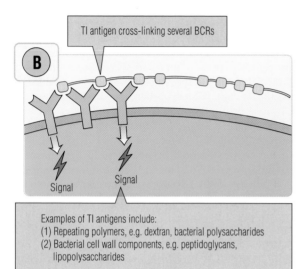

Fig. 14.10 T-independent (TI) antigens.

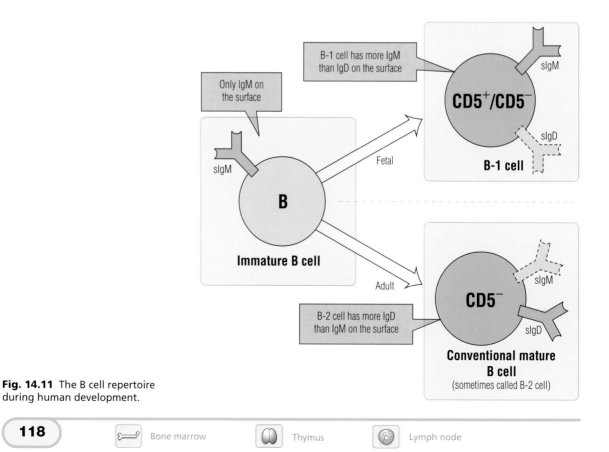

Fig. 14.11 The B cell repertoire during human development.

Bone marrow   Thymus   Lymph node

not all, B-1 cells express a surface marker called CD5 that is not found on conventional B cells.

B-1 cells comprise the majority of B cells found in the fetus and neonate. After birth, a developmental transition occurs during which B cell precursors switch from being committed to the B-1 lineage to being committed to the conventional B lineage. Unlike conventional B cells, which are constantly being renewed from bone marrow precursors, B-1 cells in the adult replenish themselves by continuing division of cells carrying surface IgM (sIgM$^+$) in peripheral tissues, thereby ensuring a persistent B-1 population long after their generation has ceased. This property likely contributes to the tendency of B-1 cells (particularly the CD5$^+$ cells) to be a frequent source for a relatively common B cell neoplasm called chronic lymphocytic leukemia (Box 14.3 and Ch. 34).

The B-1 cell receptor repertoire is rather restricted, as a result of preferential use of a few V_H genes and limited, if any, insertional diversity, caused by a lack of TdT expression in these cells. The BCRs expressed on B-1 cells are often reactive toward bacterial antigens (e.g., polysaccharides) and they frequently display polyspecificity—the ability to cross-react with multiple antigens. Hence, B-1 cells provide an important protective function against bacterial pathogens early in life until the adult repertoire develops. However, the tendency of B-1 cells to produce cross-reactive antibodies may partly explain the observation that B-1 cells are disproportionately represented among autoantibody-producing B cells. The antibodies produced by B-1 cells, sometimes called **natural antibodies**, are described further in Chapter 27.

BOX 14.3
Microarrays or gene expression profiling

Microscopy-based classification systems of lymphoid tumors are rapidly being enhanced by molecular diagnostic methods. The sequencing of the human genome and the availability of probes for the expressed human genes makes it possible to use a molecular technique called microarray analysis to compare quantitatively the expression of thousands of human genes simultaneously in, for example, normal and malignant B cells. This gene expression profiling technique has been used to subdivide a broad class of B cell lymphomas, called diffuse large B cell lymphoma (DLBCL), the most frequent type of non-Hodgkin's lymphoma, into subtypes that have different patient outcomes.

The basis of the microarray technique is the ability to construct an ordered array of DNA fragments, each from a different gene, on a single glass slide or microchip. Sophisticated fabrication techniques have been developed, and continue to be enhanced, that allow thousands of different gene sequences to be represented on a single chip or slide (the "microarray"). It is already possible to measure expression of about 50% of the human expressed genes on one microarray! Next, mRNA is prepared from the cells of interest (for example, B cell tumors

of the same diagnostic category from different patients). Fluorescent cDNA probes are prepared from the total mRNA samples from each tumor cell preparation and allowed to hybridize to the microarray under conditions similar to those used for Southern blotting. Scanning devices not unlike those used in flow cytometry (see Ch. 5) are used to quantitate the amount of fluorescent cDNA probe bound to the microarray. The amount of fluorescence is proportional to the amount of probe bound, which is proportional to the amount of expression (amount of mRNA) of that gene in that cell. Thus, the genes expressed in different types of B cell tumor can be compared.

In recent studies, most genes were found to be equivalently expressed in, for example, different B cell lymphomas of the same clinical category, but differences were detected between lymphoma samples from certain diagnostic categories, e.g., in the category called diffuse large B cell lymphoma. This suggested that the new molecular diagnostic techniques will be very useful in establishing subtypes of tumors currently thought to be of one type, and in distinguishing them from one another, ultimately helping to better detect and monitor cancer.

LEARNING POINTS

Can you now:

- Draw the different cell types in the stages of the B cell development pathway?
- Recall the time-dependent changes in cell markers during the B cell development pathway?
- Draw the order of rearrangement and expression of immunoglobulin heavy chain and light chain genes during B cell development?
- Explain the molecular basis of allelic exclusion in B cells?
- Compare and contrast T-dependent and T-independent B cell activation?
- Explain antigen-induced tolerance in immature and mature B cell populations?
- Describe receptor editing and affinity maturation in terms of B cell antigen receptor improvement?

Bone marrow   Thymus   Lymph node

T cell development

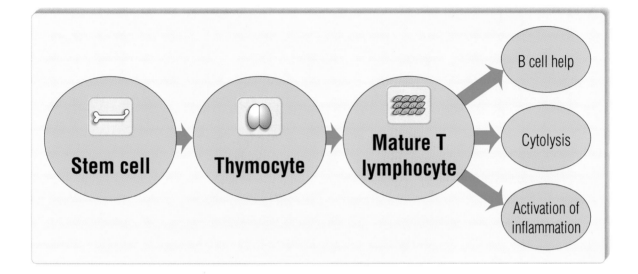

As we have already seen (Chs 7 and 10), the highly variable T cell receptor (TCR) recognizes antigen as peptide fragments bound to self-MHC molecules. The main topic for this chapter is how a diverse population of T lymphocytes with different antigenic specificities is generated. Most T lymphocytes are generated in the thymus. T cell development in the thymus is a multi-step process with several built-in checks to ensure that the appropriate differentiation has taken place. As a result of these biological checkpoints, only a small proportion of progenitor T cells, known as **thymocytes**, actually exit the thymus to the periphery as mature T cells; the vast majority (about 98%) die during the selection processes that establish the T lymphocyte repertoire. These thymic selection processes enable the host to develop a T cell repertoire that is **self-tolerant** and yet **self-restricted** (Ch. 8). This means that the mature T cells that develop are those capable of recognizing non-self antigenic peptides bound to self-MHC molecules.

Different subsets of mature T cells carry out the functions of **cell-mediated immunity** including killing virally infected cells and tumor cells, activating the bactericidal functions of macrophages, "helping" B cells and CD8+ T cells to mature into effector cells, and secreting various cytokines. This chapter, and Chapter 16, will describe how different subsets of T cells are activated to perform their effector functions.

THE THYMUS

The architecture of the thymus was described in Chapter 13, and its role as a primary lymphoid organ in Chapters 12 and 13. You should recall that the thymus is organized into three major areas: the subcapsular zone, the cortex and the medulla (Fig. 15.1). Different populations of stromal cells and thymocytes are found in each of these structurally and functionally distinct regions. The critical role of the thymus in T cell development is illustrated by the observation that individuals who never develop a thymus (complete Di George syndrome) have minimal mature peripheral T cells (Box 15.1). Despite the critical nature of the fetal thymus in establishing a peripheral T cell population, the thymus is not necessary to maintain mature antigen-specific T cells. Thymectomy has little impact on T cell responses in humans after birth unless the peripheral T cell population is eliminated and needs to be re-established, such as in the case of individuals who undergo bone marrow transplantation (Ch. 33). Also, as was noted in Chapter 13, the thymus atrophies

Material in this chapter contributed by Dr Kristen Drescher, Department of Medical Microbiology and Immunology, Creighton University School of Medicine, Omaha, Nebraska, USA.

 Blood vessel Gut Peripheral tissue

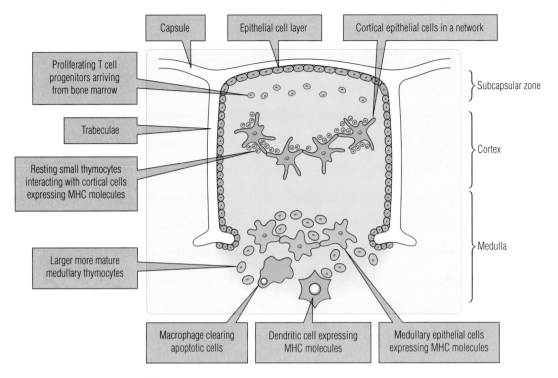

Capsule

Epithelial cell layer

Cortical epithelial cells in a network

Proliferating T cell progenitors arriving from bone marrow

Subcapsular zone

Trabeculae

Cortex

Resting small thymocytes interacting with cortical cells expressing MHC molecules

Larger more mature medullary thymocytes

Medulla

Macrophage clearing apoptotic cells

Dendritic cell expressing MHC molecules

Medullary epithelial cells expressing MHC molecules

Fig. 15.1 Simplified schematic of thymic organization.

BOX 15.1
Partial Di George syndrome

As a neonatologist, you are called to the pediatric intensive care unit to see an infant who has had a series of convulsions shown to be caused by very low calcium levels. An incidental finding on chest X-ray is that his thymus is absent. This combination is seen in the Di George syndrome, where structures derived from the 3rd and 4th pharyngeal pouches do not develop, including the thymus and parathyroid glands (which control blood calcium levels). The infant fortunately does not have some of the other anomalies associated with Di George syndrome, for example cardiac and facial defects. Further testing shows part of chromosome 22 has been deleted, confirming the diagnosis.

This male infant continues to develop fairly normally. He is observed to have a decreased number of CD3+ T cells. However, his immunoglobulin levels are normal. He handles normal childhood infections well and he is not provided any special immunological treatment.

Children with partial Di George syndrome, as in our example, tend to develop fairly normally provided they do not have other associated problems, e.g., heart defects. However, patients with complete Di George syndrome suffer from opportunistic infections (e.g., from fungi and viruses) in much the same way as do those with severe combined immunodeficiency disease (SCID; see Ch. 31).

The relatively sophisticated level of our understanding of T cell development has led some physician–scientists to attempt to reconstitute immune functions in patients with complete Di George syndrome by transplanting HLA-matched thymic tissue removed during cardiac surgery. This has met with some success in children with the complete syndrome, although only a small number of children have been treated this way and it is premature to conclude that this could become the preferred mode of treatment.

Bone marrow   Thymus   Lymph node

throughout adult life in humans. The reason for this is unknown.

Transition from thymocyte to mature T cell

In the thymus, the different stages of thymocyte development can be identified by establishing which cell surface molecules are being expressed (Figs 15.2 and 15.3). This is done with specific monoclonal antibodies using the technique of flow cytometry (Ch. 5). Specific monoclonal antibodies that recognize T cell surface molecules can be used to establish how many of a particular subset of T cells are present in the blood, to purify the subset or to block its function (Fig. 15.4). These experimental approaches have been essential to understanding T lymphocyte development, which follows the stages:

1. triple-negative (TN) cells: subcapsular zone
2. commitment to $\alpha\beta$ or $\gamma\delta$ lineage
3. double-positive cells (DP: CD4$^+$ CD8$^+$): cortex

4. selection of DP cells by MHC class I or class II: cortex
5. single-positive cells (SP: CD4$^+$ or CD8$^+$ depending on the class of MHC molecule interacted with): medulla
6. Release of SP cells as naive mature T cells: periphery.

Upon migrating to the thymus and locating in the subcapsular zone, bone marrow-derived thymocytes do not express (are said to be negative for) the cell surface molecules usually associated with T cells (e.g., CD3/TCR, CD4, CD8), and they are referred to as triple-negative (TN) cells (Fig. 15.3). At this stage, the TCR genes are in the germline (unrearranged) configuration.

As shown in Figures 15.2 and 15.3, the TN thymocyte subpopulation undergoes several important differentiation events. The TN cells become committed to the T cell lineage as TCR gene rearrangements begin to occur (described below). Another important choice that is made at this stage is commitment to either the $\alpha\beta$ or $\gamma\delta$ T cell lineage. As mentioned above (Ch. 7),

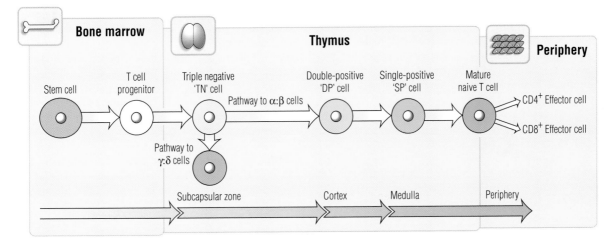

Fig. 15.2 Overview of pathway of T cell maturation.

Fig. 15.3
Order of expression of major T cell surface molecules (CD44, CD25, pTCR, CD3, CD4, CD8, TCR, etc.) during development

Stage of development	TN cell	CD4$^+$ CD8$^+$ DP cell	CD4$^+$ CD8$^-$ or CD4$^-$ CD8$^+$ SP cell	Mature naive
Surface molecule				
CD44	+	–	–	–
CD25	+	–	–	–
CD4	–	+	+ or –	+ or –
CD8	–	+	+ or –	+ or –
TCR/CD3	–	+	+	+

 Blood vessel   Gut   Peripheral tissue   **123**

Fig. 15.4
T cell surface molecules and cytokines used in identifying T cell subsets

T cell subset	CTL	T$_H$1	T$_H$2
Surface molecule			
CD3/TCR	✓	✓	✓
CD4	–	✓	✓
CD8	✓	–	–
Cytokine			
IL-2	✓	✓	✓
IL-4	–	–	✓
IFN-γ	–	✓	–

there are two major lineages of T cells expressing different types of TCR. The γδ T cells are a minor population in terms of numbers, and they are most often found in the skin and in mucosal tissue, especially the gut. The major T cell population is represented by αβ TCR-expressing T lymphocytes. Notably, both these T cell lineages derive from a common progenitor cell, with commitment to one lineage or the other being a competitive process based on which TCR genes productively rearrange first (compare with the process of immunoglobulin light chain gene expression in B cells; Ch. 14).

The next major step in the T cell development pathway is the double-positive (DP) stage (Figs 15.2 and 15.3). DP cells express both CD4 and CD8. They are found at very low levels in normal blood; most are found in the thymic cortex. The DP stage is the point at which cells are positively selected (retained) if they express a TCR that can recognize self-MHC and nega-

tively selected (deleted) if they express receptors that recognize self-peptide antigens with self-MHC molecules. Most (approximately 95%) DP cells never mature because they lack TCRs that can appropriately recognize self-MHC.

At the next step in the T cell development pathway (Figs 15.2 and 15.3), the cells migrate to the thymic medulla. At this point, depending on whether or not the TCR interacts appropriately with a class I or class II MHC molecule, the cells become single positive (SP): either CD4⁻ CD8⁺ or CD4⁺ CD8⁻. This is known as **lineage commitment**. SP cells undergo further selection and they are then released into the periphery as naive mature T cells (Figs 15.2 and 15.3).

Order of T cell receptor gene rearrangements
As shown in Figure 15.5, rearrangement of TCR genes begins at the TN stage. The β, γ and δ genes all attempt to rearrange at this stage. This involves activation of the

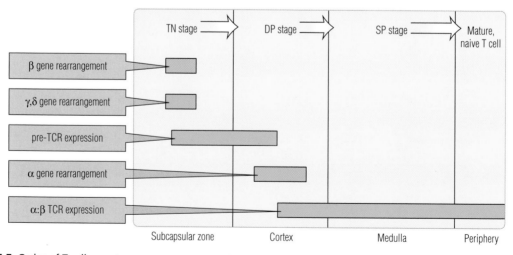

Fig. 15.5 Order of T cell receptor gene rearrangements.

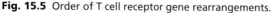

🦴 Bone marrow   🫘 Thymus   🔴 Lymph node

biochemical "machinery" described in Chapter 7, and multiple gene rearrangements. If a functional γδ receptor is produced then a γδ TCR-expressing T cell results. Those cells with γδ TCRs establish the γδ lineage. The functions of this lineage of T cells are discussed further later in this chapter.

Some of the other TN cells express a TCR β-chain. This involves TCR gene segment rearrangements, activation of recombinase genes (*RAG-1*, *RAG-2*), and other molecular events as described in Chapter 7. Once a functional TCR β-chain is expressed at the cell surface, it complexes with an invariant pre-T α-chain, and the CD3 molecule (Chs 7 and 11) to form a pre-TCR complex. Expression of the pre-TCR allows signal transduction (Ch. 11), and, in some fashion that is not yet entirely clear, this halts further β-chain rearrangements and allows proliferation of the DP-T cells. Proliferation promotes TCR α-chain rearrangement after recombinase expression. Therefore, similar to the role of the pre-BCR (Ch. 14), expression of the pre-TCR is a critical step in the pathway to assembly of an αβ TCR and formation of the αβ T cell population.

Positive selection: establishment of self-restriction

The DP cell, based on interaction with MHC molecules, may mature into an SP cell. However, most DP cells die in the cortex because they lack receptors capable of interacting with self-MHC. Cortical epithelial cells play an important role in positive selection by displaying the MHC–peptide antigen complex for the TCR. Survival (**positive selection**) of any given DP thymocyte is dependent on the ability of the TCR expressed on that cell to interact with the MHC–peptide antigen complex on the cortical epithelial cell and transduce a signal that triggers differentiation into

an SP cell. The TCR may interact with either an MHC class I or MHC class II molecule depending on its particular structure and recognition capability. Positive selection depends on the intensity of the signal generated by the TCR during the interaction. In ways that are not entirely understood, this signal influences the expression of either the CD4 or CD8 molecule on the cell surface. In a second step in the process, the combination of TCR and co-receptor (CD4 or CD8) is "double-checked". This step involves ensuring that a T cell that is CD8+, for example, expresses a TCR that preferentially recognizes non-self peptides displayed by MHC class I molecules. Only those cells with a co-receptor that matches the specificity of that cell's TCR (i.e., CD4 with a TCR that is specific for (restricted to) MHC class II molecules, and CD8 with a TCR that is specific for (restricted to) MHC class I molecules) are able to complete the maturation process and move out into the periphery. Figure 15.6 illustrates some of the steps in this positive selection process.

Negative selection: establishment of self-tolerance

The pool of cells generated by positive selection is self-MHC restricted, but it also includes self-reactive cells. These self-reactive cells must be eliminated or the host risks autoimmune disease. The process of elimination involves **negative selection** (Fig. 15.6). During negative selection, clones reactive with self-peptides are eliminated, and a state of self-tolerance is established. The process of negative selection involves encountering self-peptides displayed on MHC molecules on the surface of dendritic cells in the medulla of the thymus. Many tissue and soluble antigens are encountered in the thymus, but not all. Therefore, negative selection is not a perfect way to eliminate self-reactivity—some

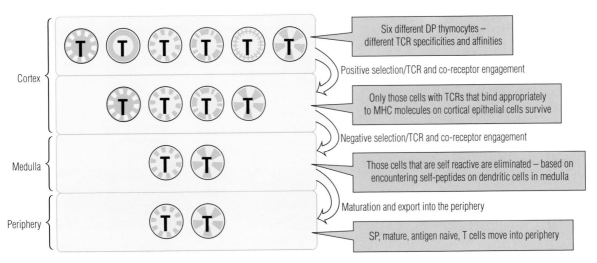

Fig. 15.6 Positive and negative selection processes.

cells with receptors reactive with self-peptides will survive.

Negative selection is mediated by signal transduction through the TCR, leading to induction of apoptosis and eventual clonal deletion. Apoptosis is the mechanism responsible for cell death induced by negative selection in the thymus. Apoptotic cells are disposed of by thymic macrophages. The apoptotic process can be visualized by TUNEL assay (terminal deoxynucleotidyl transferase-mediated dUTP nick-end labeling; Box 15.2).

It has been estimated that two thirds of the cells that survive positive selection in the cortex are subsequently deleted by negative selection in the medulla. Consequently, a very small number of the original thymocytes emerge into the periphery as mature, but still antigen-naive, T cells. **Naive** refers to the fact that these cells have not yet encountered the antigen that specifically "fits" their TCR.

T cell receptor signaling in positive and negative selection

The same molecular interaction (i.e., TCR binding to MHC–peptide antigen complex) mediates both positive and negative selection (Fig. 15.8). How can very different outcomes result from the same type of

BOX 15.2
TUNEL assay for apoptotic cells

Apoptosis is programmed cell death. While cytotoxic T cells can induce apoptosis in target cells, there is also the internally generated cell death program which can occur in most cells in the absence of injury or attack by the immune system. Apoptosis probably helps maintain homeostasis in normal tissues, and represents a mechanism to replace a small percentage of cells. Some tissues, e.g., neural tissue, where cells are not constantly regenerated, do not exhibit apoptosis, but in others, e.g., the thymus, there is a significant amount of cell death by apoptosis.

One of the changes in apoptotic cells is the activation of endonucleases and degradation of DNA into relatively small fragments. These events have been exploited to develop a morphological assay (the TUNEL assay) for apoptosis. The fragments of DNA are labeled and visualized as follows.

A purified sample of the enzyme TdT (terminal deoxynucleotidyl transferase), which has been mentioned before in terms of its role in gene rearrangement in immunoglobulin and TCR genes, is utilized to add a biotin-labeled nucleotide (usually uridine, i.e., dUTP) to the ends of the DNA fragments. The biotin is then detected using an enzyme-derivatized form of streptavidin which binds very tightly to the biotin. The enzyme coupled to streptavidin is capable of converting a colorless substrate into a colored insoluble product. The colored precipitate is only found in cells that have undergone apoptosis (see Fig. 15.7).

The example of a TUNEL assay in Figure 15.7 shows apoptosis in virally infected neural tissue from a murine spinal cord. The virus is Theiler's virus, a murine virus that causes a neurodegenerative disease similar to human multiple sclerosis. The viral infection results in cell death by apoptosis, and the apoptotic cells are the cells stained as red/black areas in the photograph.

(a)

(b)

Fig. 15.7 TUNEL histology. (a) Virally infected neural tissue. (b) (Control), uninfected neural tissue.

Bone marrow   Thymus   Lymph node

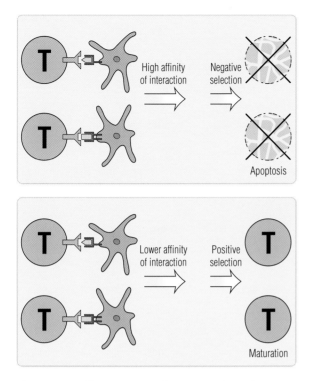

Fig. 15.8 T cell receptor signaling in positive and negative selection.

lower (but not too low!) affinity interactions between the TCR and the MHC molecule lead to positive selection and continued maturation.

THE PERIPHERY: NAIVE T CELL ACTIVATION BY ANTIGEN

The mature T cells that leave the thymus have not yet encountered the antigen that they have specificity for (sometimes referred to as their **cognate antigen**). At this stage, they are said to be naive, mature T cells. These cells may circulate from the bloodstream to the central lymphoid organs (e.g., spleen, lymph nodes, Peyer's patches) for years before they die or encounter antigen.

Antigen is usually encountered on a professional antigen-presenting cell (APC) in a secondary lymphoid organ (Ch. 13). If the TCR recognizes antigen displayed on MHC molecules (first signal) and also receives a second co-stimulatory signal (Ch. 16) the T cell is activated (Fig. 15.9; Ch. 11). The activated cells then proliferate and undergo clonal expansion and differentiation into effector cells, most of which are short lived. These effector cells are often said to be "antigen primed", and this process is referred to as "priming" the T cells. The effector T cells at this stage are also sometimes referred to as "armed" effector T cells. These primed or armed cells undergo several changes, e.g., expression of new cell surface molecules such as CD154 (CD40 ligand) and various adhesion molecules (Chs 13 and 16). The effector T cells can move into peripheral tissues and other organs to handle pathogen infection directly, or they can migrate to germinal centers to help to activate B cells with specificity for the same antigen to secrete antibody.

The end result is a vigorous T cell response and destruction of the pathogen. Most of the activated T

receptor–ligand interaction? It has been suggested that different affinities of interaction between TCRs and MHC–peptide complexes generate different intracellular signals. These signals might be quantitatively or qualitatively different. Investigations are underway to determine the nature of these signals and to establish an answer to this paradox. At the present time, one simplified interpretation of the available data would be that high-affinity interactions between the TCR and the appropriate MHC molecule lead to negative selection (deletion) of the cell expressing that TCR, whereas

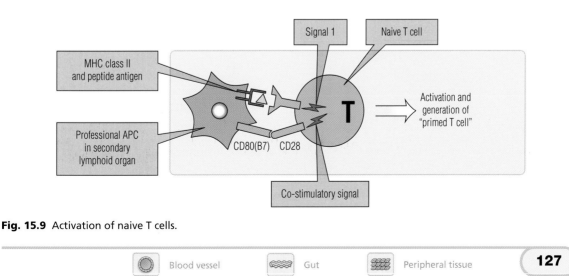

Fig. 15.9 Activation of naive T cells.

cells then die by apoptosis, restoring homeostasis to the T cell pool. A few armed effector cells mature into memory T cells which can respond faster and more effectively on re-encountering antigen (see Ch. 17).

Mature T cell responses and functions

After the naive, mature T cell has encountered its cognate antigen–MHC complex and received either a co-stimulatory signal from a professional APC or stimulation by an appropriate cytokine, it proliferates and differentiates into an effector cell. Cytokines such as interleukin (IL) 2 are also released from the T cell and contribute to the clonal expansion. The CD8+ and CD4+ T cell subsets can then develop with different effector functions.

By virtue of CD4+ and CD8+ effector T cells, the immune response can monitor extracellular pathogens (e.g., bacteria and toxins; Fig. 15.10) and intracellular pathogens (e.g., viruses; Fig. 15.11), respectively. CD4+ T cells monitor MHC class II molecules, which display peptides generated in vesicles (e.g., from extracellular pathogens taken up by phagocytosis), and CD8+ T cells monitor MHC class I molecules, which display peptides generated in the cytoplasm (e.g., from intracellular pathogens such as viruses replicating in the cytoplasm). Non-peptide antigens are dealt with by $\gamma\delta$ T cells. The clinical consequences of a failure to express MHC molecules in the thymus is illustrated in Box 15.3.

CD4+ T cells

CD4+ T cells recognize antigen displayed on MHC class II molecules (Chs 8 and 10). As is discussed in more detail in Chapter 16, CD4+ T cells may differentiate into one of two helper cell subsets (T_H1 or T_H2),

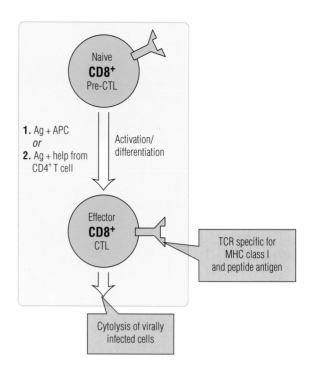

Fig. 15.11 The CD8+ T cells as effectors in intracellular infections.

depending on the cytokines present in the environment of the cell (Fig. 15.12). For example, if APCs are responding to infection by microbes and releasing IL-12, the T_H1 population of CD4+ T cells predominates. IL-12 stimulates primed CD4+ T cells to differentiate into T_H1 cells. These cells mainly have the role of activating the bactericidal function of macrophages. This is largely accomplished by the release of interferon (IFN) γ from T_H1 cells. This cytokine is a potent activator of macrophage phagocytic activity and thereby helps to enhance the destruction of bacteria and viruses present in the macrophages. T_H1 responses may be involved in exacerbations of multiple sclerosis (Box 15.4).

In contrast, an environment enriched in IL-4 (e.g., IL-4 released from mast cells on encountering a parasitic worm or allergen) preferentially stimulates the production of CD4+ T helper cells of the T_H2 subset. These cells are characterized by the release of IL-4 and IL-5, cytokines that stimulate B cells, enhance antibody class switching and promote the secretion of IgE.

Chapter 16 provides more information on the T_H1 and T_H2 subsets of CD4+ T helper cells.

CD8+ T cells (cytotoxic T lymphocytes)

The naive CD8+ T cells that emerge from the thymus are sometimes referred to as pre-CTLs (cytotoxic T lymphocytes). They require further activation and differentiation to become the effector T cells that lyse virally infected target cells and tumor cells (See Box 15.5).

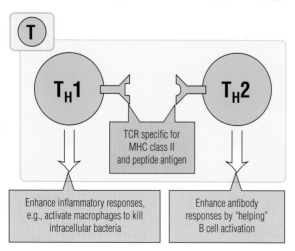

Fig. 15.10 The CD4+ T cells as effectors in extracellular infections.

Bone marrow   Thymus   Lymph node

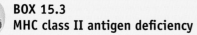

BOX 15.3
MHC class II antigen deficiency

The clinical consequences of a lack of MHC molecule expression in the thymus can be illustrated by the human immunodeficiency disease known as MHC class II antigen deficiency. Many patients with this autosomal recessive condition are of North African descent. The patients' B cells (and blood monocytes) lack MHC class II molecules on the cell surface. Those affected by this syndrome exhibit persistent problems with viral and bacterial infections. These patients also exhibit thymic hypoplasia. The lack of MHC class II molecules results in abnormal thymic selection processes and a block in CD4+ T cell development.

Laboratory analyses show that there are normal numbers of CD8+ T cells but very low levels of CD4+ T cells. The low level of CD4+ T cells creates difficulties in providing T-helper function and this probably explains the hypogammaglobulinemia in these patients which is present despite normal numbers of B cells.

Detailed molecular genetic analyses have pinpointed the genetic alterations in these patients. The mutations determined so far lie in regulatory genes that affect the expression of MHC class II genes and not in the MHC class II genes themselves.

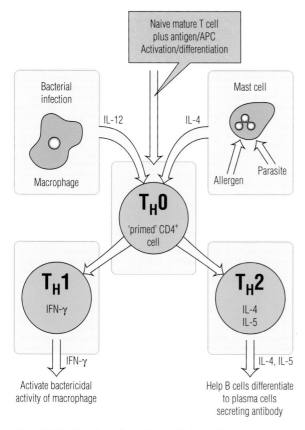

Fig. 15.12 The function of the T helper subsets T_H0, T_H1 and T_H2.

CD8+ T cells recognize antigen displayed on MHC class I molecules. Since MHC class I molecules are found on essentially all nucleated cells of the body, this means that CD8+ T cells can monitor all cells for signs of infection, but it also means that they may encounter antigen on a non-professional APC. CD8+ T cells are activated to become effector T cells either by encountering antigen on a professional APC and receiving activation signals from both MHC class I and co-stimulatory molecules (e.g., B7), or by encountering antigen on a non-APC target cell and receiving a "second signal" from cytokines released by CD4+ T helper cells.

In any event, CD8+ T cells require activation signals from antigen and either co-stimulatory molecules or cytokines to differentiate into effector CTLs with the function to lyse other cells. The cellular machinery required for cell killing and the mechanisms employed by CTLs to lyse target cells are described in Chapter 21.

The $\gamma\delta$ T cell subset

As described earlier in this chapter, $\gamma\delta$ TCR-expressing T cells are a minor population (<5%) of all T cells and represent a separate lineage from the $\alpha\beta$ T cell. The $\gamma\delta$ TCR recognizes antigen very differently from the $\alpha\beta$ TCR in that it recognizes non-peptide antigens without processing and presentation on an MHC class I or class II molecule.

The $\gamma\delta$ T cell acts as a part of the first line of defense, recognizing microbial invaders in the skin and gut mucosa predominantly. They can:

- secrete cytokines that initiate an inflammatory response
- help B cells
- activate macrophages
- lyse virally infected cells.

BOX 15.4
Influence of the pregnancy-induced reduction in T cell immune responses on multiple sclerosis

Multiple sclerosis (MS) is an inflammatory demyelinating disease of the central nervous system (CNS). The majority of patients experience relapsing–remitting disease characterized by periods of disability followed by periods of disease resolution. T cell-mediated autoimmune responses to CNS components are involved in the development of symptoms, and, while the disease is heterogeneous, the CNS lesions of many patients are infiltrated by macrophages and T cells. The T cells in the MS lesions are primarily of the CD4$^+$ T$_H$1 phenotype and investigators have postulated that modulation of the T$_H$1 response may alleviate exacerbations. A recent study of pregnant patients with MS supports this hypothesis.

A prospective study was performed to determine

the effects of pregnancy on MS. It was found that MS relapse rates were significantly decreased during the third trimester, then significantly increased at 3 months postpartum. Pregnancy is associated with a reduction in cellular immunity, i.e., a reduction in T$_H$1 type responses. Following childbirth, there is a return toward T$_H$1 type responses. Therefore, the changes in immune response during pregnancy correlate with the changes observed in disease symptoms, and support the hypothesis that modulating T$_H$1 type responses in MS patients would improve their lives. These changes in the immune response during pregnancy, when other profound endocrinological changes also take place, indicate the inter-relationship between the immune system and other physiological systems (Chs 13 and 35).

Therefore, in a functional sense, they are similar to $\alpha\beta$ T cells. However, their unique ability to recognize non-peptide antigens (such as bacterial cell wall phospholipids; Ch. 7) without processing and presen-

tation distinguishes them from $\alpha\beta$ T cells, and this enables them to have a unique protective role in the first line of defense against invading microbes.

BOX 15.5
Acute Epstein–Barr virus infection

Most people have been infected with Epstein–Barr virus (EBV). In the developing world, infection takes place in early childhood and it is usually asymptomatic. In the developed world, infection is usually delayed until adulthood and it causes infectious mononucleosis (also known as glandular fever). Symptoms of infectious mononucleosis (IM) include a sore throat, malaise, lymphadenopathy and, possibly, an enlarged spleen. There may also be malignancy associated with EBV infection, and this complication is discussed in Chapter 34.

From the point of view of the host response, acute EBV is characterized by a massive increase in the number of CD8$^+$ T cells in the peripheral blood. The increase appears to be of EBV antigen-specific T cells (Fig. 15.13). Based on recent studies using a new technique for enumerating virus-specific T cells, known as tetramer analysis (see Box 17.1), it has been suggested that the enormous expansion of T

cells during acute EBV infection may be a result of the expansion of a few dominant clones of CD8$^+$ T cells with specificity for EBV antigens—a so-called oligoclonal expansion.

The original EBV-specific CD8$^+$ T cells are generated in the thymus and clonally expanded on contact with EBV antigens in the periphery. EBV infects its target cell, the B cell, for life. Thus, EBV establishes a latent infection. Infected B cells proliferate, although very little free virus is produced. CD4$^+$ T cells also respond to acute EBV infection and produce IL-6, IFN-γ and tumor necrosis factor. These cytokines contribute to the fever and fatigue observed in these patients.

An antibody response, mostly IgM, is also mounted during acute EBV. The combination of antibody and CD8$^+$ CTL reduces but does not eliminate the infection. Finally, some of the CD4$^+$ T and CD8$^+$ T cells become memory cells and help in a future response to the virus (Fig. 15.13).

🦴 Bone marrow   🫘 Thymus   🔬 Lymph node

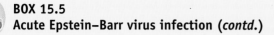

BOX 15.5
Acute Epstein–Barr virus infection (*contd.*)

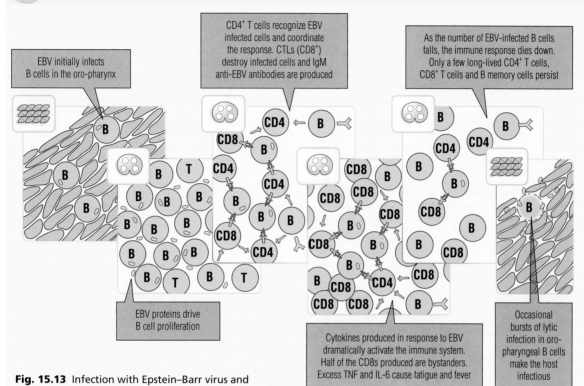

CD4+ T cells recognize EBV infected cells and coordinate the response. CTLs (CD8+) destroy infected cells and IgM anti-EBV antibodies are produced

As the number of EBV-infected B cells falls, the immune response dies down. Only a few long-lived CD4+ T cells, CD8+ T cells and B memory cells persist

EBV initially infects B cells in the oro-pharynx

EBV proteins drive B cell proliferation

Cytokines produced in response to EBV dramatically activate the immune system. Half of the CD8s produced are bystanders. Excess TNF and IL-6 cause fatigue and fever

Occasional bursts of lytic infection in oro-pharyngeal B cells make the host infectious

Fig. 15.13 Infection with Epstein–Barr virus and immune responses.

LEARNING POINTS

Can you now:

- Recall the role of the thymus in establishing the T cell repertoire?
- Draw the major steps in the pathway of T cell development and indicate the cell surface molecules that are expressed at different stages?
- List the major cell surface molecules expressed on thymocytes at different stages of development and indicate their function?

- Compare and contrast positive and negative selection?
- Draw the events involved in naive T cell activation?
- List the functional properties of different T cell subsets?
- Compare and contrast the roles of $\gamma\delta$ and $\alpha\beta$ T cells?

Blood vessel   Gut   Peripheral tissue

Cell–cell interaction in generating effector lymphocytes

16

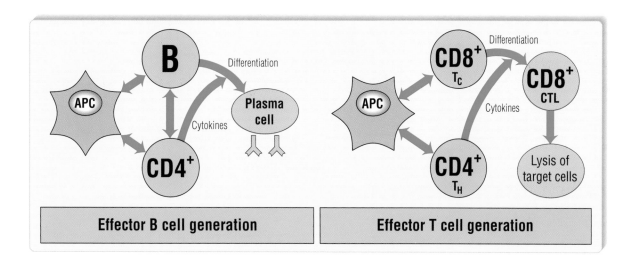

Effector B cell generation | Effector T cell generation

Some of the basic concepts of cell–cell interaction and cooperation in immune responses were introduced in Chapter 2. We also learned, in Chapters 7 and 8, how T cell receptors (TCRs) recognize antigen only when presented by MHC molecules on antigen-presenting cells (APCs) (an example of the requirement for cell–cell interaction in generating an immune response). In addition, the need for co-stimulatory signals provided by interaction with accessory cells for the full activation of B and T lymphocytes was introduced as a concept in Chapter 11 and discussed in Chapter 15. At this point, it is appropriate to bring these concepts together and to explain the critical role of lymphocyte–accessory cell interaction in generating the signals required to produce effector B cells (plasma cells) and effector T cells (T-helper cells and cytotoxic T lymphocytes (CTLs)).

Generation of stimulated (or primed) B and T cells

Foreign antigen, collected at sites of infection, is typically brought to secondary lymphoid organs, such as the spleen and lymph nodes (Ch. 13), by dendritic cells (DCs). Naive B and T cells circulate through the lymphoid organs and monitor for the presence of antigen (Ch. 13). Cytokines released by activated DCs and other APCs can function as signals of infection and

stimulate circulating leukocytes to adhere to high endothelial venules (HEVs), extravasate and transmigrate into the secondary lymphoid tissue (Ch. 12). This process brings B and T cells into proximity with APCs bearing foreign antigen and stops their migration. B cells with a B cell receptor (BCR) specific for available antigen then take up the antigen via receptor-mediated endocytosis (Ch. 10). Antigen processing takes place with the eventual display of antigenic peptides on the B cell surface in association with MHC class II molecules (Ch. 10; Fig. 16.1).

T cells constantly scan for APCs displaying appropriate MHC–antigenic peptide complexes; when they are detected, a T cell–APC conjugate forms. Contact with an MHC–foreign peptide antigen complex results in signaling through the TCR (Ch. 11), which, in addition to activating biochemical pathways in the cell, strengthens the adhesive bond between the cells by inducing expression of cell adhesion proteins. Some of the most important receptor–ligand pairs involved in the T cell–APC interaction are illustrated in Figure 16.2.

Lymphocyte–DC interactions take place in the T cell zone of a secondary lymphoid organ, e.g., of a draining lymph node (Ch. 13). At this point, we have reached the stage where there are activated B and T cells, specific for the same antigen, in the same zone of a lymph node.

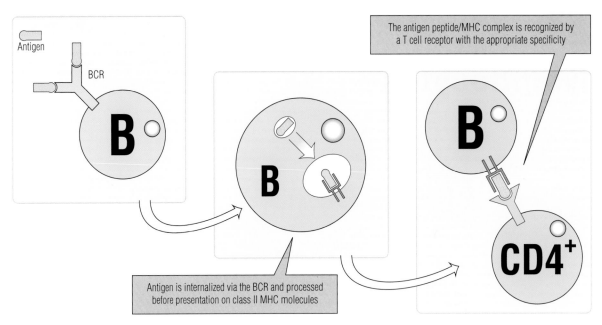

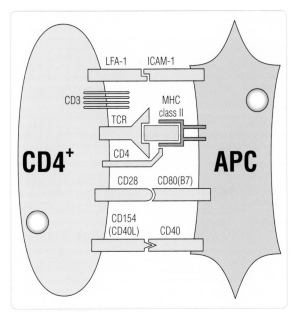

The antigen peptide/MHC complex is recognized by a T cell receptor with the appropriate specificity

Antigen is internalized via the BCR and processed before presentation on class II MHC molecules

Fig. 16.1 B cell presentation of antigen to T helper (T_H) cells.

Fig. 16.2 The major cell surface molecules involved in the interaction of T cells with antigen-presenting cells (APCs). ICAM-1, intercellular adhesion molecule 1; LFA-1, leukocyte function associated antigen 1.

Generation of effector cells

A major activity of CD4+ T helper (T_H) cells is the release of cytokines. Cytokines released from T_H cells can drive the immune response in the direction of antibody synthesis—a T_H2 response—or in the direction of

cell-mediated immunity—a T_H1 response. Box 16.1 provides a description of cytokine expression by these T helper subsets. Box 16.2 provides an example of the difference that a preponderance of cytokines from a T_H1 response rather than a T_H2 response can make to the outcome of an infection (leprosy).

CD4+ T_H interaction with B cells

B cells expressing MHC class II–antigenic peptide complexes can be recognized by CD4+ T_H cells and a B cell–T cell conjugate (Fig. 16.4) forms. The conjugate between an APC and a T cell is sometimes referred to as an **immunological synapse**. Next, there is release of cytokines from the T cell, and delivery of co-stimulatory signals from membrane-bound receptor–ligand pairs. These signals, plus signals from the BCR, cause the B cells to differentiate into plasma cells secreting IgM (a primary response).

As discussed in Chapter 12, some of the activated B cells do not differentiate into plasma cells but instead initiate formation of a germinal center in the lymphoid follicles. These B cells have received a co-stimulatory activation signal by virtue of the interaction between CD40 on the B cell and CD154 (formerly known as CD40L or CD40 ligand) on the T cell. CD154–CD40 interaction, and the resulting co-stimulatory signal delivered to the B cell, is required for the transition from a B cell producing a low-affinity IgM response to a B cell producing a high-affinity antibody of a different class (e.g., IgG). Prevention of CD154–CD40 interaction leads to greatly diminished antibody responses to typical protein antigens.

BOX 16.1
Cytokine expression by human CD4+ T cell subsets

As we have seen in Section III of this book, the activities of CD4+ T cells can be critical in mediating effector cell function in the immune response. For example, CD4+ T cells help B cells to differentiate into antibody-secreting plasma cells, and CD4+ T cells provide stimuli for the differentiation of CD8+ T cells into CTLs capable of killing virally infected cells. The CD4+ T cells mediate their activities via cytokine release and by cell–cell contact, with the involvement of receptor–ligand pairs that activate signal transduction pathways. Given that cytokine production is such an important aspect of CD4+ T cell function, extensive studies to characterize the cytokines released by CD4+ T cells have been carried out. CD4+ T cells can be separated into two distinct subsets—the T helper 1 (T_H1) and T helper 2 (T_H2) subsets—on the basis of the cytokines they express. It should be noted that these designations are based on in vitro analyses. It is also important to note that while human T cells can be separated into T_H1 and T_H2 subsets, the distinction between T_H1 and T_H2 cells in terms of cytokine profiles is less clear in humans than in mice. Figure 16.3 lists the cytokines that predominate in each subset in humans.

Cytokines such as interferon γ (INF-γ) and tumor necrosis factor β (TNF-β) enhance CD8+ cytotoxic T cells and activate macrophages and natural killer cells. IL-4 and IL-5, however, activate B cells and eosinophils and induce IgE-type responses. T_H2 cells are dominant in parasitic infections (e.g., worms). T_H1 cells are dominant in responses to microbial infection. Subset-specific cytokines can also have regulatory effects on the other subset; for example, IFN-γ inhibits the generation of T_H2 cells and IL-4 inhibits the generation of T_H1 cells.

Fig. 16.3
Cytokine expression by activated human CD4+ T cell subsets

Cytokine	T_H1	T_H2
Interferon-γ	+	–
Tumor necrosis factor β (lymphotoxin)	+	–
Interleukin 4	–	+
Interleukin 5	–	+

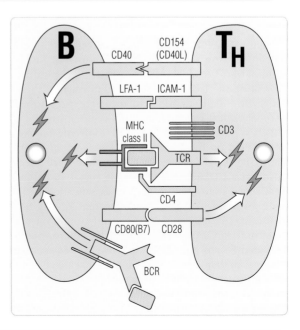

Fig. 16.4 Formation of a B cell–T cell conjugate. ICAM-1, intercellular adhesion molecule 1; LFA-1, leukocyte function associated antigen 1.

 Blood vessel ~~~ Gut ▦ Peripheral tissue

BOX 16.2
Leprosy

A few years after arriving in the Midwestern US from Asia, a 35-year-old man (A.M.) presented at the local teaching hospital emergency room with multiple nodules and lesions on the arms, hands and buttocks. These lesions had been present for more than one year but now he was also experiencing considerable loss of sensation in his hands, and had been having difficulty functioning in his job as a waiter in a busy restaurant in Chicago. A skin biopsy demonstrated acid-fast bacilli that were identified as *Mycobacterium leprae*. Further examination by hematoxylin and eosin staining of tissue taken from an arm lesion showed numerous bacteria in macrophage-like cells, as well as disseminated infection into local nerves. Leprosy was diagnosed, and treatment begun with the drugs dapsone, rifampicin and clofazimine. After about 12 months of this drug treatment regimen, A.M.'s lesions and neurological symptoms were substantially reduced. The final diagnosis was borderline lepromatous leprosy.

There are several forms of leprosy (see Fig. 25.1). Often, as in the case described, the disease is somewhere in between the two polar extremes, tuberculoid leprosy and lepromatous leprosy. The immune status of the individual seems to determine the outcome of infection by *M. leprae*. In an individual where the immune system is triggered in the direction of a T_H2-type response (i.e., antibody

production, IL-4 cytokine release and little cell mediated immunity) then lepromatous leprosy results. In this form of the disease, infection is widely disseminated, the vigorous antibody response is ineffective and the bacilli continue to grow in macrophages. In the absence of drug treatment there is a poor clinical picture with extensive damage to connective tissues and peripheral nerve tissue.

On the other hand, in an individual who triggers a T_H1 response to infection by *M. leprae* the organism is substantially localized to macrophages and bacterial growth is controlled by the T_H1 T cells that activate macrophage killing of the bacilli. In this so-called tuberculoid form of the disease there is usually a less severe clinical picture, especially if there is drug treatment. In tuberculoid leprosy there is some inflammation and granuloma formation with localized peripheral nervous tissue damage but nothing as severe as in the lepromatous form of the disease.

More often than not leprosy presents as intermediate between the two extremes of tuberculoid and lepromatous, as in the case of A.M. What produces the different forms of leprosy in different individuals is not clear. However, this organism can cause two very different disease outcomes depending on the type of immune response that is triggered in the infected host.

Figure 16.5 illustrates the steps in B cell–T cell interaction leading to a secondary immune response. Stimulation of the T cell through the TCR induces CD154 on the T cell. CD154–CD40 interaction stimulates the B cell (or APC) to induce expression of another critical co-stimulatory molecule on the B cell (APC) surface: CD80(B7). The B7 molecule interacts with CD28 on the T cell (they are a receptor–ligand pair). The signal delivered by CD28 to the T cell after it encounters CD80(B7) is the critical signal along with TCR signal transduction that causes activation of the gene for interleukin (IL) 2 and eventual T_H proliferation (Fig. 16.5). B7 molecules are only found on professional APCs (see Ch. 2) such as macrophages, activated B cells and dendritic cells. The requirement for co-stimulation via CD28 ensures that the T cell is only activated by antigens presented by APCs.

The co-stimulatory receptor–ligand pairs CD40–CD154 (CD40L) and CD80(B7)–CD28 act synergisti-

cally to enable T_H cell proliferation. A mutation in the human gene encoding CD154 exists, and this causes a syndrome known as X-linked hyper-IgM. This disease (Box 16.3) demonstrates the critical role of the CD40–CD154 interaction in the response to T-dependent antigens (Ch. 14).

Proliferation of T_H2 cells helps the germinal center B cells to differentiate into plasma cells secreting a higher affinity and different class of immunoglobulin than the low-affinity IgM typical of the primary response. For example, IL-4 released from T_H2 cells causes class switching (Chs 6 and 14) to IgE production.

The germinal center B cells are subject to rapid somatic mutation in their variable region gene segments and they undergo selection to retain those that have a higher affinity immunoglobulin. Class switching may then occur and a high-affinity immunoglobulin of the IgG, IgA or IgE type can be produced. These plasma cells then secrete antibody until the antigen is

🦴 Bone marrow   🫁 Thymus   Lymph node

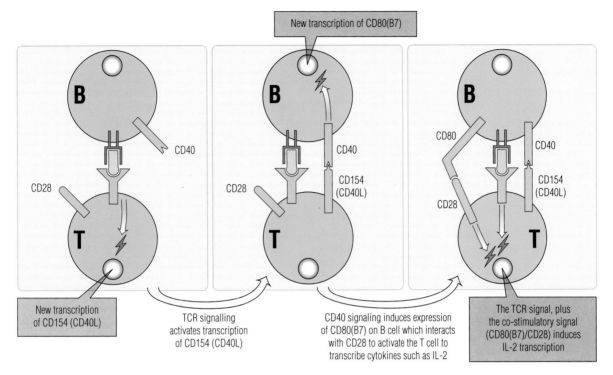

New transcription of CD80(B7)

B — CD40

CD28

T

New transcription of CD154 (CD40L)

B — CD40

CD28 — CD154 (CD40L)

T

TCR signalling activates transcription of CD154 (CD40L)

CD40 signaling induces expression of CD80(B7) on B cell which interacts with CD28 to activate the T cell to transcribe cytokines such as IL-2

CD80 — B — CD40

CD28 — CD154 (CD40L)

T

The TCR signal, plus the co-stimulatory signal (CD80(B7)/CD28) induces IL-2 transcription

Fig. 16.5 Co-stimulatory signals in B–T interactions.

BOX 16.3
B lymphocyte–T lymphocyte interaction: CD40–CD154 and X-linked hyper-IgM syndrome

A 10-month-old child had a series of bacterial chest and sinus infections since he was about 6 months of age. He was found to have low IgG and IgA but high IgM. These abnormalities are consistent with the hyper-IgM syndrome and the diagnosis was confirmed when his T cells were shown not to express CD154 (CD40 ligand). He can only produce IgM because his T cells are unable to offer appropriate help to induce B cells to switch immunoglobulin class. He was started on immunoglobulin replacement and responded well, with a decreased frequency of chest and sinus infectious. Hyper-IgM syndrome also affects T cell function: because CD154 is absent, T cells cannot communicate normally with APCs.

Boys with hyper-IgM syndrome are especially vulnerable to protozoal infections of the liver and

continued

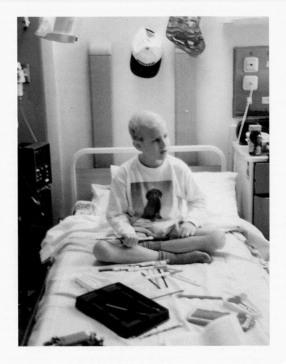

Fig. 16.6 A boy with hyper-IgM syndrome recovering from bone marrow transplant. His hair loss is a consequence of the conditioning chemotherapy required for BMT (Ch. 33).

 Blood vessel   Gut   Peripheral tissue   **137**

> **BOX 16.3**
> **B lymphocyte–T lymphocyte interaction: CD40–CD154 and X-linked hyper-IgM syndrome (*contd.*)**
>
> gastrointestinal tract. At the age of 8 years, this child showed evidence of infection with *Cryptosporidium*. Fortunately, he has a sister with an identical HLA type and she was able to act as a bone marrow donor for the patient (see Ch. 33). This is a prolonged and unpleasant procedure, but it was his only hope of improving T cell function. Over the next few months his condition improved steadily and at the age of 11 years he is competing in national skiing championships!

eliminated or until they die. Plasma cells typically survive from a few days up to a few weeks.

A few of the activated germinal center B cells become long-lived quiescent memory B cells, as described in Chapter 17. Similarly, some of the activated T cells become memory T cells (Ch. 17). Subsequent encounter with antigen by these memory cells leads to a more rapid, and more effective, secondary, tertiary, or subsequent, immune response.

CD4+ T_H interaction with CD8+ T cells

CD8+ CTLs kill virally infected cells (also known as target cells). CD8+ T cells require activation signals before they can differentiate into effector CTLs with the full range of granule enzymes etc. required to kill a target cell (see also Ch. 21). The required activation signals are recognition of antigen, i.e., MHC–viral antigenic peptide complexes, and co-stimulatory signals from virus-specific CD4+ T_H cells. This is another example of the requirement for cell–cell interaction to generate an immune response, in this case a cell-mediated immune response. As shown in Figure 16.7, CD4+ T_H cells recognize viral antigen displayed on APCs; activation of the CD4+ T_H cell causes release of IL-2, which stimulates viral antigen-specific CD8+ T cells. TCR recognition of viral antigen, plus a second signal via the IL-2 receptor (IL-2R) (Fig. 16.7), stimulates differentiation of the CD8+ T cell into an effector CTL,

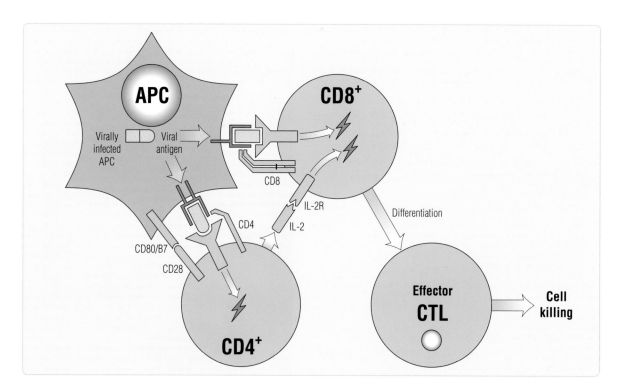

Fig. 16.7 Interaction of CD4+ T cells and CD8+ T cells in the maturation of effector cytotoxic T cells.

Bone marrow   Thymus   Lymph node

capable of cell killing on encountering a virally infected target cell. CTLs kill target cells by exchanging granule contents and eventually inducing apoptosis (see Ch. 21).

Providing the most appropriate immune response for a given pathogen

The cell–cell interaction and cooperation that we have described above allows the immune system to make the appropriate response for a particular pathogen. For example, a pathogen (e.g., a virus), multiplying in the cytoplasm of any given cell will generate peptide antigens that are carried to the cell surface by MHC class I molecules (Ch. 10). $CD8^+$ T cells with appropriate TCRs will encounter the MHC class I–viral antigen complex and be activated, eventually becoming mature effector CTLs capable of killing the virally infected cell (see Fig. 16.7).

By comparison, peptide antigens derived from pathogens growing in intracellular vesicles of macrophages, or peptide antigens derived from ingested toxins or extracellular bacteria, will be picked up and carried to the cell surface by MHC class II molecules (Ch. 10). Since MHC class II molecules are scanned by $CD4^+$ T cells, T cells of the T_H1 or T_H2 subsets may be activated. If T_H1 cells are generated then these cells will activate the bactericidal action of macrophages through release of interferon γ (IFN-γ). If T_H2 cells are activated then they can activate B cells to make antibody, which can neutralize the extracellular toxins or opsonize the extracellular bacteria. Consequently, infection by viruses or bacteria tends to result in production of cytokines that favor the generation of T_H1 cells (Fig. 16.8). The T_H1 cells are then able to activate the appropriate protective response, i.e., macrophages or CTLs. Parasitic infections (e.g., worms) generate cytokines that favor T_H2

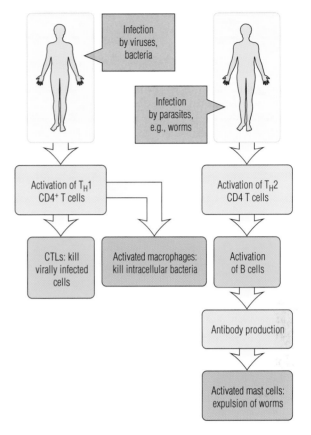

Fig. 16.8 T cell subsets and their role in responses to different pathogens.

cell production. The T_H2 cells are then able to activate B cells and eosinophils to generate an appropriate protective response. The fact that the two helper subsets mediate different immune responses forms the basis for potential immunotherapy in autoimmune disease (Box 16.4).

BOX 16.4
Immune deviation

Given that the two helper T cell subsets mediate different effector responses, considerable thought has been given to ways to regulate the balance of the T_H1 and T_H2 subsets as an immunotherapy for certain diseases, for example, to convert the T cell balance in asthma, a disease largely mediated by T_H2 responses, to one in which T_H2 cells no longer dominate. Similarly, T_H1 cells are the major effector cells in several organ-specific autoimmune diseases (see Ch. 27), and induction of more of a T_H2-type

response might aid in the treatment of these diseases. Encouraging results with this approach to immunotherapy have been obtained in some animal models. For example, administration of antibodies reactive with IL-4, resulting in changes in the balance of $T_H1:T_H2$ cytokines, improved outcomes in an animal model of the autoimmune disease systemic lupus erythematosus (SLE), which is dominated by T_H2 cells (Ch. 27). Similarly, administration of exogenous IL-4 has been shown to reduce the

continued

Blood vessel   Gut   Peripheral tissue

BOX 16.4
Immune deviation (*contd.*)

symptoms of a T_H1-dominated autoimmune disease in mice, experimental autoimmune encephalomyelitis (EAE), which is a model for multiple sclerosis, by inducing T_H2-like CD4$^+$ T cells. Much remains to be done to determine if this approach will be useful in humans. There is need for caution before immune deviation is adopted as a therapy for human disease. For one, there appears to be a more complex regulation in humans, compared with mice, with respect to T_H1 and T_H2 responses. In addition, some autoimmune diseases have both a cell-mediated and an antibody-mediated component. Hence, changing the ratio of T_H1 to T_H2 cells might only switch the dominant source of the immune-mediated damage and lead to a different type of damage.

BOX 16.5
Exploiting our knowledge of B–T cooperation to prevent bacterial meningitis with a conjugate vaccine

Until the advent, in about 1990, of national vaccination programs that utilized a conjugate vaccine, meningitis caused by the bacterial pathogen *Haemophilus influenzae* B was a serious concern. The disease peaks in infants of 10–11 months of age and in severe cases there may be neurological damage or even death. The original vaccine was a purified capsular polysaccharide, a T-independent antigen that did not function well in infants below the age of about 20 months. Consideration of the knowledge immunologists had gained about T-dependent immune responses, and about B cell–T cell cooperation in immune responses, led to the development of a vaccine where the bacterial polysaccharide was coupled covalently to a protein. This conjugate vaccine (so-called Hib vaccine) induced far better responses than the unconjugated vaccine, even in very young children. Several proteins have been used for the conjugate, including the protein component of tetanus toxoid. In countries where this conjugate vaccine is being used, the incidence of meningitis has dramatically declined. In the US, the incidence of meningitis declined by about 80% one year after introduction of the national Hib vaccination program.

The theory behind the vaccine is that B cells with immunoglobulin receptors for the bacterial capsular polysaccharide component of the vaccine take up the conjugate by receptor-mediated endocytosis. The protein component of the conjugate can then be processed and presented on the surface of the B cell associated with MHC class II molecules. The MHC class II–vaccine peptide complex can then be recognized by a T_H cell of the appropriate specificity. The T_H cell then activates the B cell to make antibody against the bacterial polysaccharide. The general principle is as illustrated in Figure 16.9, except that the "antigen" is a conjugate of a B cell epitope (the polysaccharide component) and a T cell epitope (the tetanus toxoid protein). The structure of the vaccine and its interaction with the B cell is illustrated in Figure 16.9.

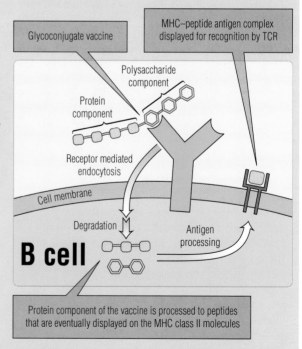

Fig. 16.9 B cell processing of a glycoconjugate vaccine.

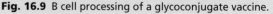

Bone marrow   Thymus   Lymph node

BOX 16.5
Exploiting our knowledge of B-T cooperation to prevent bacterial meningitis with a conjugate vaccine (*contd.*)

The conjugate Hib vaccine has been so successful that other glycoconjugate vaccines (covalent conjugates of a bacterial capsular polysaccharide antigen and a protein) have been developed, and more are in development to help control increasingly antibiotic-resistant encapsulated bacteria that cause infectious disease. For example, a pneumococcal conjugate vaccine has shown success in controlling otitis media in a trial with Finnish children, and a new typhoid vaccine has recently been reported to have been very successful in preventing typhoid fever in young children in Vietnam. These vaccines based on polysaccharide–protein conjugates offer promise of an effective response to the problem of multi-drug resistant infectious disease emerging in impoverished areas of the world and presenting a danger to everyone in this era of global travel.

LEARNING POINTS

Can you now:

- Describe how naive B and T cells are primed by cell–cell interactions with antigen-presenting cells?
- Draw the cell–cell interactions involved in the generation of plasma cells and memory B cells?

- Draw the cell–cell interactions involved in the generation of cytotoxic T lymphocytes (CTLs)?
- Describe the difference between a T_H1 response and a T_H2 response in terms of disease outcome?
- Describe how a glycoconjugate vaccine induces a protective response?

Immunological memory

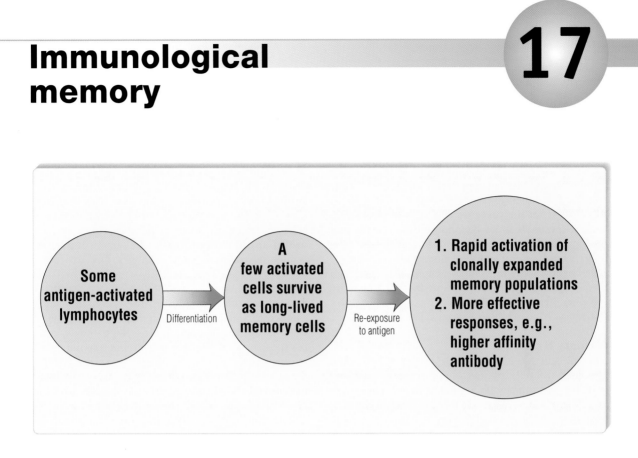

Some antigen-activated lymphocytes → *Differentiation* → A few activated cells survive as long-lived memory cells → *Re-exposure to antigen* → 1. Rapid activation of clonally expanded memory populations 2. More effective responses, e.g., higher affinity antibody

One of the hallmarks of the adaptive immune system is that it "remembers" previous encounters with antigen (Ch. 2). Immune memory is very important in protection from infectious agents. Immune memory allows the host to initiate the **secondary immune response** on subsequent encounters with a pathogen. This secondary immune response was initially discussed in Chapters 1 and 2 and allows the immune system to make a more vigorous (e.g., more antibody production) and a more effective response (e.g., higher affinity specific antibody) on re-exposure to previously encountered antigens (Figs 17.1, 1.6 and 2.5).

As described in Chapters 2 and 5, vaccination takes advantage of immunological memory. Vaccines against infectious diseases, such as smallpox and poliomyelitis, have been some of the most important achievements of medical science. Vaccines, along with improved hygiene and sanitation, have saved countless lives and they have been responsible for dramatically improving the quality of life for literally millions of people throughout the world. However, although great successes have come from taking advantage of the existence of immunological memory, we still have much to understand about how immunological memory is

Fig. 17.1
Contrasting aspects of primary and subsequent antibody immune responses. Activated B cells differentiate to become memory B cells which, on re-encountering antigen, can generate a more rapid, and more effective, protective antibody immune response.

	Primary response	Subsequent response
Time period to response (days)	5–10	1–3
Major antibody class	IgM	IgG (IgA or IgE)[a]
Affinity for antigen	Low	High

[a] Usually the antibody is IgG. However, depending on the nature of the antigen and the route of antigen entry, the response may be IgA or IgE (see Ch. 14).

Blood vessel   Gut   Peripheral tissue

established and maintained. This chapter will present a summary of what is most important about long-term immunological memory.

Long-term immunological memory

Long-term immunological memory refers to the capacity to generate an enhanced and more effective immune response to an antigen last encountered some considerable time ago. Long-term memory is thought to result from the presence of clonally expanded, antigen-specific B and T lymphocytes that persist in a resting state for many years and, in some cases, lifelong. It has been difficult to distinguish these memory cells unequivocally from other lymphocytes, although there is now general agreement that there is a memory cell phenotype with both qualitative and quantitative differences from other lymphocytes (Fig. 17.2).

Memory B cells

Naive B cells when activated by antigen differentiate into effector B cells (plasma cells) that secrete antibody (Ch. 14). In a primary response the plasma cells secrete an IgM antibody of relatively low affinity, whereas in a secondary response a higher-affinity antibody, usually of a different class (i.e., IgG, IgA, or IgE), is secreted. Somatic hypermutation takes place during the sec-

ondary response to generate a higher-affinity binding site for antigen (Chs 6 and 14).

It is thought to be likely that the memory B cell is derived from an activated B cell that has undergone genetic changes (somatic hypermutation) in variable region (V) gene segment DNA to create a more effective antibody (Fig. 17.3). Clearly then, this cell is qualitatively different from the original naive cell that first reacted with antigen. This memory cell can be distinguished from the naive B cell by the somatic mutations that have created differences in the immunoglobulin gene sequences. The memory B cell preserves the more useful antigen receptor that has been derived by sequential somatic genetic changes. On subsequent exposure to antigen, it is this memory cell that responds, not another naive cell. Evidence that this is true comes from the following observation. Individuals exposed to a pathogen early in life, e.g., measles virus, respond to the same epitopes on the pathogen when re-exposed later in life, and they do not respond to new epitopes present on the pathogen, even though they are antigenic. This observation is consistent with secondary and subsequent exposure to antigen activating pre-existing memory cells rather than inducing the differentiation of new naive cells. The advantage to the host is that a secondary response (i.e., a more rapid and higher affinity response) is generated, allowing the

Fig. 17.2
Phenotype of memory cells

	Memory cell	Naive cell	Effector cell
B lymphocytes			
Response time to antigenic stimulation	Fast	Slow	Responding
Antigen receptor: immunoglobulin class expressed	IgG (IgA or IgE)	IgM	IgG (IgA or IgE)
Affinity of antibody secreted	High	Low	Increases during response
Effector function	None	None	Antibody secretion
T lymphocytes			
Response time to antigenic stimulation	Fast	Slow	Responding
Recirculation pattern	Circulate through tissues for which they have homing receptors then migrate to site(s) of infection	Constantly circulates from blood to lymph nodes and other lymphoid organs to scan for antigen	Migrates to site(s) of infection, usually in the periphery
Effector function	None	None	Help (cytokine release), or target cell killing

Bone marrow   Thymus   Lymph node

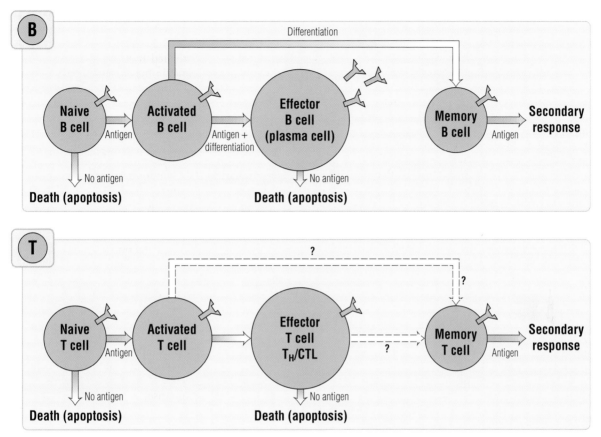

Fig. 17.3 Differentiation pathway of memory cells. T_H, T helper cell; CTL, cytotoxic T lymphocyte.

infection to be eliminated sooner than if a new primary response were generated.

Memory T cells

Unambiguously defining the memory phenotype of T cells has been much more difficult than for B cells. Part of the reason for this has been that the genes for the T cell receptor do not undergo the qualitative changes, somatic hypermutation and class switching that occur in genes for the B cell receptors (immunoglobulins). However, a memory T cell effect has been observed. There is a quicker, more efficient T cell response on subsequent exposure to antigen, and the number of T cells that respond to antigen is increased.

With respect to T cells, it has been observed that there is a subset of T cells that is similar to effector CD4+ or CD8+ T cells, but has some functional differences. This subset of T cells is activated more quickly and efficiently than naive cells are, when encountering antigen. This may be because of a lower requirement for co-stimulation, higher affinity receptors for antigen,

or both. This functional phenotype is consistent with a memory cell.

Defining marker proteins that distinguish unambiguously between naive, effector and memory T cells has been very difficult. There are differences in cell surface proteins, perhaps the most significant being changes in certain cell adhesion molecules. The adhesion molecule, L-selectin (Ch. 13), is expressed at high levels on naive T cells but is found at a much lower level on most T cells of a memory phenotype. This may help to explain the observation (Ch. 13) that T cells with a memory phenotype recirculate between blood and tissues, whereas naive T cells recirculate between blood and lymph nodes.

A relatively new technology known as the tetramer assay (Box 17.1) can visualize and enumerate T cells based on their binding to specific fluorescent MHC–peptide antigen complexes. This is being used to improve characterization of subsets of antigen-specific T cells. This technology will undoubtedly also help in the characterization of memory T cells and their distinction from naive, effector or anergic T cells.

BOX 17.1
In situ detection of T cell immunity

Extensive proliferation of CD8+ T cells is observed during early phases of infection with viruses such as Epstein–Barr virus (EBV), human immunodeficiency virus (HIV), etc. Until recently, experimental attempts to identify how much of this proliferation was a function of virus-specific T cells, as opposed to general T cell activation, led to the conclusion that about 1–5% of the activated CD8+ T cells were specific for viral antigens. However, a new technology, called tetramer analysis, which involves using fluorescent-labeled tetramers of MHC molecules (Fig. 17.4) to stain specific T cells directly, suggests that the earlier techniques provided low estimates of the number of

antigen-specific cytotoxic T lymphocytes (CTLs). Direct visualization of tetramer-stained cells by flow cytometry suggests that as much as 50–70% of the activated CD8+ T cells can be virus specific in certain situations.

Once an exact antigenic peptide/MHC molecule binding relationship has been established, tetramer–MHC complexes are prepared as follows. Soluble domains of MHC class I molecules (Ch. 8) are biotinylated on the C-terminus of the molecule. A peptide from the virus being studied that has been predetermined to bind to that MHC molecule is allowed to bind to the peptide-binding cleft of the

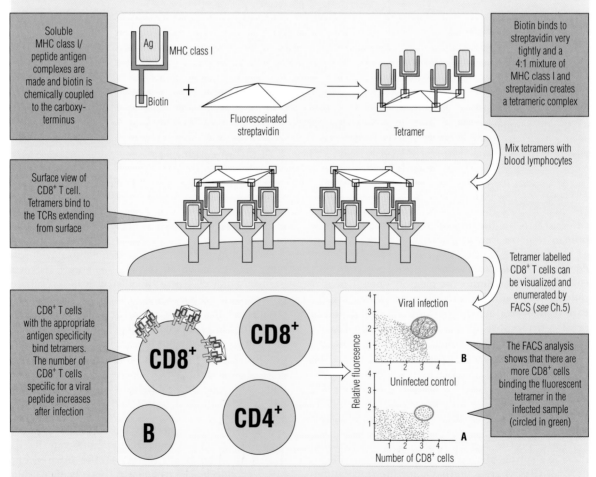

Fig. 17.4 Tetramer assay to identify T cells. Tetramers (four base units) bind to T cell receptors (TCR) thus linking the presence of TCR on a cell with fluorescent intensity. Fluorescence-activated cell sorting (FACS) can then assess cell number. There is clearly a new population of T cells in viral infection (**A**) compared with the uninfected state (**B**).

Bone marrow   Thymus   Lymph node

Role of persistent antigen in memory

Some antigens have been observed to be retained for very long periods of time. One question that arises from this observation is whether or not this residual antigen plays any role in maintaining memory cells. This is a difficult issue to resolve experimentally, but the data at present are consistent with the view that tiny quantities of residual antigen, usually present as immune complexes on follicular dendritic cells, are sometimes important in maintaining memory cells but are not essential. It has been found that certain antigen–antibody complexes, bound to Fc receptors on the surface of follicular dendritic cells, can exist for extended periods of time in vivo and may be taken up by B cells with immunoglobulin receptors specific for the antigen and processed. In some cases, this can activate the immune response more rapidly. However, it does not appear to be the case that all antigens persist for extended periods of time.

LYMPHOCYTE HOMEOSTASIS

Given that it is possible for us to retain immunological memory of every foreign antigen encounter we have ever had, then even if the number of memory cells generated in each immune response were small (and it is usually substantial!), there would eventually be an issue of availability of appropriate body sites to maintain and nurture these cells. The blood and lymphoid tissues have space for only a finite number of cells! Fortunately, like other lymphocytes, most memory cells appear to die eventually—probably by programmed cell death (**apoptosis**). The mechanisms involved in apoptosis are further described below and in detail in Chapter 21. Cell death maintains a balance (homeostasis) between the need for vast clonal expansion of lymphocytes in primary responses to new antigens, and the need for maintaining memory cells, with the limited number of suitable sites for lymphocytes.

The concept that is currently favored by immunologists with regard to lymphocyte homeostasis and the persistence of memory cells is as follows. Most activated effector cells die as antigen is eliminated. Clones of antigen-specific memory cells survive for longer periods. For these memory cells to survive they need to compete for a nurturing environment with growth factors (cytokines etc.) available. Given that these are in finite supply, it is possible that memory cells from some antigenic encounters do not survive. Conceivably, some memory cells are better adapted for survival under these conditions. For example, they have a reduced need for cytokines/growth factors and, therefore, they are more competitive in terms of ability to survive. This could mean that immunological memory of some antigens may be more stable than for others.

Apoptosis

Apoptosis is triggered through receptor–ligand interactions—mainly the Fas–Fas ligand interaction (Fig. 17.5). Binding of Fas ligand (e.g., expressed on a killer T cell) to Fas (e.g., expressed on a target cell) triggers a cascade of intracellular biochemical changes in the

○ Blood vessel   〰 Gut   ▦ Peripheral tissue

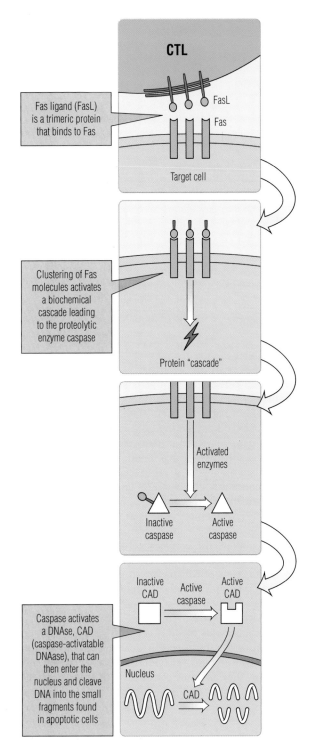

Fas ligand (FasL) is a trimeric protein that binds to Fas

CTL

FasL

Fas

Target cell

Clustering of Fas molecules activates a biochemical cascade leading to the proteolytic enzyme caspase

Protein "cascade"

Activated enzymes

Inactive caspase

Active caspase

Inactive CAD

Active caspase

Active CAD

Caspase activates a DNAse, CAD (caspase-activatable DNAase), that can then enter the nucleus and cleave DNA into the small fragments found in apoptotic cells

Nucleus

CAD

Fig. 17.5 Cell death pathway: the role of receptor–ligand interactions (Fas–Fas L) to activate caspase and, finally, caspase-activatable DNAase (CAD), which degrades DNA.

target cell. Fas interacts with several proteins in the "death pathway" eventually to activate a proteolytic enzyme known as **caspase**. Caspase is critical in activating several more proteolytic enzymes in the caspase cascade. This proteolytic cascade is somewhat analogous to the kinase cascade of cell activation (see Ch. 11). The critical step of the caspase cascade is activation of a cytoplasmic enzyme, caspase-activatable DNAse (CAD), which can then migrate to the nucleus and cleave DNA into the small fragments that are a characteristic end-point of apoptosis (Fig. 17.5 and Ch. 21).

Several genes have been found to promote cell death and there are also several genes that inhibit cell death (Box 17.2). The family of death-inhibiting genes includes the *bcl* genes. A gene, *bcl-2*, initially detected

---

BOX 17.2
Apoptosis—programmed cell death

Apoptosis is a mechanism for the elimination of excess or damaged cells. It is an evolutionarily conserved process that is initiated by the dying cell and represents a form of controlled cellular destruction. Several genes have been identified that either promote or inhibit apoptosis (Fig. 17.6). Anti-apoptotic genes could confer characteristics such as longer than usual survival. The most important of the anti-apoptotic genes appears to be *bcl-2*. Anti-apoptotic genes of the *bcl-2* type appear to work by raising the so-called apoptotic threshold of a cell, i.e., the dose of apoptosis initiator required for a cell expressing the Bcl-2 protein is greater than in the absence of Bcl-2.

The gene *bcl-2* was originally detected as a mammalian oncogene involved in a human chromosomal translocation between chromosomes 14 and 18 that is detected in over 70% of lymphomas. The chromosomal translocation results in increased expression of Bcl-2 and this imparts a relative resistance to apoptosis on the resulting B tumor cells (see also Ch. 34).

Fig. 17.6
Death-inhibiting/death-promoting genes

Anti-apoptotic (death-inhibiting) genes	Pro-apoptotic (death-promoting) genes
bcl-2	bax
bcl-X_L	bak
bcl-w	bcl-X_S

Bone marrow   Thymus   Lymph node

in a chromosomal translocation in B cell lymphomas (see also Ch. 34), is typical of the death-inhibiting or anti-apoptotic genes. One explanation that has been proposed for the survival of long-term memory cells is that they have a higher than usual level of expression of the Bcl family of proteins. This characteristic then protects them from antigen-induced cell death and facilitates their long-term survival.

LEARNING POINTS

Can you now:

- Recall examples of the major medical triumphs that resulted from artificial induction (by vaccination) of immunological memory?
- List the major differences between a primary and a secondary immune response?
- Draw a model for the differentiation pathway of memory lymphocytes?
- List the qualitative and quantitative changes that distinguish memory from naive lymphocytes?
- Draw the principal features of the apoptotic pathway?
- List the characteristics of memory cells that help to ensure their survival?

Review of immune physiology

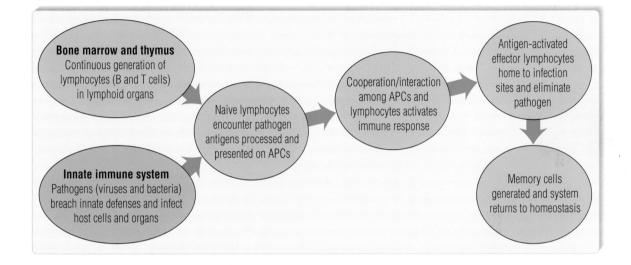

Section III has principally focused on the physiology of the adaptive immune response. After a discussion of the genes and molecules involved in antigen recognition in Section II, we moved in Section III to cells, tissues and organs and a more integrated, physiological system view of the adaptive immune response.

By this point in the book you should understand the following:

- how a repertoire of antigen receptors is developed
- how antigen-presenting cells (APCs) process and display antigens for recognition by T cells
- how naive B and T lymphocytes recognize antigen and are then activated to differentiate into effector cells
- how APCs, and B and T lymphocytes, interact and cooperate in an adaptive immune response
- how lymphocytes home to lymphoid tissues and recirculate to the periphery to protect against invading pathogens
- how memory of a prior response is maintained, allowing a more rapid and effective response on re-encountering a pathogen.

We established in Chapter 10 that antigen associates with the $\alpha\beta$ T cell receptor (TCR) only after handling by specialized APCs. The route of antigen processing (cytosolic versus vesicle bound) determines whether an antigen is presented by MHC class II molecules to a TCR on a CD4+ T helper (T_H) cell, or by MHC class I molecules to a TCR on a CD8+ cytotoxic T cell.

By themselves, the $\alpha\beta$ (or $\gamma\delta$) TCR protein chains, and the membrane-bound immunoglobulin molecule, are poor receptors, i.e., they are ineffective at delivering a message to the interior of the cell that a stimulus (antigen) has been received. Chapters 11 and 16 described:

- the structure and function of the B cell receptor (BCR) and the TCR
- the role of co-receptor, and co-stimulatory, molecules in optimizing the function of the antigen receptors
- the connection between the antigen receptors and the signal transduction machinery of B and T lymphocytes.

We have also described how our growing knowledge of how antigen interacts with the BCR and the TCR, and of how lymphocytes are activated, is leading to the design of new inhibitors of lymphocyte proliferation (e.g., altered peptide ligands (Boxes 8.2 and 11.1)) that can function as partial agonists or antagonists and regulate lymphocyte activation in disease situations. There is considerable hope that these "designer drugs" may improve on existing drugs, such as ciclosporin, which are used for immunosuppression after transplantation (see Chs 11 and 33).

Chapters 14 and 15 discuss how the repertoire of B and T cell specificities is developed. We learned that there are orderly processes of gene rearrangement that take place in different cell types during B and T cell development in the adult bone marrow and thymus, respectively. How thymocytes and B cell precursors mature into T and B effector cells with an appropriate repertoire of antigen receptors was also described. There are many similarities in the development of B and T lymphocytes and their respective repertoires of antigen-specific receptors. The greatest difference between the two lineages is that the BCR is subject to continued improvements after exposure to antigen. Thus, the processes of somatic hypermutation (affinity maturation) and class switching are utilized to generate a higher affinity, more effective, antibody molecule during the immune response. Although the TCR does not change in structure during an immune response, clonally expanded memory T cells are better able to mount a faster and more effective response by having a lower threshold for activation when they encounter antigen, e.g., after memory T lymphocyte circulation to the peripheral tissues (Ch. 17).

Studies of the adaptive immune response have shown that not only must the lymphoid cells cooperate to mount an effective immune response (Ch. 16) but also that any immune response takes place in a physiological system of organs and tissues connected by the lymph and blood (Chs 12 and 13) and, consequently, is subject to influence by other organ systems. Lymphocytes recirculate throughout the body, homing to particular lymphoid organs and moving out of the blood into sites of infection as they respond to cytokines and other molecules released from, or expressed on the cell surface of, activated lymphoid and other cells (particularly APCs). Cell adhesion molecules (Ch. 13) are particularly important in the trafficking of lymphocytes—the constant patrolling of lymphocytes, particularly naive T lymphocytes, in search of antigen.

Chapter 17 describes immunological memory and also pointed out the existence of mechanisms that maintain lymphocyte homeostasis. Unless there is a response to antigen (e.g., during an infection), the number of lymphocytes in a human is maintained within a relatively narrow range. There are ordered pathways to generate new lymphocytes when they are required (Chs 12, 14 and 15), and there are ordered and regulated pathways for lymphocyte death. Chapter 17 briefly describes the process of programmed cell death (apoptosis) and explains how this may be balanced by anti-apoptotic molecules encoded by the so-called death-inhibiting family of *bcl* genes. This topic will be expanded on in Chapter 34.

The immune response takes place in an organism, and the immune system has to be integrated with the other physiological systems. The immune system does not work alone, and there is still much to understand about the immune response in the context of the whole organism. It seems likely that such an integrative view will be important for further medical advances based on exploiting our knowledge of immunology. This integrated view of the immune system will be a topic for Section V, but the topic of connections between different aspects of the immune system will also be central to the next section of the book (Section IV), which will otherwise predominantly describe **innate immunity**.

To aid in learning a complex subject like immunology, we generally break up the topic into pieces. However, as students of human immunology we have to remember to put the pieces back together again! As in other things, the whole of immunology is definitely more than the sum of the parts. One way in which to demonstrate that this is true is to consider the connections between the innate and adaptive immune response. For some time immunologists who studied aspects of the adaptive immune response, such as B cell ontogeny, or TCR gene rearrangement, carried out their research largely oblivious to the results of studies of the innate immune response, for example, studies of the activation of neutrophils, or studies of the details of the inflammatory response in constitutive defense reactions to microbes. However, the two aspects of the immune response, adaptive and innate, are interconnected in important ways. The innate response complements the adaptive response. For example, the innate response includes physical barriers and first line of defense responses to external pathogens (Ch. 2). If the defenses of the innate system are breached, then the adaptive system is triggered. However, the innate response is not separate from the adaptive response. Rather there are overlapping and connecting molecules (e.g., cytokines) and cells (e.g., macrophages) that integrate the two. It is perhaps more appropriate to view the adaptive and innate responses as stages, but somewhat seamless stages, of the same system, where a primary adaptive immune response generally depends on prior activation and participation of the innate immune system.

As will be developed more fully in the next section, an excellent example of the connection between the innate and adaptive systems is the role played by the pattern-recognition molecules (PRMs), such as the Toll-like receptors (Box 18.1), of the innate system. The concept of PRMs was introduced in Chapter 2 in connection with mannan-binding lectin and the lectin pathway of complement activation. PRMs can bind to molecules that are shared among infectious microbes but are not found in vertebrates, e.g., the complex carbohydrates called mannans found in the cell walls of yeasts, and the lipopolysaccharide (LPS) cell wall components of Gram-negative bacteria. Mammals use several pattern-recognition molecules, such as complement components and lung surfactant protein, for innate host defense reactions (Ch. 19). These molecules (PRMs) distinguish between mammalian self and

Bone marrow   Thymus   Lymph node

microbial non-self in a non-microbe-specific way (see Box 18.1 and Ch. 2).

It is the coordinated action of the innate and adaptive immune responses that counters attacks by pathogens. The next section of the book will describe the innate response in more detail. It ends with a review of the coordinated innate and adaptive response to microbes (Ch. 23).

BOX 18.1
The role of Toll-like receptors as a link between the innate and adaptive immune systems

Certain pattern-recognition molecules (PRMs) found on antigen-presenting cells (APCs) function as receptors for pathogen-specific molecules, such as LPS, and transduce activation signals (**danger signals**; see Chs 19 and 20) on binding these molecules (Fig. 18.1). The activated APCs then send signals (cytokines, etc.) that alert and activate lymphocytes. The PRMs that do this were identified as macrophage cell surface molecules after a search for mammalian equivalents of molecules called Toll receptors, which have critical roles in the immune systems of insects (Ch. 20). The fruit fly, *Drosophila melanogaster*, and other insects have well characterized innate immune systems that confer resistance to microbial infections. A major aspect of host defense in *Drosophila* is release of antimicrobial peptides. During the response to infections in *Drosophila*, a protease cascade generates a ligand for a transmembrane receptor protein known as Toll. The Toll receptor then triggers biochemical events leading to activation of the transcription factor NF-κB (Ch. 11), new gene transcription and synthesis of antimicrobial peptides. Humans have been shown to possess molecules that are homologs of Toll, e.g., the molecule referred to as hTLR (for human Toll-like receptor). Human APCs have several Toll-like receptors. They function as PRMs and bind entities such as lipopolysaccharide (LPS). LPS binding triggers the Toll-like receptor, then the cytoplasmic domain of the TLR initiates a signaling cascade that leads to the production of cytokines (e.g., IL-6 and IL-8) and co-stimulatory molecules (e.g., CD80 (B7), the ligand for CD28—see Ch. 16) by APCs (Fig. 18.1) The cytokines attract antigen-specific lymphocytes and the co-stimulatory molecules on APCs help to activate the lymphocytes and bring the adaptive immune response into play.

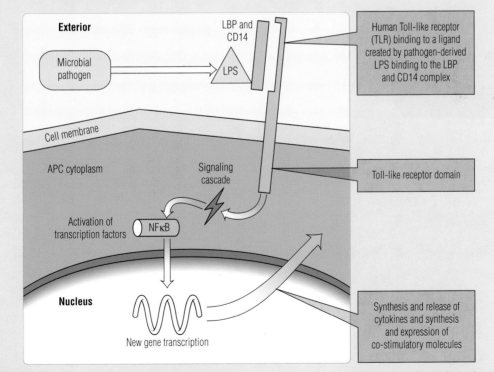

Fig. 18.1 Toll-like receptors in activation of antigen-presenting cells (APC) by microbes. LPS, lipopolysaccharide; LBP, LPS-binding protein; NFκB, nuclear factor kappa **B**.

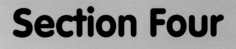

Section Four

Innate immunity

Constitutive defenses including complement

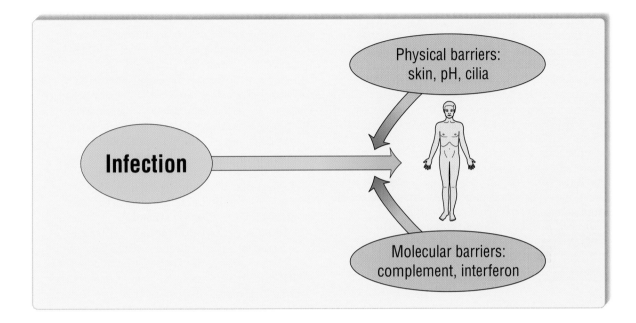

The innate immune system is a series of non-specific defenses in constant readiness to fight off infection. The innate system differs in a number of ways from the adaptive immune system (Fig. 19.1). The way innate immune systems operate and interact with the adaptive system is dealt with in the next four chapters.

The innate immune system has two key roles:

- it provides a very rapid response to infection (described in this chapter)
- it uses danger signals to alert the adaptive immune system that infection is taking place (Ch. 20).

Fig. 19.1
Differences between the innate and adaptive immune systems

Innate system	Adaptive system
Preformed (constitutive) or rapidly formed components	Relies on genetic events and cellular growth
Responds within minutes to infection	Response develops over days
No specificity; the same molecules and cells respond to a range of pathogens	Very specific; each cell is genetically programmed to respond to a single antigen
Uses pattern-recognition molecules	Uses antigen-recognition molecules
No memory; the response does not change after repeated exposure	Immunological memory; on repeated exposure the response is faster, stronger and qualitatively different
An old system, seen in all members of the animal kingdom	Evolved in early vertebrates
Rarely malfunctions	Frequently malfunctions, causing autoimmunity and immunodeficiency

BARRIERS TO INFECTION

The skin and respiratory and gastrointestinal tracts have evolved as specialized barriers to infection.

Skin

Although many organisms live on the surface of the skin, the dense outer layer of dead keratinocytes prevents penetration of these organisms into deeper tissues. The deeper-layer living keratinocytes are active components in the innate immune system. These keratinocytes secrete cytokines such as interleukin 8 (IL-8) and tumor necrosis factor (TNF) if they are damaged in any way. These cytokines are responsible for the inflammation that occurs following exposure to, for example, ultraviolet light.

Skin also contains **Langerhans cells**, which are sentinel cells of the dendritic cell lineage. Following exposure to microorganisms, these cells migrate to the local lymph node and present antigen to T cells.

The skin is typical of innate immune system components in its ability to respond rapidly to stimulation and to activate and inform the adaptive immune response.

Respiratory tract

From the point of view of the innate immune system, the respiratory tract is divisible into upper and lower segments. The upper airway begins at the nose and ends in the bronchioles and is protected by the **mucociliary escalator**. Mucus secreted by goblet cells forms a fine layer lining the airway and trapping microorganisms. Cilia waft the mucus towards the mouth and nose, where trapped organisms are cleared by sneezing or coughing. Mucus secretion is abnormal in cystic fibrosis and cilia are defective in primary ciliary dyskinesia (see Box 19.1).

In the lower respiratory tract (terminal bronchioles and alveoli), layers of cilia and mucus can obstruct oxygen diffusion. The main defenses here are **surfactants** secreted by type II pneumocytes. Surfactants are a mixture of proteins and phospholipids that prevent alveoli from collapsing during expiration. Surfactant also contain pathogen-binding proteins, which are members of the **collectin** family (Fig. 19.2). The collectins have globular lectin-like heads that can bind to sugars on microorganisms and long collagen-like tails that bind to phagocytes or complement. These molecules have a **pattern-recognition** role.

Both segments of the respiratory tract are also reliant on immunoglobulins, as shown by the frequency of respiratory infections in patients with antibody deficiency.

BOX 19.1
Ciliary dyskinesia

A 4-year-old boy has had a series of acute chest infections. Initially he was well between these attacks. At the time of presentation he coughs up infected sputum every day. This chronic infection of the airways is called **bronchiectasis**. An unexpected finding is that his heart is on the right hand side (**dextrocardia**).

Electron microscopy of a nasal biopsy shows that the cilia on the respiratory epithelium are abnormal, diagnostic of **primary ciliary dyskinesia**. This causes dextrocardia in about 50% of cases because normal cilia are required to position the heart during embryonic life. Patients with primary ciliary dyskinesia also suffer from infertility because of the role of cilia in the genital tract. The combination of dextrocardia and bronchiectasis is referred to as Kartagener's syndrome.

Secondary ciliary dyskinesia is much more common, for example cigarette smoke paralyses cilia for several hours. Some bacteria secrete toxins that paralyze cilia, enabling them to colonize the respiratory tract.

pH

The low pH of the stomach is one of the main defenses against infection of the gut. For example, patients unable to secret gastric acid have a high risk of salmonella infection.

EXTRACELLULAR MOLECULES OF THE INNATE IMMUNE SYSTEM

The innate immune system relies on families of proteins that can provide a very rapid response to infection. The **type I interferons** (IFN) are produced locally in response to infection and directly inhibit the growth of pathogens. **Collectins, complement** and the **C reactive protein** are constitutively produced proteins, although they are found at higher levels during infections, and bind onto microorganisms.

Type I interferon

Cells treated with IFN become resistant to viral infection; IFN interferes with viral replication. The antiviral effects are most potent with type I IFN (IFN-α and IFN-β) and less so with IFN-γ. IFNs, especially IFN-γ, also activate the immune response.

🦴 Bone marrow   🫘 Thymus   ⬤ Lymph node

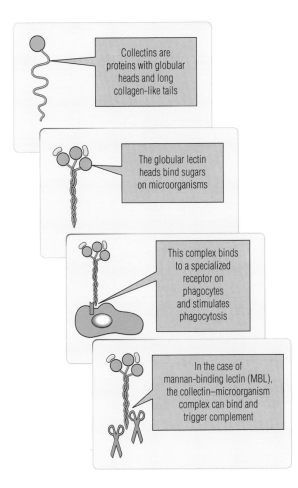

Fig. 19.2 The collectin family includes surfactant proteins and mannan-binding lectin (MBL); both are important pattern-recognition molecules. C1q is a related protein. These proteins have both lectin-like and collagen-like domains. Lectins are sugar-binding proteins that can bind to microorganisms. The collagen-like domains bind to cellular receptors or activate complement.

Type I IFNs are secreted by a wide range of cells in response to double-stranded RNA. Double-stranded RNA is not present in mammalian cells but is produced by viruses during intracellular infection of cells. Type I IFNs have a range of actions (Fig. 19.3):

- inhibition of viral replication by activation of two intracellular enzyme pathways that degrade the viral genome and inhibit transcription of viral messenger RNA
- activation of natural killer cells (Ch. 21)
- stimulation of activity of TAP (transporter associated with antigen presentation) peptide transporters and proteasomes (Ch. 10); both of these increase the availability of peptides for binding to MHC class I and promote the effects of CD8$^+$ T cells.

Within hours of viral infection, type I IFN secretion is induced, inhibiting viral replication and arming natural killer cells to destroy infected cells. Even though IFNs improve antigen presentation on MHC class I, primary T cell and antibody responses may take

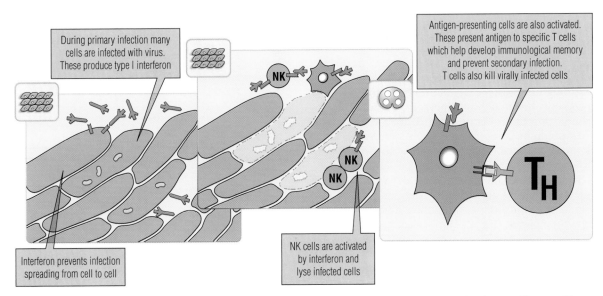

Fig. 19.3 Type I interferons include α, β and γ forms. Inferferon γ has more potent immunostimulatory effects and less potent direct effects on viral replication. NK, natural killer.

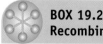

BOX 19.2
Recombinant interferons

Recombinant interferons (IFNs) can be synthesized in high quantities in mammalian cells and have been tested in a range of diseases.

IFN-α is useful in viral hepatitis infection. In hepatitis B, IFN-α improves liver function and reduces viral replication in 40% of patients. Treatment is less successful in hepatitis C infection, where only 20% of patients respond.

The benefits of IFN-α are mediated mainly by its antiviral effects and partly through stimulation of the adaptive immune system.

IFN-α has also been used to treat malignancies, most often chronic myeloid leukemia. The exact mode of action is unclear, although interferon seems to induce either apoptosis or maturation of malignant cells.

IFN-β is useful in some patients with multiple sclerosis. This is an autoimmune disease that is caused by T cells attacking nervous system proteins

(see Box 15.4). IFN-β may dampen down the response in multiple sclerosis to nervous system antigens, which seems to contradict its physiological function. Another possibility is that IFN-β prevents infections that may otherwise trigger exacerbations of the disease.

There are three problems with IFN treatment:

- IFN treatment usually induces influenza-like symptoms, for example, fever and headache
- Patients can produce neutralizing antibodies, which prevent IFN from working. Even though recombinant interferons use human amino acid sequences, proteins produced in non-primates are coated in sugar molecules in a conformation that differs from primate sugars and these sugars can be recognized by the human immune system
- IFNs are expensive, especially when only a minority of patients respond.

as long as a week to develop. Consequently, IFNs provide a rapid response that bridges the period required to initiate the innate immune response.

During infections, macrophages and other innate immune system cells secrete other cytokines such as IL-1, IL-6 and TNF. These cytokines activate the specific immune system and cause the **acute phase response** (see below).

IFN-α is used to treat viral hepatitis and IFN-β is used in multiple sclerosis (Box 19.2).

Complement

Although there are a large number of complement components with difficult names, the overall system is simple and easy to understand. There are nine basic complement components, C1 to C9. When they become activated, complement components are split into small and large fragments; the small fragments are referred to as C3a, C4a, etc. Three different activators detect pathogens and activate a key component, C3, which is required to switch on three different types of effector molecule (Fig. 19.4).

Complement can be activated by interactions between antibody and antigen. Complement facilitates the effects of antibody and is so named because antibody alone will not kill most bacteria; these molecules are required to complement the bactericidal effects of antibody.

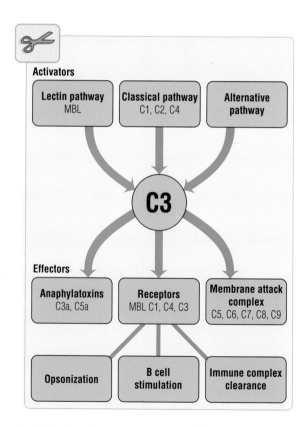

Fig. 19.4 Overview of complement. MBL, mannan-binding lectin.

Bone marrow   Thymus   Lymph node

Activation of complement

There are three ways in which C3 can be activated (Fig. 19.5).

Lectin pathway. Mannan-binding lectin (MBL) is a collectin that is able to bind, through its lectin portions, onto carbohydrates present on bacteria. Although MBL has no enzyme activity of its own, after the lectin portions bind to bacteria, the MBL collagen-like domain indirectly activates the next complement components C2 and C4, which together activate several hundred C3 molecules.

The classical pathway. This is so named because it was discovered first, although it was probably the last to evolve. The classical pathway is triggered by immune complexes of antibody and antigen. C1 is the initiating protein and is able to recognize the Fc portion of immunoglobulin molecules when sufficient Fc portions are in close enough proximity. This is most likely to occur when an antigen binds several immunoglobulin molecules. Because it has five Fc portions, IgM is particularly good at C1 binding. C1 also has no enzyme activity, but after binding to an Fc, it is able to activate C2 and C4, which in turn activate multiple C3 molecules.

The alternative pathway. C3 is not a stable molecule and is constantly undergoing spontaneous low-level activation. Spontaneous activation of C3 is most likely to happen on surfaces, although normal cells express surface complement inhibitors, that prevent C3 activation. The surfaces of pathogens lack complement inhibitors. Any cell surface that is not protected by complement inhibitors will be attacked by complement. Alternative pathway complement activation has proven to be a special challenge in the transplantation of organs from other species (see Box 19.3).

Summary of activation. The alternative pathway activates complement on the surface of *any* cell that lacks complement inhibitors, while the lectin and classical pathways provide focused complement activation to molecules that have been bound by MBL or antibody. Deficiencies in any of these pathways will produce defective immune responses, the symptoms varying with the site of the defect (see Box 19.4).

Amplification steps

Each complement component is constantly present in blood and, on activation, becomes capable of activating several downstream components. Complement activators are sensitive to small signals, such as very few bacteria, and the subsequent amplification steps ensure a dramatic, but usually local response. This is obtained through the enzyme activity of complement components throughout the complement cascade: C2, C4, C3, C5 and C6. These molecules are activated by cleavage into small and large fragments (Fig. 19.6). The large fragments may become enzymes themselves and cleave and activate the next molecule in the cascade. These

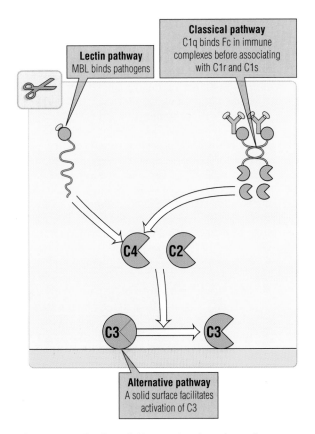

Fig. 19.5 Activation of C3 can take place through any one of three pathways.

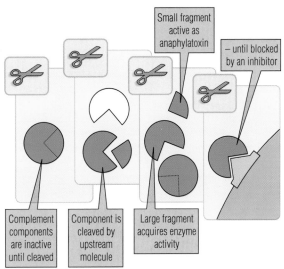

Fig. 19.6 After cleavage, fragments of complement components C2, C4, C3, C5 and C6 acquire enzyme activity and activate downstream components.

 Blood vessel   Gut   Peripheral tissue

fragments may also interact with inhibitors that switch off the amplification steps.

The small fragments of C3 and C5 have biological activity and are known as **anaphylatoxins** (see below).

Complement effectors

Activation of complement produces a number of effector molecules: the anaphylatoxins, fragments binding and activating complement receptors and the membrane attack complex.

Anaphylatoxins. The activation of complement components C3 and C5 produces small fragments C3a and C5a. Because they have a low molecular weight, these peptides diffuse away from the site of complement activation and cause the effects shown in Figure 19.7. The C2a low-molecular-weight peptide has marked effects, increasing vascular permeability.

Complement receptors. There are several complement receptors (CR) present on a variety of cells; these bind early complement components (MBL, C1, and activated C4 and C3). Complement receptors serve the following functions (Fig. 19.8).

- Opsonization. This is the process by which bacteria and other cells are made available for phagocytosis. Molecules that help to bind pathogens to phagocytes and stimulate phagocytosis are known as **opsonins**. Because so much activated C3 is produced during complement activation, it is the most important opsonin and binds to three different receptors present on a range of phagocytes. IgG can also act as an opsonin, when it binds to Fc receptors on phagocytes. Because

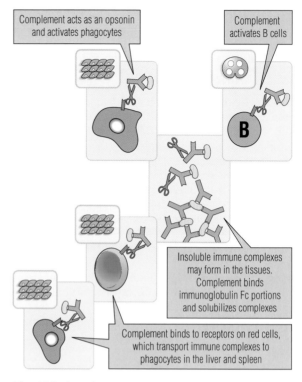

Fig. 19.8 Complement receptors.

phagocytes do not have Fc receptors for IgM, complement-mediated opsonization is particularly important during a primary antibody response, when an IgM response dominates.
- B cell stimulation. Binding of C3 to the CR2 receptor on B cells provides co-stimulation and decreases the B cell activation a hundred-fold (Ch. 11). CR2 has been subverted by the Epstein–Barr virus (Ch. 34), which uses it as its receptor.
- Immune complex clearance. Immune complexes are insoluble lattices of antigen bound to antibody that can form in tissues or in the blood. These trigger inflammation, and immune complex disease (Ch. 29) will occur if they are not removed. Complement helps to remove immune complexes in two ways:
  — large insoluble complexes are particularly difficult to remove from tissues; high numbers of activated C3 interrupt the lattice of the immune complex making them soluble
  — C4 and C3 present in solubilized immune complexes can bind onto complement receptor CR1 on red cells, which transport the immune complexes to organs rich in fixed phagocytes, such as the liver and spleen. Using their own complement and Fc receptors, these phagocytes remove the immune complexes from red cells,

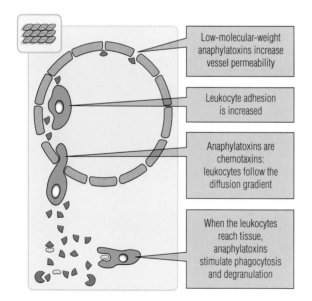

Fig. 19.7 Anaphylatoxins.

phagocytose and destroy them. The red cells are not harmed by this process.

Patients with complement deficiency are at high risk of disease caused by immune complexes, such as SLE (see Box 19.4).

Membrane attack complex. Activated C3 activates the final part of the cascade of complement components C5–C9. These components form the membrane attack complex. C5 and C6 have enzyme activity, which allows components C7, C8 and C9 to insert themselves into the plasma membrane of the target cell. A group of 10 to 16 molecules of C9 form a ring, which creates a pore in the plasma membrane (Fig. 19.9). This allows free passage of water and solutes across the membrane, killing the cell. The membrane attack complex attacks pathogens directly but in humans only appears to be crucial for defenses against *Neisseria*.

Figure 19.10 summarizes how complement is involved in the response to bacterial infection.

Complement inhibitors

Complement tends to undergo spontaneous activation, especially by the alternative pathway. Excessive complement activation is undesirable because it causes inflammation and widespread cell death. To prevent inadvertent complement activation, eight complement inhibitors exist. Their site of action is shown in Figure 19.11.

The importance of these inhibitors is indicated by the fact that deficiency can lead to illness, for example hereditary angioedema (Box 19.5). Another important implication for complement inhibitors is that they are species specific and this provides a challenge for scientists attempting to make xenotransplantation a more useful therapy (Box 19.3).

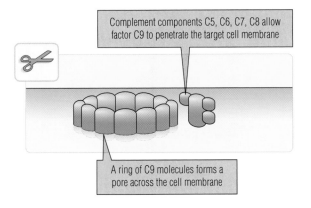

Complement components C5, C6, C7, C8 allow factor C9 to penetrate the target cell membrane

A ring of C9 molecules forms a pore across the cell membrane

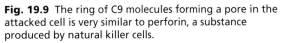

Fig. 19.9 The ring of C9 molecules forming a pore in the attacked cell is very similar to perforin, a substance produced by natural killer cells.

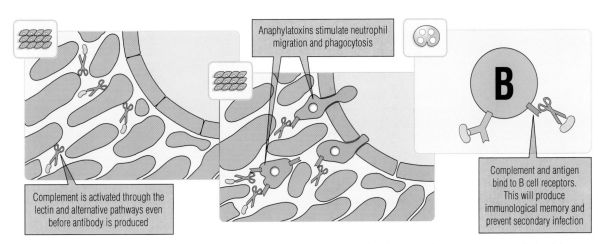

Anaphylatoxins stimulate neutrophil migration and phagocytosis

Complement is activated through the lectin and alternative pathways even before antibody is produced

Complement and antigen bind to B cell receptors. This will produce immunological memory and prevent secondary infection

Fig. 19.10 Complement is particularly important in dealing with bacterial infections. There are some parallels with the ways by which interferons inhibit viral infections. Both complement and interferon can directly attack pathogens and each recruits different cells of the innate and adaptive immune response.

 Blood vessel   Gut   Peripheral tissue

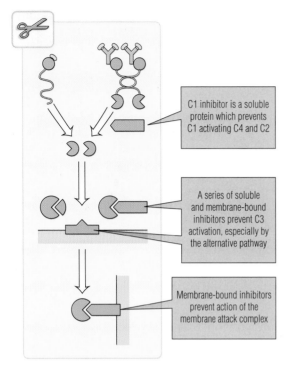

Fig. 19.11 Complement inhibitors.

C1 inhibitor is a soluble protein which prevents C1 activating C4 and C2

A series of soluble and membrane-bound inhibitors prevent C3 activation, especially by the alternative pathway

Membrane-bound inhibitors prevent action of the membrane attack complex

BOX 19.3
Molecular incompatibility

Organs from animals such as pigs could relieve the shortage of human donor organs. Kidneys transplanted from pigs to primates die within minutes. This is in part mediated by alternative pathway complement activation. Pig cells act as a surface on which the spontaneous activation of C3 is promoted. Although pig cells express complement inhibitors, these will not inhibit human complement. Thus molecular incompatibility leads to widespread complement activation and destruction of the kidney.

To overcome molecular incompatibility, nuclear transfer and cloning techniques are being used to insert human complement inhibitor genes into pigs. Although there are other problems to overcome in xenotransplantation (see Ch. 33), these technologies promise to prolong the survival of transplanted pig organs.

BOX 19.4
Complement deficiency

The complement deficiencies are rare and the symptoms produced depend on the site of the defect (Fig. 19.12).

Deficiencies in the early lectin and classical pathways cause type III hypersensitivity (immune complex disease) because immune complexes cannot be solubilized or transported to phagocytes (Ch. 29). Deficiency of early complement components can cause the autoimmune disease systemic lupus erythematosus (SLE). Low levels of early complement components also cause recurrent bacterial infection, partly because the innate immune system clears opsonized bacteria and partly because complement is involved in initiating antibody production.

Deficiencies of the membrane attack complex lead to a specific higher risk of infection with *Neisseria* species. In these patients, *Neisseria meningitidis* infection may present atypically and may be recurrent.

Low levels of complement are more usually the result of consumption rather than reduced production of complement components in the liver. Complement is consumed when immune complexes are produced, for example during infections or autoimmune diseases.

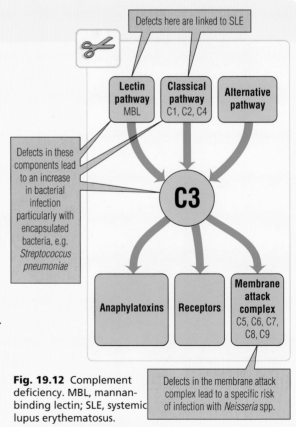

Defects here are linked to SLE

Defects in these components lead to an increase in bacterial infection particularly with encapsulated bacteria, e.g. *Streptococcus pneumoniae*

Lectin pathway MBL

Classical pathway C1, C2, C4

Alternative pathway

C3

Anaphylatoxins

Receptors

Membrane attack complex C5, C6, C7, C8, C9

Defects in the membrane attack complex lead to a specific risk of infection with *Neisseria* spp.

Fig. 19.12 Complement deficiency. MBL, mannan-binding lectin; SLE, systemic lupus erythematosus.

Bone marrow   Thymus   Lymph node

BOX 19.5
Hereditary angioedema

A 7-year-old girl presents with airway obstruction following a dental procedure. She has had bouts of unexplained severe abdominal pain throughout life. Her C4 level is low, although C3 is normal. A sample is analyzed for levels of C1 inhibitor, which is found to be very low.

Hereditary angioedema is an autosomal dominant disease caused by deficiency of C1 inhibitor, allowing the early classical pathway to activate inappropriately after minimal stimulation. The activation of complement is aborted at the level of C3, because an appropriate surface for complement activation is missing. C4 and C2 are cleaved in this process and excessive amounts of the C2a kinin are produced. The result is increased capillary permeability at any site, causing painful, and sometimes life-threatening, swelling.

Purified C1 inhibitor can prevent and treat attacks of hereditary angioedema. An alternative is to give anabolic steroids, which increase C1 inhibitor levels.

BOX 19.6
C reactive protein

C reactive protein (CRP) binds to phospholipids on the surface of bacteria (such as pneumococci). CRP then acts as an opsonin stimulating phagocytosis. CRP also activates the complement system through the lectin pathway. CRP production is increased dramatically during inflammation through the actions of TNF. The clinical value of CRP is its role as an **acute phase protein**. The early response to infection is known as the **acute phase response** (Box 19.7).

BOX 19.7
Acute phase response

Early in infections, metabolism is switched to fighting the microorganism, for example, increasing the body temperature impairs pathogen reproduction. Fever is part of the acute phase response to infection (see Ch. 20).

The acute phase response is triggered by the release of IL-1, IL-6 and TNF from macrophages. These cytokines stimulate the production of a series of proteins:

- innate immune system molecules: C3, C4 and CRP
- adaptive immune response molecules: polyclonal production of immunoglobulins
- damage-limiting proteins: α1-antitrypsin, haptoglobin
- clotting factors: fibrinogen.

The acute phase response is often used to distinguish inflammation from other types of clinical problem. For example, a young child with abdominal pain may have symptoms because of constipation (does not need an operation) or appendicitis (needs an operation!). Surgeons use the acute phase response to distinguish between the two conditions; the acute phase response is activated during appendicitis, but not constipation. CRP is a particularly good indicator of inflammation; for example, levels are increased 1000-fold early in appendicitis and fall rapidly after the appendix has been removed. CRP is also increased by non-infectious problems. For example, CRP is increased in the autoimmune disease rheumatoid arthritis and provides a good way of monitoring disease activity and response to treatment.

The increased synthesis of the proteins mentioned above increases plasma viscosity, which is reflected by an increased **erythrocyte sedimentation rate**. Measuring the erythrocyte sedimentation rate is one of the simplest ways of showing an acute phase response. The erythrocyte sedimentation rate takes longer than CRP to become abnormal during an inflammatory response.

LEARNING POINTS

Can you now:

- List the differences between the innate and adaptive immune response?
- Explain how interferons work and list their roles in treatments?
- Draw a diagram of the complement system?
- List the consequences of complement deficiencies?
- Describe how the acute phase response can be measured?

Bone marrow   Thymus   Lymph node

Phagocytes

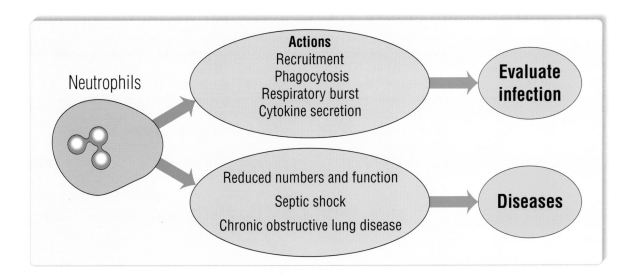

Phagocytosis is the internalization of particulate matter by cells into cytoplasmic vesicles. Phagocytosis is triggered by a number of specific activation events. Phagocytes contain lysosomes: granules containing enzymes that fuse with the vesicles and degrade the particulate matter. In addition, activation of phagocytes initiates the respiratory burst, which is necessary to kill phagocytosed organisms. Phagocytes are, therefore, mainly concerned with clearing pathogens, such as bacteria, protozoans and fungi, and cellular debris.

Phagocytic cell types

Phagocytes are bone marrow-derived (myeloid) cells. A range of phagocytic cells have evolved in humans, each with specific functions.

Neutrophils

Neutrophils are the most numerous white cells in blood (Fig. 20.1a). Neutrophils migrate rapidly into sites of infection, where they kill pathogens. Pus

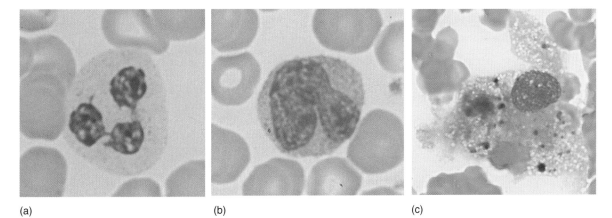

(a)   (b)   (c)

Fig. 20.1 Phagocytic cells. (a) Neutrophils have a very distinct appearance because of their granules, which contain proteolytic enzymes. They can easily be counted by automated instruments when the acute phase response is being measured. (b) Monocytes are immature macrophages (c) which have a much more distinctive appearance.

BOX 20.1
Neutropenic sepsis

A 12-year-old girl has been receiving cytotoxic chemotherapy for acute lymphoblastic leukemia. Although the leukemia has been showing signs of going into remission, she has become neutropenic (neutrophils were less than $0.5 \times 10^3/\mu l$). Early in the evening, she complained of shivering and chills and was found to be pyrexial (have a high fever). Within half an hour she collapsed and was found to have the features of shock (tachycardia and hypotension) along with warm peripheries. When she is examined by the physician, there are no signs of focal organ involvement (such as pneumonia) and a diagnosis of **neutropenic sepsis** complicated by **septic (endotoxic) shock** is made.

Blood culture is taken (these later grow *Escherichia coli*) and she is started on broad-spectrum antibiotics and fluid replacement. She gradually improves over the next 12 hours.

Neutrophils play a crucial role in the early part of bacterial infection. When neutrophils are present and can function normally, they limit infection to the site of entry and produce pus. This creates physical signs such as pneumonia or abscess formation. In neutropenic patients, the innate immune response cannot localize infection, which rapidly spreads to the blood and then to other tissues. Other parts of the immune system are able to function normally; for example, this patient was able to mount an acute phase response with fever and rigors. Septic shock (Box 20.6) is an exaggerated part of the normal innate response to infection.

This story illustrates how important it is to respond promptly to very early symptoms of infection in neutropenic patients.

formed at the site of infection is largely composed of dead neutrophils. Neutrophils play a crucial part in early defenses against bacterial infections; consequently, patients with defective neutrophils or low levels of neutrophils (**neutropenic**) are at particular risk of serious bacterial infection (Box 20.1).

Monocytes/macrophages

Monocytes (Fig. 20.1b) are also myeloid cells but are very different from neutrophils (Fig. 20.2). Monocytes in the blood are immature cells migrating to their site of activity. Monocytes migrate into a range of tissues where they mature into macrophages and take on a number of specialized forms. All macrophage forms have long life spans, surviving in the tissue for months or years.

Tissue macrophages. These are found in a wide range of sites. They are large cells with specialized granules and cytoplasmic compartments. In some tissues (bone marrow, lymph nodes) these active macrophages are referred to as **histiocytes**.

Giant and epitheloid cells. In sites of chronic inflammation, macrophages undergo further maturation and become giant cells or epitheloid cells, under the influence of T cell cytokines. Epitheloid and giant cells are characteristic of granuloma formation (Ch. 22) and participate in prolonging the inflammatory response by presenting antigen to T cells and by secreting cytokines. Unlike neutrophils, macrophages live for many years and pus is not formed during this type of inflammation.

Fixed macrophages. These specialized phagocytes line

Fig. 20.2
Differences between neutrophils and monocytes/macrophages

Neutrophils	Macrophages
Rapid increase in production during the acute phase response	Slight increase in blood levels during inflammation
Only found in inflamed tissues	Found in healthy tissues
Single mature form	Variety of mature forms
Rapidly form pus	Slowly form granuloma—with T cell help
Short lived—die after phagocytosis	Long lived—survive after phagocytosis

sinusoids in the spleen and liver. In the liver, these macrophages are referred to as **Kupffer cells**. Their role is to phagocytose circulating particulate matter (Fig. 19.9) and, in some situations, phagocytose entire cells (see hemolytic anemia in Ch. 27).

Alveolar macrophages. These contribute to the lung's innate defenses. They are involved in disease processes such as chronic obstructive pulmonary disease (Box 20.2).

Glial cells. These are long-lived macrophages resident in the nervous system. They are involved in clearing dead neuronal cells.

Osteoclasts. The most specialized macrophages are the osteoclasts in bone, which participate in regulating calcium metabolism by resorbing bone and releasing calcium into the blood.

Phagocyte production

Neutrophils and monocytes are produced from the same precursor cells in the bone marrow (Fig. 20.4) (see Ch. 12). Many more neutrophils are produced each day than monocytes. This rapid production is especially vulnerable to the effects of cytotoxic drugs, which can give rise to neutropenia and vulnerability to infection (Box 20.1). Production of these cells is stimulated by **colony stimulating factors** (CSFs), which are produced by tissue macrophages as part of an acute

BOX 20.2
Chronic obstructive pulmonary disease

A 58-year-old man complains of increasing breathlessness for 5 years. He has smoked 1 pack of cigarettes a day for 40 years. Chest X ray film shows hyperexpanded lungs and respiratory function tests show air flow limitation that is not improved by bronchodilators. A diagnosis of chronic obstructive pulmonary disease (COPD) is made. A trial of oral corticosteroids is given for 2 weeks. There is no improvement in his respiratory function tests. He is, however, able to stop smoking and general measures are taken to improve his respiratory health.

COPD is the fourth largest cause of death in the USA, affecting over 14 million patients. COPD consists of two elements; **chronic bronchitis** and **emphysema**. In chronic bronchitis, the airways are inflamed, with increased mucus secretion, and there are repeated bronchial infections. The infections may partly be a consequence of cilial paralysis caused by cigarette smoke.

There is also a reduction in the number of functioning alveoli. The residual alveoli are distended with trapped air (Fig 20.3). These are the characteristic changes of emphysema. Emphysema is probably a result of proteolytic enzymes released by macrophages and neutrophils in the airways and alveoli. Smoking stimulates secretion of chemokines by local fibroblasts, which attract macrophages into the airways. The macrophages secrete excessive amounts of a **metalloproteinase**, elastase, which attacks elastin and destroys alveolar walls. Stopping smoking prevents further damage to alveoli and there is a possibility of improvements in respiratory function. Although corticosteroids inhibit macrophage function, they have little effect in established emphysema, because the damage has already been done.

Emphysema is rare in non-smokers. One possible cause is deficiency of α_1-antitrypsin, an inhibitor of metalloproteinases. In these patients, metalloproteinase activity is unopposed by the inhibitor and widespread alveolar destruction takes place. Patients with α_1-antitrypsin deficiency also develop cirrhosis, probably because of the effects of metalloproteinase on the liver. Metalloproteinases are also involved in damaging joints in rheumatoid arthritis (Ch. 29).

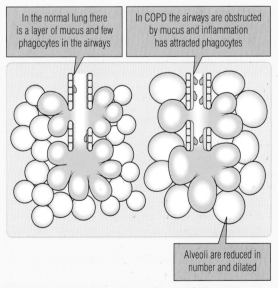

In the normal lung there is a layer of mucus and few phagocytes in the airways

In COPD the airways are obstructed by mucus and inflammation has attracted phagocytes

Alveoli are reduced in number and dilated

Fig. 20.3 Increased mucus and proteolytic enzyme production represent the inappropriate response of the innate immune system to cigarette smoke.

and integrins such as intercellular adhesion molecule (ICAM).

Chemokines are low-molecular-weight *chemo*tactic cyto*kines* that direct cells to specific sites. There are a dozen or so chemokines and a similar number of chemokine receptors. Macrophages at the site of infection secrete chemokines, such as interleukin (IL) 8. These modify neutrophil integrins to make the neutrophils more adherent. This allows them to bind to endothelium and undergo diapedesis (passage through intact vessel walls into tissues) (Ch. 13). The final chemokine-mediated step is **chemotaxis**: the directional migration of cells along a gradient of chemokines. The net result of chemokine secretion is the attraction of neutrophils into tissues. Interestingly, the same chemokines that attract neutrophils into inflamed tissue stimulate the departure of local dendritic cells for lymph nodes in order to stimulate the adaptive immune system.

Anaphylatoxins (Ch. 19) produced by activation of the complement cascade are also chemotactic for phagocytes.

To summarize, resident macrophages at the site of infection secrete cytokines and chemokines, which stimulates neutrophil production, neutrophil and endothelium expression of selectins and integrins, neutrophil adherence to endothelium in local vessels and, finally, chemotaxis to the site of infection.

Receptors on phagocytes

Phagocytes are activated by signals acting through receptors on the phagocyte membrane during their journey through the tissues and their encounters with pathogens or damaged cells (Fig. 20.6).

- Receptors for chemokines and cytokines; these direct phagocytes to the site of inflammation and, once there, prepare them for action.
- Pattern-recognition molecules recognize families of pathogens and induce macrophages to transmit a danger signal that infection is taking place (Box 20.3; see also Box 18.1).
- Receptors for complement components; complement may bind onto pathogens and cellular debris (Ch. 19). Opsonized bacteria generally stimulate an inflammatory response, for example when they are being phagocytosed by neutrophils inside an abscess. By comparison, immune complex clearance by fixed macrophages in the liver and spleen takes place with no inflammation.
- Receptors for apoptotic cells (see Box 21.6). Cells that have undergone apoptosis have done so as part of a physiological process and are phagocytosed without eliciting an inflammatory response.

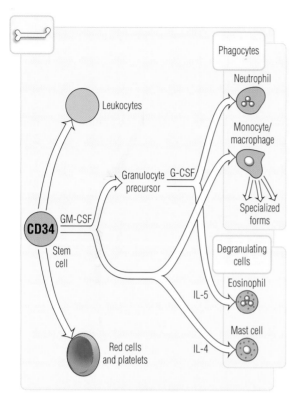

Fig. 20.4 Neutrophil production is increased during the acute phase response by granulocyte colony-stimulating factor (G-CSF). Production of eosinophils and mast cells, which are discussed in Chapter 25, is promoted by interleukin (IL) 4 and 5, respectively. GM-CSF, granulocyte–macrophage colony-stimulating factor.

phase response. CSFs ensure that neutrophils are produced in increasing numbers during infection. Recombinant granulocyte CSF (filgrastim, lenograstim) can be used to boost neutrophil numbers, for example following bone marrow transplant.

Phagocyte recruitment

Monocytes constantly migrate into healthy tissue and differentiate into the specialized macrophages mentioned above. Macrophages remain in a resting state unless they are stimulated by signals binding to their receptors, described below. Although neutrophils make up the majority of phagocytes circulating in the blood, they are absent from normal tissues and will only migrate into inflamed tissue (Fig. 20.5). Resident macrophages detect infection and recruit neutrophils to sites of inflammation using signals similar to those already discussed in Chapter 13 in relation to lymphocyte trafficking. For example, cytokines produced by local macrophages stimulate endothelial cells in local capillaries to increase expression of P selectin

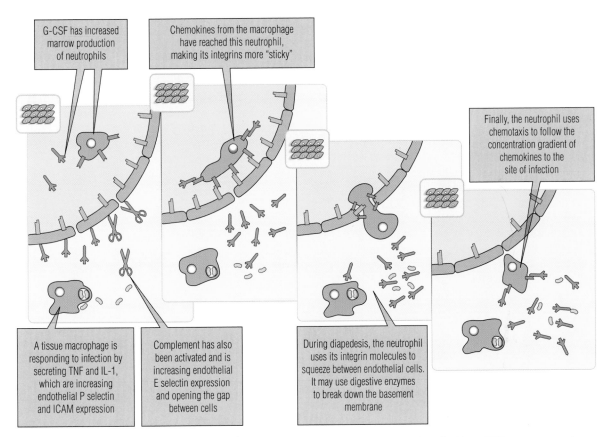

Fig. 20.5 Neutrophil migration. G-CSF, granulocyte colony-stimulating factor; IL-1, interleukin 1; TNF, tumor necrosis factor; ICAM, intercellular adhesion molecule.

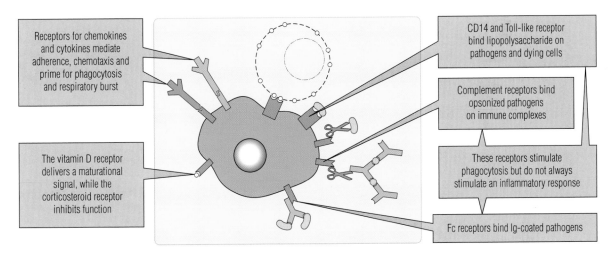

Fig. 20.6 Phagocyte receptors. LPS, lipopolysaccharide.

- Receptors for immunoglobulin. Phagocytes can recognize immunoglobulin through their Fc receptors and IgG can then act as an opsonin.

Actions of phagocytes

Once they have arrived in the tissues and been stimulated through their receptors, phagocytes kill and clear pathogens through phagocytosis, respiratory burst and

 Blood vessel Gut [Peripheral tissue icon] Peripheral tissue

BOX 20.3
Macrophage pattern-recognition molecules

Phagocytes have pattern-recognition molecules for microbial components. These are not specific for particular organisms but rather recognize families of pathogens.

One of the most important recognition molecules is for lipopolysaccharide (LPS). LPS is an **endotoxin**—toxins released when bacteria die—as distinct from **exotoxins**, produced by living bacteria. LPS is a component of the cell wall of Gram-negative bacteria and is one of the most potent stimuli in biology. LPS is often responsible for septic shock (Box 20.6). LPS is recognized by one type of phagocyte **Toll-like receptor**, which is specific for all Gram-negative bacteria that contain LPS. Other Toll-like receptors recognize sugars present on mycobacteria. Toll-like receptors are very ancient molecules—the original Toll protein with similar functions and roles to Toll-like receptors is found in fruit flies! There are at least 10 Toll-like receptors expressed by macrophages and each of these transmits a **danger signal** that infection is taking place (see Box 18.1).

Other types of molecule recognize DNA base pair combinations that are found much more frequently in bacteria than in human cells, for example cytosine and guanosine together. Thus, pattern-recognition molecules recognize motifs that characterize pathogens and inform the innate immune system of infection.

BOX 20.4
Evasion of phagocyte killing

Several bacterial species have evolved mechanisms for evading phagocytosis and its consequences (Fig. 20.7).

Pneumococci produce a large polysaccharide coat around their cell wall, which evades complement. Although C reactive protein (Ch. 19) binds pneumococci, it is only a weak opsonin. For reliable phagocytosis, pneumococci must be coated with antibody. This is why this is such a major pathogen in patients with antibody deficiency.

Mycobacteria, such as *M. tuberculosis*, have waxy coats that block the effects of phagocyte enzymes. They also secrete catalase, which prevents the effects of the respiratory burst. How macrophages control mycobacteria without killing them is discussed in Chapter 22.

Listeria causes meningitis, particularly in pregnant women. Listeria secretes listeriolysin, which punches holes in the phagolysosome walls. The bacteria can then escape into the cytoplasm, where they are not exposed to the toxic products of the metabolic burst or to proteolytic enzymes.

Other ways by which organisms evade the immune system are described in Chapter 24.

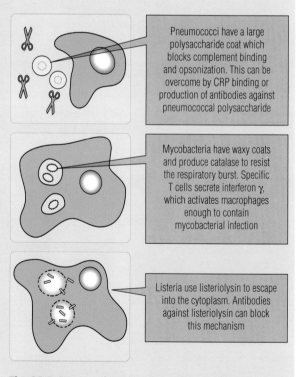

Pneumococci have a large polysaccharide coat which blocks complement binding and opsonization. This can be overcome by CRP binding or production of antibodies against pneumococcal polysaccharide

Mycobacteria have waxy coats and produce catalase to resist the respiratory burst. Specific T cells secrete interferon γ, which activates macrophages enough to contain mycobacterial infection

Listeria use listeriolysin to escape into the cytoplasm. Antibodies against listeriolysin can block this mechanism

Fig. 20.7 Some pathogens escape the innate phagocytic killing mechanisms. In these situations, the adaptive immune system produces antibodies or T cells to facilitate killing, or at least containment of pathogens. CRP, C reactive protein.

Bone marrow   Thymus   Lymph node

the release of proteolytic enzymes. A number of pathogens have developed defense mechanisms to avoid destruction by phagocytes (Box 20.4).

Phagocytosis

Phagocytosis is a metabolically active process that is triggered by binding through one of the receptors mentioned above. Phagocytosis is most effectively triggered by pathogens that have been opsonized by complement or IgG (Fig. 20.8). A **phagosome** is formed by the ingestion of particulate matter.

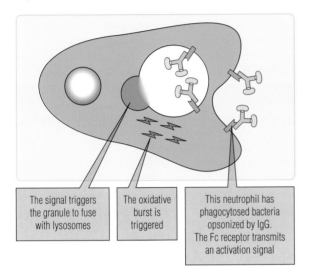

The signal triggers the granule to fuse with lysosomes

The oxidative burst is triggered

This neutrophil has phagocytosed bacteria opsonized by IgG. The Fc receptor transmits an activation signal

Fig. 20.8 Phagocyte killing.

Respiratory burst

Following phagocytosis, three interrelated enzyme pathways are activated that produce toxic molecules which further damage pathogens (Fig. 20.9). The enzymes produce hydrogen peroxide (phagocyte NADPH oxidase), hypochlorous acid (bleach; myeloperoxidase) and nitric oxide (inducible nitric oxide synthetase).

The phagocyte NADPH oxidase enzymes are defective in a type of primary immunodeficiency, chronic granulomatous disease (Box 20.5). Myeloperoxidase is one target of the autoantibodies antineutrophil cytoplasmic antibodies (ANCA) (see Fig. 28.9).

Nitric oxide is a special molecule because as well as being toxic to pathogens it also acts as an important messenger. Nitric oxide is constitutively produced at low levels by neuronal and endothelial cells and has a role as a neurotransmitter and in maintaining vascular tone. Phagocytes can produce high levels of nitric oxide when inducible nitric oxide synthetase is activated. High levels of nitric oxide reduce vascular tone and cardiac output and contribute to the low blood pressure of septic shock (Box 20.6). There is also evidence that nitric oxide acts as a messenger molecule and can promote the effects of T cells, contributing to chronic inflammation.

Proteloytic enzymes

Macrophages contain enzymes in lysosomes, which can be regenerated during the long life of these cells. In neutrophils, the proteolytic enzymes are contained in granules, which give the cell its characteristic appearance.

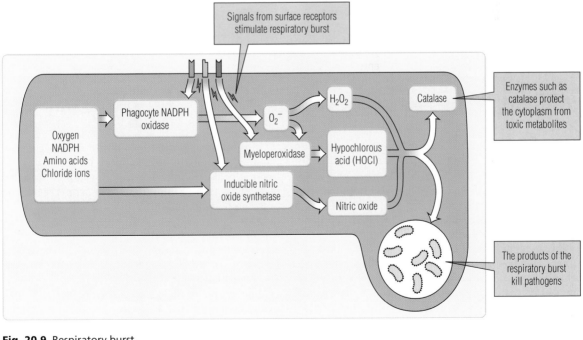

Signals from surface receptors stimulate respiratory burst

Oxygen
NADPH
Amino acids
Chloride ions

Phagocyte NADPH oxidase

O_2^-

H_2O_2

Catalase

Enzymes such as catalase protect the cytoplasm from toxic metabolites

Myeloperoxidase

Hypochlorous acid (HOCl)

Inducible nitric oxide synthetase

Nitric oxide

The products of the respiratory burst kill pathogens

Fig. 20.9 Respiratory burst.

BOX 20.5
Chronic granulomatous disease

A 4-year-old boy presents with a high fever and signs of fluid in the left pleural cavity. A sample from the pleural cavity shows pus, from which *Staphylococcus aureus* is grown.

The child has a history of growth retardation and perianal abscesses. He has no siblings and the only family history is of the death of a maternal uncle from infection in his teens.

Blood examination shows a marked neutrophilia of $23 \times 10^3/\mu l$ when the normal range is $3–6 \times 10^3/\mu l$. A nitro blue tetrazolium (NBT) test is carried out to determine whether his neutrophils are capable of mounting a respiratory burst (Fig. 20.10). The patient's neutrophils are unable to oxidize NBT, consistent with a diagnosis of chronic granulomatous disease (CGD).

CGD is a primary immunodeficiency affecting neutrophil function. This disease is characterized by recurrent bacterial and fungal infections in the presence of a neutrophilia. It is caused by mutations in the genes for NADPH oxidase or its regulatory proteins. CGD is usually X-linked. Although neutrophils are produced in abundance and are able to migrate to sites of infection, they cannot produce superoxide radicals and kill pathogens. Neutrophils are recruited to the site of infection and, as they die, contribute to the pus. The consequence is pus-filled lesions in response to trivial infections. The term *granulomatous* in this context is, therefore, a misnomer; these are abscesses not granulomata. True granulomata are described in Chapter 22.

Infection in children with CGD can be prevented by the use of prophylactic antibiotics and antifungal agents, although other approaches, such as bone marrow transplant, have been tried.

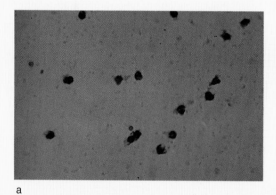
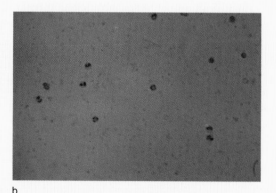

a   b

Fig. 20.10 The nitro blue tetrazolium test. (a) Neutrophils from a normal donor; the stimulated normal neutrophils oxidize the dye to produce a black color. (b) Neutrophils from a patient with chronic granulomatous disease are unable to oxidize the dye.

Macrophages contain enzymes in lysosomes. Neutrophils cannot regenerate granules and when these have been used up, the cell dies. The main enzymes present are proteolytic and are able to digest bacteria in the acid pH of the lysosomes.

In the case of macrophages, the digested peptides can be presented to T cells.

The proteolytic enzymes are usually held retained in lysosomes. Enzymes that leak out of phagocytes are usually prevented from damaging tissues by enzyme inhibitors, such as α_1-antitrypsin. When enzymes are produced excessively, in response to inappropriate stimuli, or when inhibitors are absent, diseases such as emphysema may occur (Box 20.2).

Other substances are released into the phagosome, including **defensins** and **lactoferrin**. Defensins are low-molecular-weight peptides that punch holes in bacteria. Lactoferrin binds onto iron, depriving bacteria of this important nutrient.

Inflammatory signaling

Neutrophils and macrophages produce inflammatory mediators called **prostaglandins** and **leukotrienes**. These are discussed in Chapter 21.

Although neutrophils secrete chemokines and nitric oxide, their short life span prevents them from contributing to a stable, long-lasting inflammatory lesion. Instead, a short-lived lesion is produced, usually with

Bone marrow   Thymus   Lymph node

BOX 20.6
Septic shock

Septic shock is an acute state of hypotension caused by the effects of bacterial endotoxins. The shock is a result of decreased vascular tone and impaired cardiac output. Septic shock is common in neutropenic patients but may be seen in patients with normal immune responses when overwhelmed by infection, for example after a ruptured bowel. Most cases are caused by Gram-negative organisms and LPS is typically the endotoxin implicated.

Endotoxin release triggers the innate immune response when macrophages are directly activated through Toll-like receptors. Consequences of macrophage activation include the secretion of tumor necrosis factor (TNF), prostaglandins and nitric oxide. The TNF triggers more nitric oxide production by smooth muscle and endothelial cells. The very high levels of nitric oxide are responsible for the decreased vascular tone and cardiac output (it should be remembered that normal levels of nitric oxide help maintain vascular tone). Endothelial cell activation may also trigger the clotting cascade.

Septic shock is complicated by widespread organ failure, especially when the clotting cascade is also activated. The mortality from septic shock is over 70%. Attempts at blocking the effects of gross activation of the innate immune system have largely been unsuccessful (Fig. 20.11).

Toxic shock syndrome is a different entity, mediated by cytokines secreted from T cells (Box 7.2).

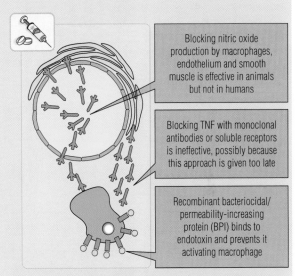

Blocking nitric oxide production by macrophages, endothelium and smooth muscle is effective in animals but not in humans

Blocking TNF with monoclonal antibodies or soluble receptors is ineffective, possibly because this approach is given too late

Recombinant bacteriocidal/permeability-increasing protein (BPI) binds to endotoxin and prevents it activating macrophage

Fig. 20.11 All three approaches to preventing septic shock have failed in clinical trials, possibly because the innate immune system has already mediated its damage by the time symptoms develop; consequently the therapeutic agents may have been given too late.

pus formation. This type of response may be termed a **pyogenic** (pus-forming) reaction.

By comparison, macrophages have a key role in stimulating chronic inflammation, largely through secretion of soluble messengers with local and systemic effects. Macrophages are also important antigen-presenting cells because they process antigen, secrete cytokines and express high levels of co-stimulatory molecules and MHC class II molecules (see Chs 16 and 8, respectively). If antigen is not cleared, the inflammation becomes chronic and a **granuloma** is the result. Granulomata are discussed more fully in Chapter 22, but Figure 20.12 shows how mediators produced by macrophages and T cells contribute to chronic inflammation.

Acute phase response

Macrophages secrete IL-1, IL-6 and TNF after they have recognized pathogens using pattern-recognition molecules. These cytokines increase production of complement and arm the adaptive immune system (Ch. 19). TNF has direct effects on metabolism. It increases the breakdown of fat in the body's stores, and weight loss

is often a dramatic consequence of activation of the immune system.

IL-1, IL-6 and TNF also affect the central nervous system through receptors in the hypothalamus. The main response is an increase in body temperature, which is seen very rapidly after the beginning of the response to infection. The role of increased body temperature is to inhibit the replication of viruses and bacteria.

Through the acute phase response, the innate immune system acts as a sensory system and has profound effects on the nervous system and the metabolism (see also Ch. 35).

Phagocyte defects

Primary disorders of phagocytes are rare but include important problems such as chronic granulomatous disease (Box 20.5). Secondary phagocyte defects are much more common. The most important is neutropenia, where numbers of neutrophils are reduced, usually as a result of drug treatment (Box 20.1). Phagocyte function is impaired secondary to a number of other

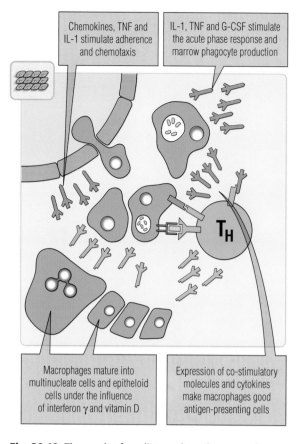

Fig. 20.12 The result of mediator release by macrophages can be granuloma formation. A granuloma is a site of chronic inflammation in which macrophages may mature into giant cells or epitheloid cells. Lymphocytes are also present and support macrophages by secreting interferon γ. TNF, tumor necrosis factor; IL-1, interleukin 1; G-CSF, granulocyte colony-stimulating factor.

Labels within Fig. 20.12:
- Chemokines, TNF and IL-1 stimulate adherence and chemotaxis
- IL-1, TNF and G-CSF stimulate the acute phase response and marrow phagocyte production
- Macrophages mature into multinucleate cells and epitheloid cells under the influence of interferon γ and vitamin D
- Expression of co-stimulatory molecules and cytokines make macrophages good antigen-presenting cells

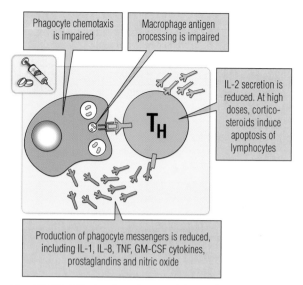

Fig. 20.13 Effects of corticosteroids on phagocyte function. IL-1, interleukin 1; IL-8, interleukin 8; TNF, tumor necrosis factor; GM-CSF, granulocyte–macrophage colony-stimulating factor.

Labels within Fig. 20.13:
- Phagocyte chemotaxis is impaired
- Macrophage antigen processing is impaired
- IL-2 secretion is reduced. At high doses, corticosteroids induce apoptosis of lymphocytes
- Production of phagocyte messengers is reduced, including IL-1, IL-8, TNF, GM-CSF cytokines, prostaglandins and nitric oxide

disorders, such as diabetes and renal failure, and during corticosteroid treatment (Fig. 20.13).

MOLECULAR RECOGNITION BY THE INNATE AND ADAPTIVE IMMUNE SYSTEMS

It is useful at this point to consider the ways in which the two arms of the immune system recognize different molecules. This is summarized in Figure 20.14. It is important to understand that although the adaptive

Fig. 20.14
Molecular recognition in the innate and adaptive immune systems

Innate system	Adaptive system
Pattern-recognition molecules	Antigen-recognition molecules
Collectins (mannan-binding lectin, surfactant), complement C1, C reactive protein and Toll-like receptors	Use hypervariable regions in immunoglobulin and T cell receptor
Receptors use germline genes	Receptor genes created through recombination
Probably fewer than 100 receptors exist, each recognizes entire classes of pathogen	Possibility of up to 10^{16} different receptors
Pattern-recognition molecules detect danger signals, for example, lipopolysaccharide, mannan and other molecules unique to pathogens	Recognizes conformational structures (immunoglobulin) or short peptides bound to MHC molecules (T cell receptor)
Can only recognize molecules on pathogens	Cannot distinguish host from pathogens

Bone marrow   Thymus   Lymph node

immune system can recognize many millions of possible antigens, MHC molecules, T cell receptors and immunoglobulin molecules themselves are incapable of distinguishing self from non-self. This means that if the adaptive immune system was able to initiate a response autonomously, it could react to self peptides and initiate autoimmunity (Ch. 27). By comparison, the pattern-recognition molecules used by the innate system can only recognize pathogen molecules. Recognition systems, such as the Toll-like receptors on macrophages deliver danger signals. These stimulate macrophages to express increased amounts of MHC molecules, co-stimulatory molecules such as B7 and to secrete cytokines. Only then can T cells respond to antigen. *Thus the innate immune system alerts the adaptive system.*

Many students make the mistake of believing that the more recently evolved adaptive immune system acts autonomously of the older innate system. We have seen now that this is not correct. Antigen-presenting cells must first detect invading pathogens before they can co-stimulate T cells.

LEARNING POINTS

Can you now:

- List the differences between the roles of neutrophils and macrophages?
- List the different types of macrophage and their specialist functions?
- Describe how the innate immune system directs the adaptive system?
- Describe two kinds of problem that arise when there are quantitative and functional phagocyte defects?
- Describe how phagocytes may contribute to problems such as septic shock and emphysema?

Killing in the immune system

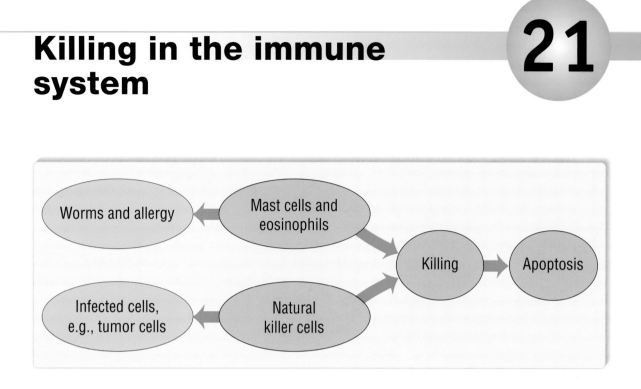

The immune system has to destroy a wide range of pathogens and uses the mechanisms shown in Figure 21.1 to achieve this. In this chapter, we introduce three further types of killing cell in the innate immune system (mast cells, eosinophils and natural killer (NK) cells) and apoptosis, a generic killing mechanism.

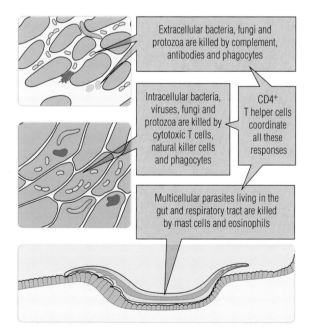

Fig. 21.1 Targets for killing by the immune system. In immunodeficiency states, the type of defect is reflected by the infections patients develop. For example, antibody-deficient patients suffer mainly bacterial infection.

Response to parasite worms

During human evolution, parasitic worms were a major threat to the species. Probably because of improved sanitation, worms are no longer considered a problem to people in the developed world, although a third of the world's population is still infested with these parasites. Worms come in a variety of shapes and sizes (from 1 mm to 1 m) and tend to have complicated life cycles involving eggs, larvae and adult forms. Adult worms generally live inside the gut. Worms have evolved a range of powerful strategies for evading the immune response (Fig. 21.2). Mast cells and eosinophils evolved to respond to worms living in the gut. Essentially, on activation these cells discharge toxic substances into the gut lumen, increase mucus secretion and cause smooth muscle contraction, resulting in expulsion of the worm; these responses are summarized in Figure 21.2. The same mechanisms evolved in the airways.

Mast cells

Mast cells are derived from an unknown precursor cell in the bone marrow, under the influence of T helper 2 (T_H2) cytokines interleukin (IL) 3 and 4. Rather like macrophages, mast cells home into a range of normal tissues, including the submucosa, skin or connective tissue (Fig. 21.3). Recruitment to these front-line sites is increased during worm infestations.

Like macrophages, mast cells reside in the tissues for several weeks. During this time mast cells produce granules containing a range of mediators. They also acquire IgE on their specialized Fc receptors (FcεRI).

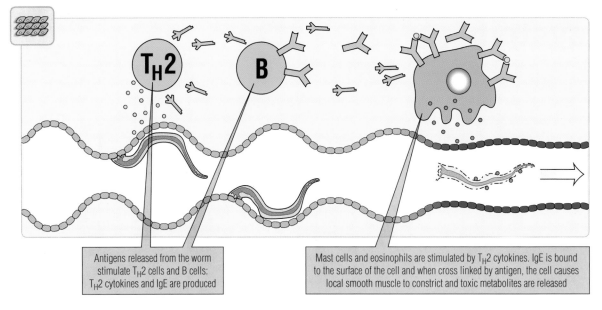

Antigens released from the worm stimulate T_H2 cells and B cells: T_H2 cytokines and IgE are produced

Mast cells and eosinophils are stimulated by T_H2 cytokines. IgE is bound to the surface of the cell and when cross linked by antigen, the cell causes local smooth muscle to constrict and toxic metabolites are released

Fig. 21.2 Summary of the response to a gut-dwelling worm.

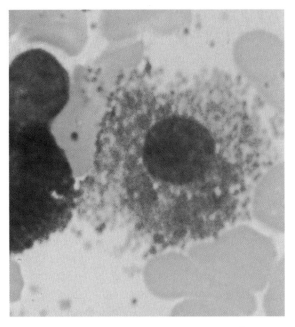

Fig. 21.3 Mast cell. The granules in this mast cell contain cytokines, histamine and proteolytic enzymes.

FcεRI have a very high affinity for IgE and so even IgE produced at very low level elsewhere in the body will bind onto mast cells. Consequently, the mast cells can bind a range of IgE molecules against a number of different antigens. Mast cells become activated when these surface IgE molecules are crosslinked by antigen

(Fig. 21.4). Mast cell FcεRI are different from other types of Fc receptor; they bind immunoglobulin that is not bound to antigen and do not induce activation until they have been crosslinked by antigen. Mast cells are also activated by anaphylatoxins C3a and C5a (Ch. 20) and by a number of drugs, including opiates.

Mast cell activation results in degranulation and release of preformed substances from the granules and activation of arachidonic acid metabolism to produce a range of freshly made mediators.

Granule contents

Mast cell enzymes. Mast cell granules contain a number of proteolytic enzymes including tryptase and chymotrypsin. These enzymes increase mucus secretion and smooth muscle contraction in, for example, bronchi. In addition, they cleave and activate components of the complement and kinin pathways, which promote inflammation.

Histamine. Histamine causes smooth muscle contraction in the gut and lungs in an attempt to expel worms. Histamine increases vascular permeability and provides a chemotactic signal to attract more white cells to the site of worm infestation. Histamine causes marked itching in the skin, possibly to draw the attention of an infested host to the presence of skin parasites.

Cytokines. Like activated macrophages, mast cells produce a range of cytokines to promote and extend the inflammatory response. Tumor necrosis factor (TNF) is preformed and present in granules and will activate local endothelium to enhance diapedesis of more inflammatory cells. Mast cells also produce other cytokines after

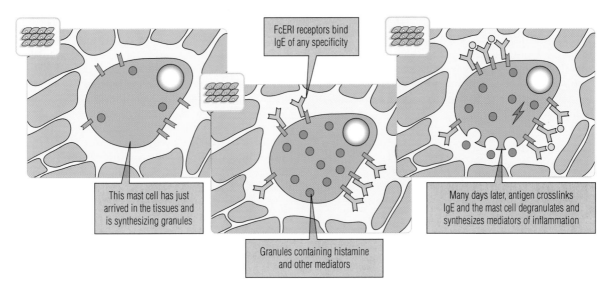

Fig. 21.4 Mast cell activation.

stimulation, and, unlike those produced by macrophages, these stimulate T_H2 responses. IL-4 activates T_H2 cells and IL-3 and IL-5 stimulate eosinophil production and activation. IL-4 and IL-5 also skew the adaptive immune response away from a T_H1 response.

Arachidonic acid metabolites

Metabolites of arachidonic acid metabolism are produced by mast cells and also by phagocytes. Arachidonic acid metabolism is activated by mast cell exposure to antigen and can follow two different pathways (Fig. 21.5).

- The cyclo-oxygenase pathway produces **prostaglandins**, which act within seconds to stimulate vasodilatation, increased vascular permeability and constriction of smooth muscle in the gut and bronchi. Prostaglandins may have other slower effects, such as inhibiting T_H1 cells.

- The lipo-oxygenase pathway produces **leukotrienes**. These have rather slower effects than prostaglandins but contribute to bronchial and gut smooth muscle contraction. In addition, leukotrienes act as chemotactic stimuli for neutrophils and eosinophils and thus contribute to increasing the cellularity of the immediate reaction and converting it to a delayed or chronic reaction.

Mast cells reside in a number of tissues that are at the front line for parasitic infection. The secretory activities of mast cells depend on their site; mucosal mast cells secrete mainly leukotrienes, while those in connective tissue secrete mainly histamine. Although activation of mast cells is dependent on preformed IgE antibodies, they respond very rapidly to antigen stimulation. The immediate response is caused by histamine, proteolytic enzymes and prostaglandins and consists of smooth muscle contraction, increased

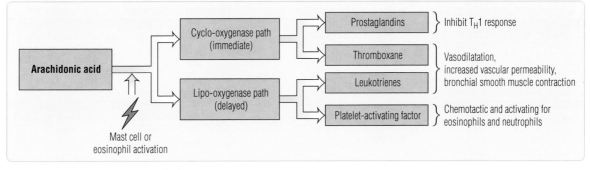

Fig. 21.5 Arachidonic acid metabolism.

vascular permeability and mucus secretion. The cytokines and leukotrienes promote a late-phase response to antigen. This is characterized by an influx of eosinophils and T_H2 cells. This late-phase inflammation may become chronic but is distinct from the granulomata, which are characterized by the presence of macrophages and T_H1 cells.

Eosinophils

Eosinophils are broadly similar to mast cells; however two factors make them unique: they are specifically recruited to tissues during some types of inflammation and their granules contain particularly toxic substances.

Eosinophils are derived from precursors similar to neutrophils and their production is stimulated by IL-3 and IL-5. Eosinophils are normally present in blood in small numbers, but their numbers increase dramatically in response to IL-3 and IL-5 secreted by T_H2 cells and mast cells (Box 21.1). Eosinophils are recruited to parasite-infested sites by the chemokine **eotaxin** produced by epithelium and leukotrienes produced by mast cells. The causes of eosinophilia are discussed in Box 21.1.

BOX 21.1
Eosinophilia

A 43-year-old man has returned from working as an overseas aid worker in South East Asia, where he has been involved in developing sewerage schemes (Fig. 21.6). On his return home he is required to undergo a medical examination during which he is found to have a raised eosinophil count of $2.5 \times 10^3/\mu l$ (the eosinophil count is normally below $0.35 \times 10^3/\mu l$) (Fig. 21.7) and to have abnormal liver function tests.

Although allergy is the commonest cause of eosinophilia in the developed world, this patient has no signs or symptoms of allergies such as asthma, rhinitis or eczema. Neither does he have any features of the cancers, for example lymphoma, sometimes associated with eosinophilia. A liver biopsy is performed and this shows parasite eggs surrounded by granulomata. A diagnosis of the parasitic worm infection, **schistosomiasis,** is made and the patient responds well to treatment.

Schistosoma mansoni is a common parasite in some parts of the world. Humans are infected when larvae penetrate the skin from contaminated water supplies. Adult worms live in the portal veins and discharge eggs, which may lodge in the liver. Mast cells and eosinophils are able to kill schistosomiasis worms and their eggs, using the mechanisms described above. The marked eosinophilia is a reflection of the activation of these cells. As the eggs disintegrate they release peptides that are processed and recognized as conventional antigens by T_H1 cells. Untreated schistosomiasis leads to chronic inflammation in the liver and is one cause of liver cirrhosis. It is not yet clear if this damage is caused by the eosinophil response to adult worms, the T_H1 cell response to worm eggs, or a combination of both.

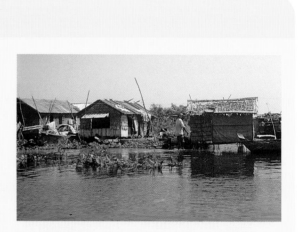

Fig. 21.6 In this village in Cambodia, human feces is dropped straight into the water supply. The plant growing in the lake is water hyacinth, which provides the home for the snail that is the host to schistosomes. In this kind of environment, mast cells and eosinophils provide important defenses for the human population.

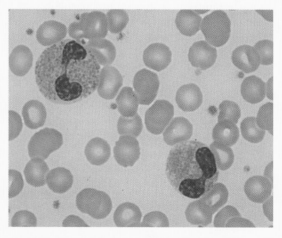

Fig. 21.7 Eosinophils. The multilobed nuclei of these cells indicate how closely related they are to neutrophils.

Eosinophils are activated by cytokines, chemokines and perhaps crosslinked IgE on FcεRI. Activated eosinophils release the same mediators as mast cells (except histamine) and, in addition, three special mediators:

- a peroxidase that is released onto the surface of parasites and then generates hypochlorous acid
- major basic protein which damages the outer surface of parasites (and host tissues!)
- cationic protein which damages the parasite's outer surface and acts as a neurotoxin, damaging the simple nervous system of the parasite.

Immediate (type I) hypersensitivity

Because the effects of eosinophil or mast cell degranulation are so rapid, this type of response is sometimes referred to as immediate (type I) hypersensitivity, although the cytokines and other mediators released can also set up delayed and chronic inflammatory responses.

People living in the developed world are no longer challenged by worms. In these populations, mast cells and eosinophils cause immediate hypersensitivity in response to innocuous antigens such as pollens—the hallmarks of allergy (Ch. 25). Eosinophils and mast cells secrete a wide range of mediators, many of which are targets in the treatment of allergy; these are discussed in Box 21.2.

Natural killer cells

NK cells have two important roles. As their name suggests, they are excellent killers of cells infected by some viruses, but, like macrophages, they have an additional role of stimulating the adaptive immune response. NK cells are part of the innate immune system and fill a potential gap in the specific immune response. Some infectious agents, notably members of the herpesvirus family, downregulate MHC expression on infected cells to evade detection by T cells (Box 21.3). Similarly, some tumor cells have acquired mutations that result in decreased MHC expression and are able to evade tumor-specific T cells. NK cells appear to have evolved to recognize and kill cells with low MHC expression.

NK cells develop and acquire their receptors in the bone marrow. Although they are not generated in the thymus they share some characteristics with T cells. For example they share some T cell surface molecules (such as CD2) and have a similar appearance to lymphocytes (an alternative name for NK cells is large granular lymphocyte; Fig. 21.10). NK cells also use the same generic killing mechanisms as cytotoxic T cells. However, NK cells do not have rearranged T cell receptor molecules and are thus classified as belonging to the innate immune system. NK cells also share some characteristics of macrophages; they are capable of recognizing antibody coated target cells, but they do not kill these by phagocytosis.

NK cells arise from the same lymphoid progenitor cells as T and B cells, although it is not clear how their production is regulated. NK cells constitute about 5–15% of lymphocytes in peripheral blood. They are activated by cytokines (Fig. 21.11), but killing itself is regulated by signaling through special receptors.

BOX 21.2
Drug treatment of allergy

Allergy is discussed in detail in Chapter 25, but it is useful now to discuss possible treatments. General measures in the treatment of allergy include identifying and avoiding possible antigens (known as **allergens**). Figure 21.8 illustrates some of the drugs aimed at inhibiting the synthesis of the immunological mediators or blocking their receptors. Corticosteroids are widely used and can prevent the immediate hypersensitivity reaction in allergy and the chronic inflammation that occurs as a delayed response. See Chapter 25 for a fuller discussion of their effects.

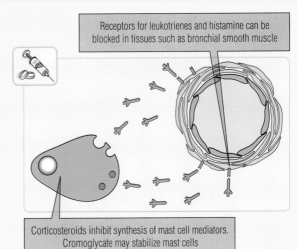

Receptors for leukotrienes and histamine can be blocked in tissues such as bronchial smooth muscle

Corticosteroids inhibit synthesis of mast cell mediators. Cromoglycate may stabilize mast cells

Fig. 21.8 Drug treatment of allergy.

**BOX 21.3
Herpes viruses**

Most cells infected with viruses, for example influenza, are killed when cytotoxic T lymphocytes recognize viral peptides bound to MHC. Herpes viruses, in contrast, inhibit MHC expression. This evasion mechanism prevents cytotoxic T cell recognition but NK cells are still able to recognize and kill cells infected with herpes simplex, for example (Fig. 21.9). Other herpes viruses have more tricks up their sleeve. Cytomegalovirus produces a viral protein that mimics MHC class I and stimulates expression of HLA-E (which is unable to present antigenic peptides), effectively inhibiting NK cells. Epstein–Barr virus secretes a protein homologous to the Bcl-2 molecule, which does not block NK activity but can prevent the infected cell from undergoing apoptosis.

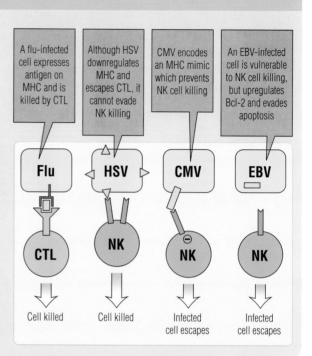

Fig. 21.9 Methods used by herpes viruses to avoid killing. Flu, influenza, HSV, herpes simplex virus; CMV, cytomegalovirus; EBV, Epstein–Barr virus; CTL, cytotoxic T cells; NK, natural killer.

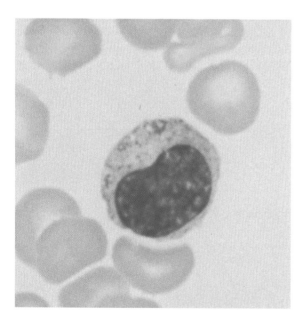

Fig. 21.10 The granules in natural killer cells contain perforin and granzyme.

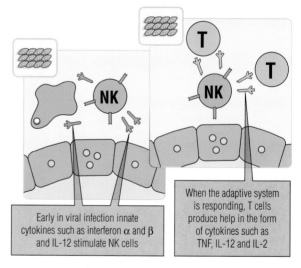

Fig. 21.11 Cytokine regulation of natural killer (NK) cells. Like T cells, NK cells proliferate in response to interleukin (IL) 2; this is exploited in the generation of lymphokine activated killer cells (Box 21.4). TNF, tumor necrosis factor.

Antibody-dependent cellular cytotoxicity

In NK cells, a special Fc receptor, FcγRIII, recognizes IgG-bound viral antigen on the surface of infected cells and triggers killing. IgG-mediated NK killing is referred to as antibody-dependent cellular cytotoxicity and is illustrated in Figure 21.12. FcγRIII is also expressed by

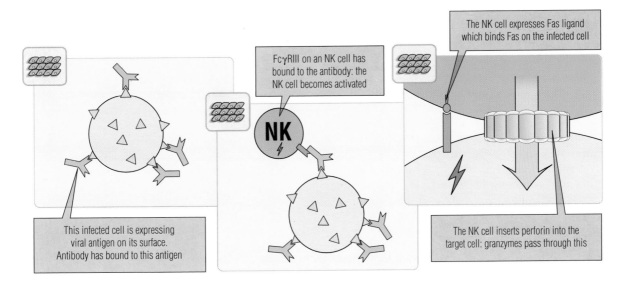

Fig. 21.12 Antibody-dependent cellular cytotoxicity. Binding of antibody to FcγRIII stimulates the natural killer (NK) cell. This process is similar to opsonization by IgG (Fig. 20.8).

some macrophages, in which case IgG acts as an opsonin and triggers phagocytosis.

Natural killer receptors

NK cells are able to recognize and kill cells that express lower than normal levels of MHC. To do this, NK cells have two types of specialized receptor for MHC. **Killer inhibitory receptors** (KIRs) recognize specific MHC α-chains. **NKG2/CD94** recognizes the non-classical HLA-E molecule. Both types of receptor are special because they can inhibit killing. When an NK cell encounters a virally infected cell, two outcomes are possible (Fig. 21.13).

- The NK cell recognizes that the cell is infected, using an innate immune system pattern-recognition molecule. The NK cell uses its receptors to check that MHC is present on the surface of the cell. If MHC is present at an adequate level, the receptor delivers a negative signal, which prevents the NK killing. Because the virally infected cell expresses MHC, it will in any case be killed by a CTL.
- If the NK recognizes that a cell is infected by a virus and confirms that levels of MHC are reduced, it will go ahead and kill the target cell.

The balance between the stimulatory and inhibitory signals determines the outcomes of NK cell activation; NK preferentially kill cells with absent MHC expression.

Cells may have absent MHC expression because of viral infection or because of mutation in cancer cells (Box 21.4). The absence of MHC expression may allow

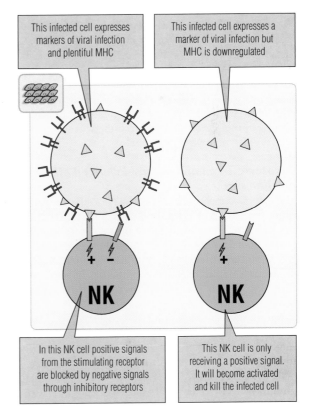

Fig. 21.13 Natural killer (NK) receptors that inhibit killing may have a role in the treatment of a variety of diseases in the near future.

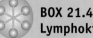

BOX 21.4
Lymphokine activated killers

NK cells are known to play a role in defenses against tumors, particularly when tumor cells have downregulated MHC expression. Because NK cells proliferate in response to IL-2, attempts have been made to generate large numbers of NK cells ex vivo by stimulating fresh NK cells with recombinant IL-2. This technique is successful in so far as large numbers of cells can be generated in this way. The cells produced are called LAK cells (lymphokine activated killers; lymphokine is an old name for cytokine). When re-infused back into cancer patients there are two major problems:

- there are considerable side-effects, most notably because of the large amounts of cytokines produced by the LAK cells, which can cause severe hypotension
- the LAK cells were only effective in a minority of tumors, probably because tumors mutate to develop several ways of evading the immune response.

LAK cells are therefore not an attractive type of cancer immunotherapy; some other approaches are discussed in Chapter 34.

---

such cells to escape killing by cytotoxic T cells, which recognize MHC class I. NK cells overcome this potential flaw in the immune response by killing cells with absent MHC expression. This type of killing is especially important when interferon γ is present; this cytokine maximizes MHC expression by normal cells and at the same time increases NK cell activity.

NK cells have one more important role. They are the major cell of the immune system in the pregnant uterus. Uterine NK cells clearly have a role in preventing viral infection of the uterus and fetus during pregnancy. They have the added advantage of not attacking fetal tissue even though it expresses foreign (paternal) HLA molecules. NK cells are inhibited by cells which express normal levels of MHC regardless of whether it is host or from another individual.

Cytotoxic T cell and natural killer cell effector mechanisms

The cytotoxic mechanisms used by NK cells are identical to those used by cytotoxic T cells. Both populations use perforin, granzyme and Fas ligand expression and secretion of TNF, all of which can induce programmed cell death: **apoptosis**. NK cells and cytotoxic T cells also secrete immunoregulatory cytokines, such as interferon γ, which promote the T_H1 inflammatory response.

Apoptosis is an important event, triggered by a range of stimuli and has significance not just in clearing infected or tumorous cells, but in the shaping of the immune response. This is discussed in Box 21.5.

Perforin. Perforin is contained within the cytotoxic granules of NK cells and cytotoxic T cells. Perforin polymers form a pore that is inserted into the target cell membrane, rather like the complement membrane attack complex (Fig. 19.9). These pores allow salts and water to flow into the target cell and, more impor-

tantly, give granzyme access to the cytoplasm.

Granzyme. Granzyme is three separate proteolytic enzymes that enter the target cell. As well as degrading host cell proteins, they specifically activate the **caspase** enzyme system (see below) which results in apoptosis.

Fas ligand. Fas ligand is a potent inducer of apoptosis and is used by NK cells and cytotoxic T cells to kill infected or tumor cells. Fas is a member of the same family of receptors as the TNF receptor (Fig. 21.15). Fas and Fas ligand are expressed on cells of the immune system during activation. Fas ligand expression is increased on cytotoxic T cells and NK cells when they become activated. Fas ligand binds Fas on a target cell, which then undergoes apoptosis through the mechanisms described in Box 21.6. T cells may also express Fas and become targets of Fas-mediated killing. For example, cells in immunoprivileged sites, such as the testis, express Fas ligand. Any T cell that accidentally ends up in the testis will be exposed to Fas and will undergo apoptosis. T cells sometimes use Fas/Fas ligand during complex interactions that result in them killing one another—so-called fratricide. This kind of mechanism may seem obscure but is used to destroy autoreactive T cells.

Fas ligand appears to be mainly involved in killing. It does not have the other more general effects of TNF receptor, for example, promoting inflammation or causing weight loss.

NK cells secret cytokines that stimulate T_H1 responses. Although NK cells are very effective at killing in their own right, they also activate the adaptive immune response. Macrophages behave in a similar way and this is exactly what we expect from cells of the innate immune system. Both types of cell recognize families of pathogens rather than specific antigens. They attempt to eradicate the pathogen but also activate the adaptive immune system.

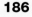 Bone marrow   Thymus   Lymph node

BOX 21.5
Apoptosis in the immune system

Apoptosis is the process of programmed cell death, where cells are deliberately killed as a part of physiological processes. The end result of apoptosis is that the cell's DNA is broken down to 200 base pair fragments. Apoptotic cells are recognized by phagocytes, which usually clear the cell remains without stimulating inflammation. By comparison, **necrosis** is the inadvertent death of cells, usually caused by exposure to metabolic insults such as hypoxia or toxins. Necrosis does not result in DNA fragmentation and often results in an inflammatory response.

Apoptosis is an important physiological process affecting many body systems. During embryonic life, for example, apoptosis is involved in remodeling tissues, such as the developing vascular system. In this way, apoptosis determines the shape of the developing fetus.

Apoptosis has a number of very important roles in shaping the adaptive immune repertoire. Autoreactive T and B cells undergo apoptosis very soon after they are generated in the thymus and bone marrow. Autoreactive lymphocytes that escape these central processes are forced to undergo apoptosis in the periphery. Finally, after an immune response to a pathogen, redundant lymphocytes are also cleared by apoptosis. Each of these uses different mechanisms (Fig. 21.14), but the result is that the specificities of the immune response are shaped by apoptosis.

Apoptosis is also involved in some pathological processes; for example, there is evidence that one of the ways CD4+ T cells are destroyed by HIV infection is through induction of apoptosis. When apoptotic debris is not cleared adequately by phagocytes, it can become immunogenic. This can lead to the production of autoantibodies, for example against DNA, and this may generate autoimmune disease, for example systemic lupus erythematosus. On the other hand, clones of B cells that have increased levels of Bcl-2 through mutations or chromosome translocations may be protected from apoptosis and can develop into a B cell malignancy (Ch. 34).

Fig. 21.14
Apoptosis in the immune system

Area involving apoptosis	Target	Mechanism
Negative selection in the thymus	T cells	
Peripheral T cell tolerance	Autoreactive T cells	Lack of co-stimulation?
At the end of an immune response when only a few cells are required to maintain memory	Responding T cells	Cytokine starvation leading to reductions in Bcl-2
Negative selection of B cells in bone marrow	B cells	
Low-affinity antibody production	B cells	Changes in Bcl-2
Peripheral B cell tolerance	Autoreactive T cells	Fas
Blocking T$_H$2 responses	B cells	FasL expressed on T$_H$1 cells
Protection of immune privileged sites	T cells	Cells (e.g., testicular cells) express FasL, which kills incoming T cells
Intracellular infection	Any cell	Fas, tumor necrosis factor, granzyme
Malignancy	Malignant cell	Fas, tumor necrosis factor, granzyme

NK cells secrete interferon γ when they encounter target cells. This cytokine stimulates T$_H$1 cells and inhibits T$_H$2 cells. A T$_H$1 response is especially effective at dealing with intracellular infection and can provide immunological memory to guarantee a strong response should the host be exposed to the same pathogen again.

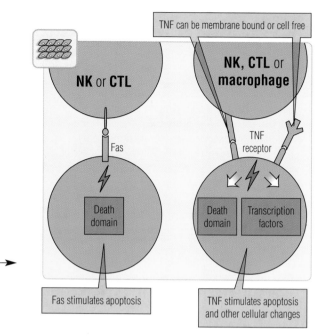

Fig. 21.15 Fas and tumor necrosis factor (TNF) receptor can both induce cell death.

BOX 21.6

BOX 21.6
Intracellular mechanisms of apoptosis

Apoptosis can occur as a result of a wide range of stimuli. For example, radiation and high-dose corticosteroids can induce apoptosis of T cells without involving any specific surface receptors. Another way T and B cells can undergo apoptosis is when the T or B cell receptor is bound during cell maturation, in either the thymus or bone marrow. Receptor ligation then activates enzymes that cause the cell to undergo apoptosis. This is how negative selection is carried out, removing autoreactive T and B cells.

In this chapter, we are most interested in apoptosis that has been induced through the ligation of receptors such as Fas or the TNF receptor (Fig. 21.16). Fas and TNF receptor both have cytoplasmic tails (called death domains) which can activate the series of caspase enzymes. Caspases are proteolytic enzymes which cleave proteins after aspartic acid residues. The final result of activation of the caspase is activation of a specific DNAase, which cleaves the target cell's DNA into 200 base pair fragments. Caspases are also activated when NK or cytotoxic T cells inject granzyme into the cell.

Another early effect of apoptosis is the disruption of mitochondria. Mitochondria become leaky and the release of mitochondrial products further activates caspases. Bcl-2 binds to and stabilizes mitochondria and prevents up-regulation of apoptosis. Falling IL-2

levels reduce the intracellular concentration of Bcl-2 and can make apoptosis more likely to occur. This happens at the end of a successful immune response when antigen levels are falling and IL-2 secretion is diminished.

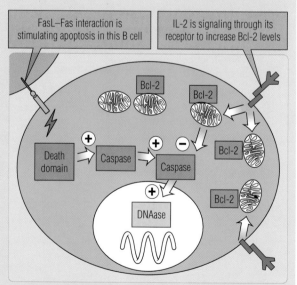

Fig. 21.16 Whether or not this B cell undergoes apoptosis is determined by the balance of signals through Fas, caspases, interleukin 2 (IL-2) and Bcl-2.

Bone marrow   Thymus   Lymph node

LEARNING POINTS

Can you now:

- Identify the type of infection that mast cells and eosinophils respond to?
- List the contents of mast cell and eosinophil granules?
- Describe the consequences of arachidonic acid metabolism?
- Identify the specific infectious problems that natural killer cells respond to?
- Describe natural killer cell receptors?
- List NK cell killing mechanisms?
- Draw the mechanism of apoptosis?

Blood vessel   Gut   Peripheral tissue

Inflammation

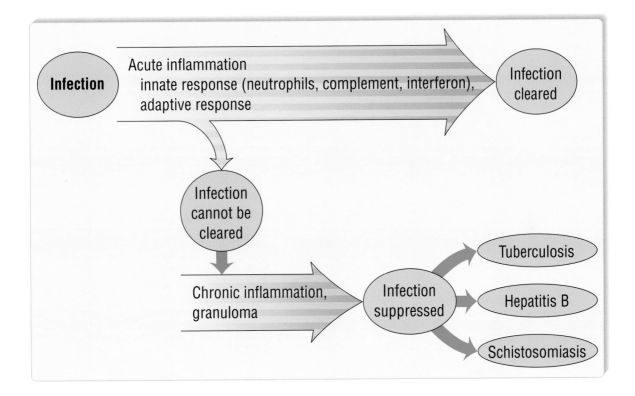

Types of inflammation

Inflammation is clinically defined as the presence of redness, swelling and pain. Histologically it is defined as the presence of edema fluid and the infiltration of tissues by white cells. There are many causes of inflammation; for example, a burn will cause an acute inflammatory response and although this is triggered by a physical stimulus, it is at least partially mediated by immunological mechanisms such as the release of tumor necrosis factor (TNF) from damaged tissues (Box 22.1).

If the offending stimulus cannot be rapidly removed, the inflammation tends to become chronic. Figure 22.1 shows some infections that result in either chronic or acute inflammation.

Acute reactions to bacteria result in pus formation; they are **pyogenic**. Chronic bacterial infections may lead to the formation of **granuloma**; collections of specialized macrophages surrounded by T cells. This occurs in tuberculosis (Box 22.2). Chronic viral infection leads to more diffuse inflammation, although macrophages and T cells are still present. This typically occurs in infections with hepatitis B virus, where acute inflammation occurs initially as a result of antiviral activity and chronic inflammation can follow as the inflammatory response continues in a failed attempt to eliminate the pathogen. This chronic stage results in damage to the host organs (Box 22.3). Acute inflammation mediated by mast cells is characterized by edema; when it becomes more long lasting, eosinophils enter the inflamed tissue. There is considerable overlap between the different types of inflammation as shown in Figure 22.7. A good example of overlapping chronic inflammation is schistosomiasis, discussed in Chapter 21. Inflammation mediated by mast cells and eosinophils is discussed in Chapter 21.

Pus formation can develop over a few hours. Granulomata take 2 to 3 days to develop because of the time it takes for the T cell response to evolve. Granulomatous reactions are sometimes referred to as **delayed hypersensitivity**. Tuberculosis elicits a typical delayed hypersensitivity reaction (Box 22.2). Granuloma development requires T cell involvement and, therefore, has characteristics of adaptive immunity,

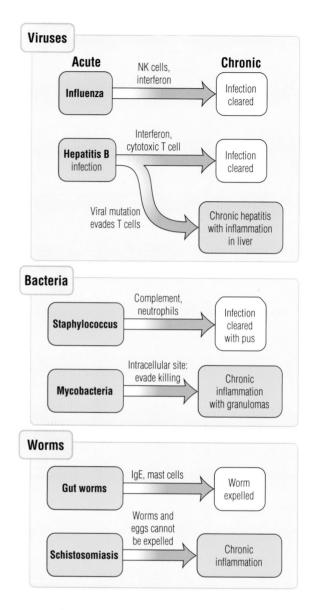

Fig. 22.1 Acute or chronic inflammation depends on pathogen and host factors. In hepatitis B virus infection, both viral mutations and host HLA type may determine whether chronic inflammation occurs. NK, natural killer.

such as antigen specificity and recall responsiveness. For example, delayed hypersensitivity can be used to test immunological memory and skin testing using tuberculin as an antigen is frequently used to check for recall immunity against *M. tuberculosis* (Box 22.4). Similar skin tests exist for other infections, for example leprosy and leishmaniasis. These skin tests should be distinguished from skin prick testing, used to diagnose immediate hypersensitivity in allergy.

Cytokine network in inflammation

Cytokines are required to initiate acute inflammation and maintain chronic inflammatory responses. These responses require help from CD4+ T cells and the interaction between these and either macrophages or eosinophils is sometimes referred to as the **cytokine network**.

Chapter 20 described how macrophage cytokines and mediators initiate immune responses that eventually lead to granuloma formation. Macrophages secrete interleukin (IL) 1, TNF and granulocyte–macrophage colony-stimulating factor (GM-CSF) which activate the acute phase response and promote marrow production of neutrophils and monocytes. Macrophage-produced TNF and IL-1 increase adherence of leukocytes to local endothelium and these leukocytes then follow the chemotactic signal of chemokines also produced by macrophages. Macrophages also produce cytokines that act on T cells, including IL-1, IL-12 and IL-18. IL-1 is a general activator of T cells and, along with co-stimulatory molecules such as CD40, activates all classes of T

Bone marrow   Thymus   Lymph node

cell. IL-12 and IL-18 preferentially activate T_H1 and natural killer (NK) cells, respectively.

In response to these macrophage-derived cytokines, T_H1 and NK cells secrete interferon γ and more TNF. The major effects of the former are to:

- increase expression of MHC on macrophages and other local cells
- increase macrophage antigen processing through proteosomes
- induce macrophage maturation
- increase NK cell activity
- inhibit T_H2 cells
- cause mild antiviral effects (Ch. 19).

The effects of interferon γ on macrophages are to stimulate T_H1 cell activity further through antigen presentation and cytokine production. The exchange of cytokines between macrophages and T cells generates a strong positive feedback loop between these two populations and skews the immune response towards a T_H1 pattern (Fig. 22.2).

TNF, produced by macrophages and T cells, has a number of important roles in the developing inflammatory response. However, high local levels of TNF can cause tissue destruction and TNF has potent systemic effects, for example weight loss. The TNF genes are polymorphic (Ch. 8) and these polymorphisms have been investigated as the basis for person-to-person variations in the immune response (Box 22.1).

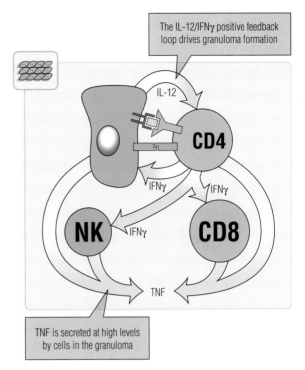

Fig. 22.2 The cytokines interleukin 12 (IL-12), interferon γ (INFγ) and tumor necrosis factor (TNF) drive granuloma formation. Mutation or polymorphisms in the genes for these cytokines or their receptors affect how chronic inflammation develops.

BOX 22.1
Polymorphisms in the gene for tumor necrosis factor

Many human genes are polymorphic, in other words their sequences differ from one person to another. Polmorphisms affect more than 1% of a population, while mutations are much rarer. Many polymorphisms do not affect function, for example eye color does not affect vision.

TNF has a special role in the response to infections and is also implicated in some autoimmune diseases. The TNF gene contains polymorphisms in both structural and regulatory sequences, which affect the level at which TNF is secreted. Considerable research has been done on how TNF polymorphisms affect the risks of specific diseases.

Septic shock is caused, at least in part, by macrophage secretion of TNF in response to bacterial endotoxin (Box 20.6). Septic shock is likely to occur in severely injured patients, in whom Gram-negative septicemia may develop. The presence of different TNF polymorphisms does not affect the risk of severely injured patients developing septicemia;

however, once septicemia has developed, they do affect the risk of developing septic shock.

In patients living in malarious areas, the presence of different TNF polymorphisms does not affect the risk of developing malaria, but they may affect the risk of life-threatening complications of malaria.

TNF polymorphisms do not affect the risk of developing infection but may modify the complications of established infection: they modify the type of inflammation that occurs when infection is taking place. It is hoped that these genetic data will be useful in predicting when drugs that block the effects of TNF may be beneficial. But, as we have explained in Chapter 20, TNF-blocking agents do not improve outcomes in septic shock, perhaps because they have been given too late. TNF polymorphisms have also been linked to autoimmune diseases such as rheumatoid arthritis (Ch. 30). This research led the way to the important discovery that blocking TNF in rheumatoid arthritis can improve symptoms dramatically.

BOX 22.2
Tuberculosis

In the late twentieth century, tuberculosis (TB) was thought to be under control. However, it has re-emerged as a major threat to global health, partly because of its link with HIV infection and partly because of the development of drug-resistant strains.

Mycobacterium tuberculosis stimulates macrophages by binding a specific Toll-like receptor that recognizes mycobacterial lipoproteins. This stimulates phagocytosis and secretion of inflammatory mediators such as interleukin 12 and nitric oxide. Mycobacterial peptides presented by macrophages elicit strong T_H1-type responses. The most important of these are secretion of TNF and interferon γ, which stimulate the formation of granuloma during primary infection.

Mycobacteria have a range of mechanisms for evading killing (Ch. 21). Because it is hard to kill them, macrophages seal off mycobacteria inside phagosomes. This sealing off process requires help from T cells, in the form of T_H1 cytokines such as interferon γ. Figure 22.3 shows the difference between healthy and impaired responses to mycobacteria.

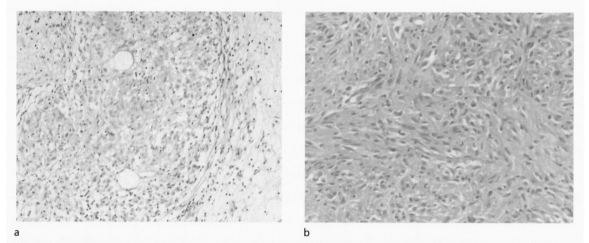

a   b

Fig. 22.3 Healthy and impaired responses to mycobacteria. (a) In a patient with tuberculosis and a normal immune response, there are very few mycobacteria and plentiful macrophages, giant cells and T cells; this is a granuloma (see also Fig. 20.12). (b) In a mycobacterial infection in a patient with AIDS, there are many more mycobacteria and few T cells and macrophages. (Courtesy of Dr Lucy Harbin, St Mary's Hospital, London.)

Initial exposure to TB results in primary infection. In most patients with primary TB, mycobacterial growth is contained within the granuloma. Here macrophages mature under the influence of interferon γ into giant cells and epitheloid cells. Granulomata seal off infected macrophages so well, that occasionally the center of a granuloma becomes hypoxic and the cells may become necrotic. The necrotic area resembles cheese and this caseous necrosis is a hallmark of TB infection.

Less than 10% patients with primary TB have any symptoms and even fewer develop widespread infection. In very young or immunodeficient patients, primary TB is not contained within the granuloma. In these patients there may be widespread infection (miliary TB) or spread to the meninges (Fig. 22.4). Even when infection is contained and controlled in the lungs, many mycobacteria may survive inside macrophages or other cells for several years.

Post-primary (re-activation) TB occurs in about 10% of patients, especially if macrophage function is moderately impaired. This commonly happens when patients are treated with high doses of corticosteroids or if there is malnutrition (for example in alcoholics). Reactivation of TB is also a common problem in HIV infection, when there is damage both to macrophages and to the T_H1 cells which secrete interferon γ.

Bone marrow   Thymus   Lymph node

BOX 22.2
Tuberculosis (*contd.*)

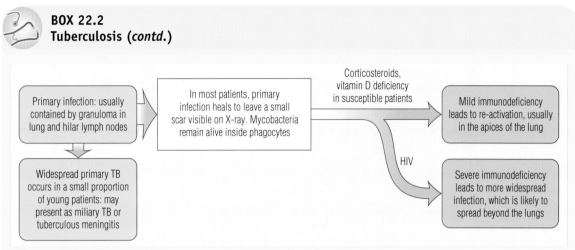

Fig. 22.4 Infection with *Mycobacterium tuberculosis* can have a number of short- and long-term outcomes.

The feedback loop ultimately comes to a halt when phagocytes have cleared all residual antigen. Thus stimulation of T cells ceases and the level of interferon γ falls. Co-stimulation by macrophages is reduced; the result is that T cells will die through apoptosis.

"Overzealous" inflammation

During inflammation, granuloma formation and cytokines may have negative effects. The negative effects of TNF have already been mentioned. An example of an overzealous response is excessive granuloma formation in the lung in response to *M. tuberculosis*, which may produce necrotic lesions that subsequently cavitate. These cavities are produced when necrotic material is coughed up, which allows the mycobacteria contained to be spread from person to person. These infectious patients are described as having "open TB".

Another mycobacterium, *M. leprae*, can also stimulate the granulomatous reaction that controls the mycobacterial infection; hypersensitivity to *M. leprae* is discussed in Chapter 25. This form of leprosy is known as tuberculoid leprosy (Ch. 25).

BOX 22.3
Hepatitis B and chronic hepatitis

Hepatitis B infection is a major global infection; there are perhaps 350 million infected individuals across the world. The virus causes hepatitis, often leading to cirrhosis and liver cancer. Hepatitis B virus only replicates in hepatocytes but does not damage these cells directly; the virus is not cytopathic.

The immune response to hepatitis B virus is important at two different stages. Antibodies to the hepatitis B virus surface protein (HBsAg) can protect from infection; these antibodies are often the result of vaccination and this is discussed in Chapter 24. Cellular immunity is important in people who do not have protective antibodies and in whom virus is already replicating in hepatocytes. Hepatitis B virus is susceptible to the antiviral effects of interferons (recombinant interferons are described in Box 19.2). During hepatitis B infection, the specific immune system responds to infection with a T_H1-type response (as you would expect for a viral infection) and hepatitis B specific CD4+ and CD8+ T cells migrate to the liver. These cells secrete interferon γ and there is evidence that the antiviral effects of this cytokine inhibit viral replication. Although nearly all infected patients develop transient hepatitis, which is life threatening in less than 1%, the majority of infected patients (80–90%) manage to suppress viral replication through the antiviral effects of interferon γ. Unlike the type I interferons, interferon γ has potent stimulating effects on inflammation and an

continued

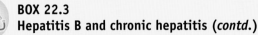

BOX 22.3
Hepatitis B and chronic hepatitis (*contd.*)

inflammatory response develops, during which hepatocytes are damaged by the immune response, rather than by the virus itself. The result is acute hepatitis. In the majority of patients, viral replication is controlled. Although virus is not eradicated, ongoing T cell responses are enough to minimize virus replication so that, for example, the patient stops being infectious to other individuals (Fig. 22.5).

In about 10–20% of infected people, the virus is not cleared through these means. This can happen when, for example, the initial innoculum of virus was particularly large. Alternatively, the virus may mutate so that antigenic epitopes change and the virus evades the immune response. Host factors, for example the HLA type, may affect the risk of not

clearing virus. In these individuals, the inflammatory response persists, although it is unable to inhibit viral replication completely. Unlike TB, chronic hepatitis B infection does not produce granulomata. In these patients, production of interferon γ is a double-edged sword; it is the best hope of inhibiting viral replication but will promote a chronic inflammatory response. This results in chronic active hepatitis. The recruitment of natural killer cells, macrophages and T cells that are not even specific for hepatitis B virus eventually leads to chronic inflammation inside the portal areas. The resulting tissue destruction causes scarrings that can lead to liver cirrhosis and, through unknown mechanisms, can set the scene for liver cancer.

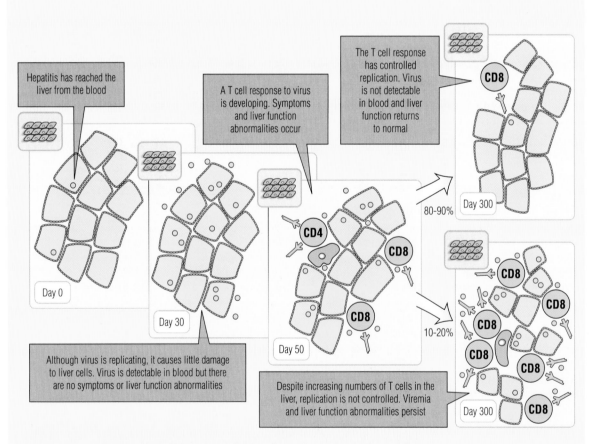

Fig. 22.5 The outcome of hepatitis B virus infection depends on immunological factors.

Bone marrow   Thymus   Lymph node

BOX 22.3
Hepatitis B and chronic hepatitis (*contd.*)

An understanding of hepatitis B infection has helped to develop strategies for preventing and treating this serious infection (Fig. 22.6).

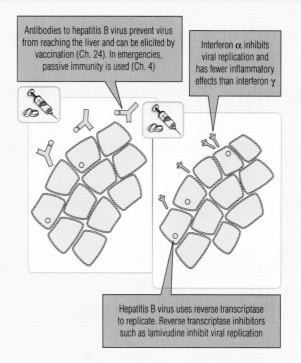

Antibodies to hepatitis B virus prevent virus from reaching the liver and can be elicited by vaccination (Ch. 24). In emergencies, passive immunity is used (Ch. 4)

Interferon α inhibits viral replication and has fewer inflammatory effects than interferon γ

Hepatitis B virus uses reverse transcriptase to replicate. Reverse transcriptase inhibitors such as lamivudine inhibit viral replication

Fig. 22.6 Hepatitis B virus infection can be prevented or treated in a number of ways.

Fig. 22.7
Types of inflammation

	Acute inflammation (pyogenic)	Chronic inflammation (granulomatous)	Acute inflammation (immediate hypersensitivity)	Chronic inflammation (eosinophil mediated)
Typical triggers	Staphylococci	Mycobacterial infection, hepatitis B	Worms	Worms
Initiating cell	Macrophage	Macrophage	?	?
Effector cell in innate system	Neutrophil	Macrophage, natural killer cell	Mast cell	Mast cell, eosinophil
Effector cell in adaptive system	None involved	T$_H$1 cell	T$_H$2 cell, B cell	T$_H$2 cell, B cell
Mediators	Complement, GM-CSF, TNF, chemokines	TNF, IL-12, IL-18, interferon γ, chemokines	Histamine, mast cell granule contents	IL-3, IL-4, IL-5, leukotrienes, chemokines
Systemic effects	Acute phase response; neutrophilia	Acute phase response; chronic effects of TNF; neutrophilia may be present	May lead to anaphylaxis (Ch. 26)	Eosinophilia, raised IgE
Type of lesion	Pus formation, abscesses	Granuloma may be present	Edema, mucus, smooth muscle contraction	Diffuse inflammation in mucosa or skin

GM-CSF, granulocyte–macrophage colony-stimulating factor, IL, interleukin; TNF, tumor necrosis factor.

Blood vessel   Gut   Peripheral tissue

BOX 22.4
Delayed hypersensitivity skin testing

Delayed hypersensitivity skin testing is most frequently carried out with intradermal injection of tuberculin: a sterile mixture of proteins and lipoproteins derived from *Mycobacterium tuberculosis*. This type of skin test is also known as the **Mantoux** or **Heaf test,** depending on the type of injection technique used. The reaction starts when specific Toll-like receptors on dermal macrophages recognize the mycobacterial lipoproteins and in response secrete TNF and chemokines, which increase the expression of local endothelial adhesion molecules (Fig. 22.8). At the same time local dendritic cells leave the site of injection and migrate to draining lymph nodes.

The migrating dendritic cells are loaded with mycobacterial antigens. This antigen can be presented to T cells in the draining lymph node, but only if adequate numbers exist from a primary response. Remember that the number of T cells for a

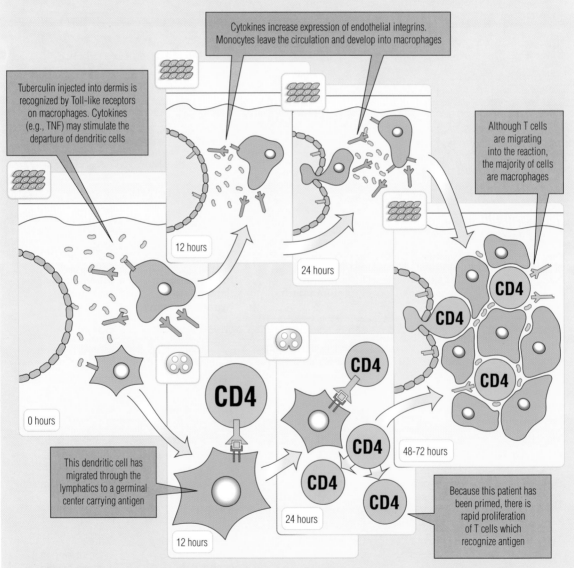

Cytokines increase expression of endothelial integrins. Monocytes leave the circulation and develop into macrophages

Tuberculin injected into dermis is recognized by Toll-like receptors on macrophages. Cytokines (e.g., TNF) may stimulate the departure of dendritic cells

Although T cells are migrating into the reaction, the majority of cells are macrophages

12 hours

24 hours

CD4

CD4

0 hours

CD4

CD4

CD4

48-72 hours

CD4

CD4

This dendritic cell has migrated through the lymphatics to a germinal center carrying antigen

Because this patient has been primed, there is rapid proliferation of T cells which recognize antigen

24 hours

12 hours

Fig. 22.8 Reactions occurring after an injection of tuberculin. After 48 hours, macrophages and T cells are accumulating in the dermis.

Bone marrow   Thymus   Lymph node

BOX 22.4
Delayed hypersensitivity skin testing (*contd.*)

specific antigen increases during the acquisition of immunological memory. The activated T cells will subsequently migrate to the site of injection and interact with local activated macrophages. Macrophages will also accumulate and mature as a result of cytokines secreted by the T cells. When a strong response (Fig. 22.9) is produced at 48 hours, over 80% of the cells present are activated macrophages.

Delayed hypersensitivity tests assess immunological memory for specific antigens; the intensity of the response depends on the extent of T cell priming and the ability to make a T cell recall response. T cell priming is bought about by primary TB infection or TB vaccine. TB vaccine is a live attenuated mycobacterium, BCG, and is used routinely in many parts of the world, but not in the USA because of concerns about its efficacy.

Interpretation of the skin test depends on whether the individual has been primed. Healthy individuals who have been vaccinated with BCG produce a moderate response to tuberculin testing at 48 hours. A response in an unvaccinated

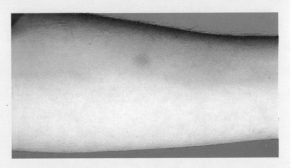

Fig. 22.9 This is a positive tuberculin skin test, 48 hours after injection, showing delayed hypersensitivity. The individual had a TB vaccine 20 years earlier and this reaction confirms sustained immunity.

individual may suggest recent exposure to TB. For this reason, tuberculin skin testing is sometimes used in screening for infection in persons exposed to patients with TB. Finally, absence of a response in a patient who is known to have had BCG vaccine may suggest immunodeficiency, for example secondary to HIV infection.

LEARNING POINTS

Can you now:

- Define inflammation?
- Describe the outcomes of tuberculosis infection?
- Describe the consequences of hepatitis B infection and how these are affected by the immune response?
- Draw the cytokine network?
- Write the sequence of cellular events in delayed hypersensitivity skin testing?

Review of innate immunity

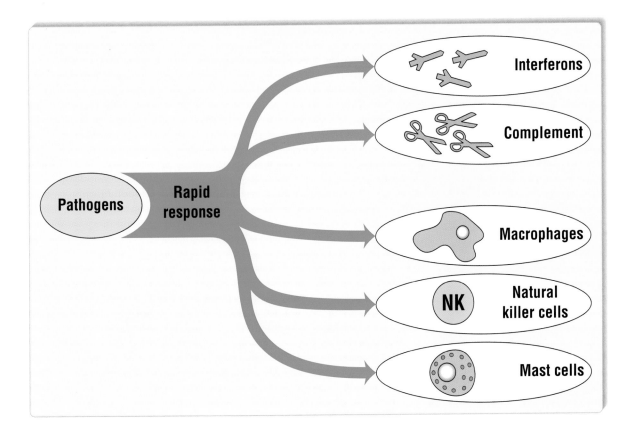

The earliest chapters of this book described the adaptive immune response before moving on to the innate immune response. In fact, in evolutionary terms, the innate system has been around a lot longer than the adaptive system. By now you will also understand that the innate system is the more rapidly responding of the two systems and is often required to activate the adaptive immune response.

In this chapter we first review how the molecular and cellular components of the innate system respond to infection together and then review how the innate and adaptive systems are integrated (Fig. 23.1).

Molecular components of the innate immune system

Interferons (IFN) α and β are secreted by a wide range of cells in response to viral infection. Cells secrete these interferons in response to double-stranded RNA, characteristic of viruses. IFN-α and IFN-β inhibit viral replication and have some weak effects activating natural killer (NK) cells.

Complement is present in the body at all times. Complement is activated independently of the adaptive immune system by molecules that recognize either sugar motifs on bacteria (ligand pathway) or pathogen surfaces that lack complement inhibitors (alternative pathway). Complement can also be activated by antibody–antigen complexes (classical pathway). Complement has several effects:

- it punches holes in bacteria: the membrane attack complex
- it releases low-molecular-weight molecules that trigger inflammation: anaphylatoxins
- it stimulates phagocytosis: opsonization
- it can activate B cells.

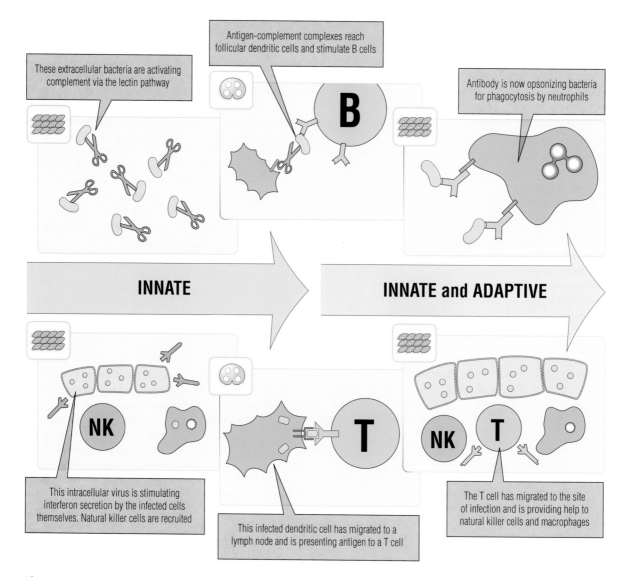

These extracellular bacteria are activating complement via the lectin pathway

Antigen-complement complexes reach follicular dendritic cells and stimulate B cells

Antibody is now opsonizing bacteria for phagocytosis by neutrophils

INNATE

INNATE and ADAPTIVE

This intracellular virus is stimulating interferon secretion by the infected cells themselves. Natural killer cells are recruited

This infected dendritic cell has migrated to a lymph node and is presenting antigen to a T cell

The T cell has migrated to the site of infection and is providing help to natural killer cells and macrophages

Fig. 23.1 The innate and adaptive immune systems interact during infections. NK, natural killer.

The production of complement and other proteins that bind bacteria, such as C reactive protein, is increased during infections. Along with fever, this reaction is part of the acute phase response.

Cells of the innate immune system

Macrophages recognize pathogens using Toll-like receptors, which bind families of pathogen-specific molecules. Macrophages also recognize pathogens that have been opsonized by complement. Once activated, macrophages phagocytose pathogens, which they then kill using the respiratory burst and proteolytic enzymes. Macrophages secrete cytokines with diverse effects, such as attraction of other white cells (notably neutrophils) to sites of infection and initiation of the acute phase response. Finally, activated macrophages are able to present digested peptides to T cells in the grooves of MHC molecules.

NK cells are especially good at recognizing pathogens that have downregulated MHC molecules which would otherwise evade killing by cytotoxic T cells. The typical target of an NK cell is a cell infected with some families of viruses. NK cells use Fas ligand, perforin and granzyme to kill target cells.

Bone marrow   Thymus   Lymph node

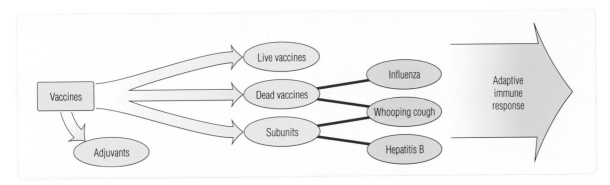

Fig. 23.2 Common features of cell recognition methods.

Interferon, complement, macrophages and NK cells have several features in common (Fig. 23.2):

- they recognize patterns on pathogens or target cells
- they respond to families of pathogens rather than specific organisms
- they act much more quickly than the adaptive immune system
- they can act independently of the adaptive immune system

- they can activate the adaptive immune system
- they can be activated by the adaptive immune system.

Mast cells differ from these systems in that they require the adaptive immune system (IgE) to respond to pathogens such as worms. Along with the related eosinophils, they release toxic compounds onto the surface of their targets. In general, their targets are parasites, which are too large to be phagocytosed.

Section Five

Immune system in health and disease

Infections and vaccines

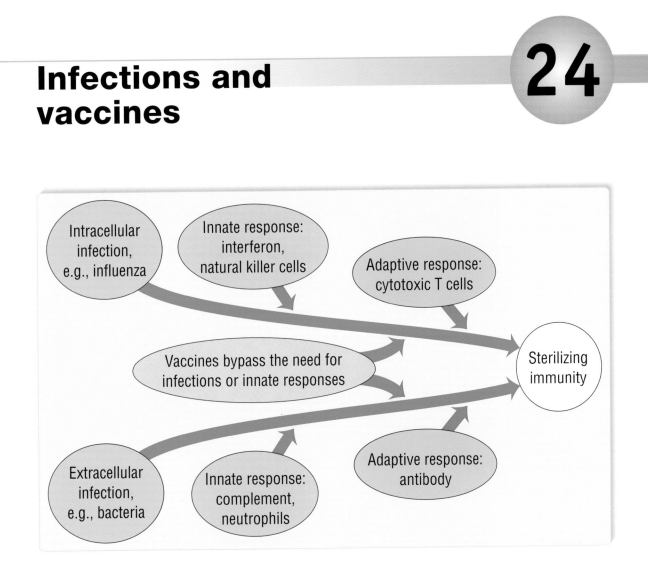

Mechanisms of immunity

The vast majority of primary infections are completely cleared by the immune system to achieve a state of sterilizing immunity. In addition, immunological memory develops: subsequent exposure to the same pathogen elicits a memory response by the adaptive immune system so that infection is prevented or symptoms reduced.

After maternal antibody has been lost, early childhood is characterized by a series of primary infections while effective immunological memory is developed. Vaccination can act as a substitute for primary infection, allowing immunological memory to develop without a symptomatic primary infection. Vaccines are a success story; smallpox is one lethal infection that has been completely eradicated by vaccination. Many other infections (polio, diphtheria and pertussis) have become relatively rare.

Before we discuss vaccines in detail, we need to mention **passive immunotherapy**. This is the transfer of adaptive immunity—usually antibodies—from one individual to another. Passive immunotherapy is often used to give protective antibodies to an individual who has been exposed to a pathogen. Examples include an individual exposed to hepatitis B (Box 4.2) or tetanus (Box 29.2). In these situations it is possible to give both passive immunotherapy (to reduce the immediate risk of infection) and the vaccine (to induce immunological memory and reduce the risk of future infection).

In this chapter, hepatitis B, influenza and whooping cough are used to illustrate how the immune system responds to infections and how vaccines can prevent infection.

Types of vaccine

Protocols currently in use involve a variety of different types of vaccine (see Fig. 24.1). The antigens in vaccines can be live organisms, dead organisms or subunits of organisms.

Fig. 24.1

Vaccine protocols. In general, live vaccines elicit the strongest responses whilst subunit vaccines have the fewest side-effects. This timetable does not include boosters, which are given from time to time

	Developing world protocol	US protocol	Non-US protocol
Infancy (first two years of life)	Diphtheria, Pertussis, Tetanus Hepatitis B (endemic areas)	Diphtheria, Pertussis, Tetanus Haemophilus Hepatitis B	Diphtheria, Pertussis, Tetanus Haemophilus Meningococcus
	Polio Tuberculosis Measles Yellow fever (endemic areas)	Polio Measles, Mumps, Rubella Varicella (chicken pox)	Polio Measles, Mumps, Rubella
Childhood and adolescence			Tuberculosis Rubella
Adulthood (selected individuals, e.g., occupational risk, overseas travel)	Hepatitis A Hepatitis B Influenza Cholera Paratyphoid	Hepatitis A Hepatitis B Influenza Cholera Paratyphoid	Hepatitis A Hepatitis B Influenza Cholera Paratyphoid
	Yellow fever	Yellow fever	Yellow fever

■ Live attenuated organisms

☐ Killed organism, toxoid and subunit vaccines

Live vaccines

Live vaccines were the first to be discovered and they are still the most effective; for example the very successful vaccines against smallpox and polio are live vaccines. Live vaccines use organisms that have been **attenuated** (i.e. weakened) so that, although they replicate in the vaccinee, they do not cause disease. Attenuation has been conventionally carried out by growing the organism in special conditions in vitro. In the future, more live vaccines are likely to be attenuated by direct manipulations of their genomes.

Live vaccines are very effective for three reasons (Fig. 24.2):

- they replicate and thus deliver sustained doses of antigen
- they replicate intracellularly so they deliver antigenic peptides to MHC class I and thus stimulate cytotoxic T cells (CTLs)
- they replicate at the anatomical site of infection, further focusing the immune response.

Attenuated live vaccines can cause serious infections in two situations. In patients with immunodeficiency they can cause infection despite attenuation. Occasionally the viruses in live vaccines may spontaneously revert to the virulent **wild-type** organism. Attenuated polio vaccine differs from the wild-type virus in only 10 base pairs. Such small differences make it easy for the virus to mutate back to the virulent form. Polio virus that has reverted from the attenuated to the virulent form has been identified in water supplies. As a result of concerns raised by this finding, the US has started to use killed polio vaccine once more.

Killed organisms

Killed organisms are generally not as effective as live vaccines at eliciting a protective immune response, although they are theoretically much safer. However, a killed pertussis (whooping cough) vaccine has been blamed for some side-effects (Box 24.1). A pertussis subunit vaccine is now preferred in some countries, although it may not offer as good protection as the intact, killed vaccine.

Subunit vaccines

Subunits are components of pathogens and induce predominantly antibody responses. Hepatitis B vaccine is a subunit antigen that has been produced using recombinant techniques (Box 24.2). Up to now, hepatitis B vaccine has been very effective. Failure to develop pro-

Bone marrow   Thymus   Lymph node

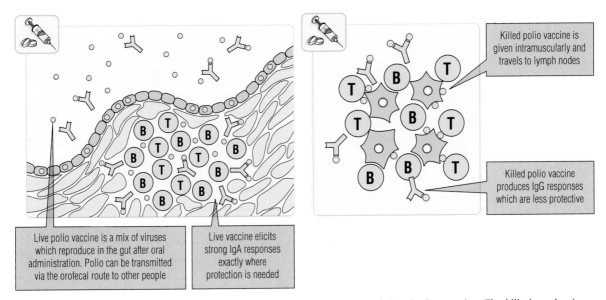

Live polio vaccine is a mix of viruses which reproduce in the gut after oral administration. Polio can be transmitted via the orofecal route to other people

Live vaccine elicits strong IgA responses exactly where protection is needed

Killed polio vaccine is given intramuscularly and travels to lymph nodes

Killed polio vaccine produces IgG responses which are less protective

Fig. 24.2 The killed polio vaccine would probably not have been as successful as the live vaccine. The killed vaccine is reserved for use in immunodeficient individuals.

tection from hepatitis B following vaccination can be a result of host or viral factors.

Host factors. Some HLA alleles, for example DR3, are associated with poor response to hepatitis B vaccine. It is likely that these alleles do not bind epitopes present in the vaccine peptide.

Viral factors. Hepatitis B is prone to undergo gradual mutation. In the face of widespread immunity to HBsAg (hepatitis B surface antigen), viral strains with mutations in this protein are at an advantage and can escape vaccine-induced immunity. These strains were very rare when the vaccine was first introduced, but the mutations are present in up to a third of all viral isolates in the very countries where widespread vaccination has been successful.

Possible solutions are to use either a larger peptide or a mixture of peptides. These approaches decrease the chances of particular HLA alleles being unable to bind epitopes and they may reduce the risk of successful viral mutations.

Toxoids are another type of subunit vaccine. They are bacterial exotoxins that have been chemically altered to make them safe, although they retain their antigenicity. The neutralizing antibodies produced block the effects of the toxins. Tetanus toxoid is a good example of this approach. Subunit and toxoid vaccines are generally of low immunogenicity compared with intact organisms and they may need **adjuvants** in order to work effectively. An adjuvant is given along with an antigen to provide a variety of non-specific stimuli to the immune system, which enhances the amount of antibody produced. For example, inorganic salts based on aluminum hydroxide (alum) that bind proteins and elicit an inflammatory response are used as adjuvants in some subunit vaccines. Alum is the only adjuvant currently licensed for human use.

Other vaccines

Subunits and dead pathogen vaccines can be very good at eliciting antibody responses. They are not so good at eliciting CTL responses because they cannot enter the intracellular pathways for presentation to T cells. CTL responses are particularly important in dealing with intracellular infections such as HIV. Various developmental vaccine techniques aim to elicit strong CTL responses by inserting pathogen genes into cells in the hope that these will be expressed, processed and displayed on MHC class I (Fig. 24.4).

Immunostimulatory complexes (ISCOMs). These micelles of lipid and subunit antigen have two special advantages over conventional vaccines:

- the antigen penetrates the cell wall (Fig. 24.4) and is delivered to the antigen-presenting pathways. In this way, subunit antigen can stimulate T cells including CTL
- ISCOMs can be used for mucosal vaccines (for example, through the nose) and induce widespread mucosal immunity in the gut and respiratory tract (see Box 13.3).

Viral vectors. Viruses that are safe for humans can be used as vectors to take the required sequence into the cells for expression. Retroviruses and adenoviruses are being used as experimental vectors.

DNA vaccines. In this experimental approach, the gene for the immunogenic protein is coated onto gold

BOX 24.1
Whooping cough

A 3-year-old boy presents with a 4 week history of coughing attacks. Each coughing attack lasts several minutes and it is terminated by vomiting. These features are typical of whooping cough and, indeed, because of parental concerns, this child did not receive whooping cough vaccine.

The causative bacterium, *Bordetella pertussis*, kills about 1 in 1000 infected children by damaging the airways. The specific immune response to pertussis is almost entirely antibody mediated. Antibodies prevent the bacteria from attaching to epithelium and neutralize the toxins produced (Fig. 24.3).

Pertussis vaccine does not entirely prevent the infection but it does protect children from the severe complications. The original pertussis vaccine is a killed whole organism. This "cellular" vaccine is very effective and protects over 90% of vaccinees from severe complications. However, the vaccine was thought to cause neurological disease in a tiny proportion of children. The cellular vaccine is still used in the UK, but not in children with progressive neurological disorders.

Because of the anxieties about side-effects, a subunit vaccine was developed and is in widespread use in the US. This "acellular" vaccine is made up of pertussis toxins and may be less protective than the killed pertussis vaccine.

Many parents in the UK and the US do not allow their children to receive either type of vaccine, because of perceived fears concerning risk. However, there is no good evidence that pertussis causes severe

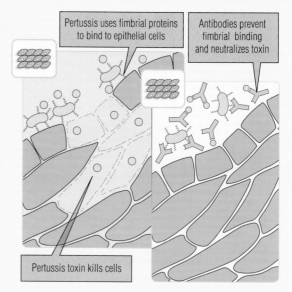

Fig. 24.3 These antibodies against pertussis are typical of neutralizing antibodies. They prevent molecular interactions that are required in disease processes.

problems in children who have been vaccinated.

The moral of the pertussis story applies to all vaccines used in childhood. It is paradoxical that the success of vaccines in reducing the number of childhood infections means that many parents, clinicians and the media have forgotten how dangerous these infections can be. For example, prior to the introduction of measles vaccine in the UK, 3000 children died each year of measles.

---

microspheres and injected directly into cells (e.g., of the skin). In mice, this has resulted in antibody production, indicating that the genes were transcribed (see also Box 10.2).

How organisms evade the immune response

It has proved very difficult to produce really effective vaccines, offering life-long immunity, for some infections because the pathogens have evolved powerful ways of evading the adaptive immune response (Fig. 24.5).

RNA viruses, such as influenza (Box 24.3) and HIV (Ch. 32), tend to mutate rapidly and their antigens can change, thus evading immunological memory (see Fig. 24.7).

Some DNA viruses, for example herpesviruses, evade the adaptive immune response by downregulating

MHC expression and the innate response is required for their control (natural killer cells). Because there is no immunological memory for the innate system, it is hard to prime these responses and protect individuals from infection (see Fig. 24.7).

Pneumococcus (*Streptococcus pneumoniae*) and *Haemophilus* sp. evade the innate response (opsonization by complement and phagocytosis) by producing a large polysaccharide coat. Polysaccharides are very poor immunogens, largely because they rely on the response of T-independent B cells (Chs 14 and 16) and do not make good vaccines. To overcome this, effective vaccines contain polysaccharide that has been chemically conjugated to a peptide antigen: tetanus toxoid is often used. T cells responding to the peptide then provide help for B cells responding to the polysaccharide (Fig. 24.8; see also Box 16.5). Other ways by which organisms evade phagocytosis are mentioned in Box 20.4.

BOX 24.2
Hepatitis B

Hepatitis B infection can result in irreversible liver damage and liver cancer (hepatoma). The hepatitis B vaccine was one of the first recombinant subunit vaccines and consists of a peptide derived from the hepatitis B surface antigen, HBsAg, grown in yeast cells. This vaccine elicits IgG antibodies, which are neutralizing; they prevent the virus from entering hepatocytes. The recombinant vaccine is very safe and protects 80–90% of vaccinees. This level of protection is adequate when vaccine campaigns aim to reduce the pool of infection in a community. For example, in developing countries where hepatitis B is very common, protecting the majority of the population is enough to slow down epidemics—so called **herd immunity**. In these countries, hepatitis B vaccination programs have almost eradicated hepatoma—the first example of a vaccine being successful at preventing cancer.

In other situations, the aim is to guarantee 100% protection to specific high-risk individuals (for example, medical students!).

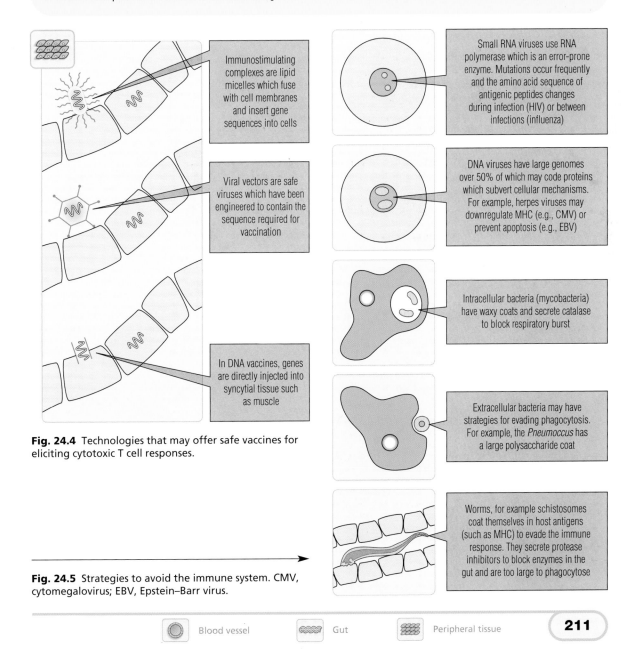

Fig. 24.4 Technologies that may offer safe vaccines for eliciting cytotoxic T cell responses.

Immunostimulating complexes are lipid micelles which fuse with cell membranes and insert gene sequences into cells

Viral vectors are safe viruses which have been engineered to contain the sequence required for vaccination

In DNA vaccines, genes are directly injected into syncytial tissue such as muscle

Small RNA viruses use RNA polymerase which is an error-prone enzyme. Mutations occur frequently and the amino acid sequence of antigenic peptides changes during infection (HIV) or between infections (influenza)

DNA viruses have large genomes over 50% of which may code proteins which subvert cellular mechanisms. For example, herpes viruses may downregulate MHC (e.g., CMV) or prevent apoptosis (e.g., EBV)

Intracellular bacteria (mycobacteria) have waxy coats and secrete catalase to block respiratory burst

Extracellular bacteria may have strategies for evading phagocytosis. For example, the *Pneumoccus* has a large polysaccharide coat

Worms, for example schistosomes coat themselves in host antigens (such as MHC) to evade the immune response. They secrete protease inhibitors to block enzymes in the gut and are too large to phagocytose

Fig. 24.5 Strategies to avoid the immune system. CMV, cytomegalovirus; EBV, Epstein–Barr virus.

Blood vessel   Gut   Peripheral tissue

BOX 24.3
Influenza

Influenza causes many thousands of deaths every year. Influenza is an RNA virus that uses a protein called hemagglutinin to bind sugars on respiratory epithelial cells. Influenza is cytopathic: it causes damage to the cells it infects. The presence of double-stranded RNA stimulates respiratory tract cells to secrete interferon-α within a few hours of viral infection, which inhibits viral replication (Box 19.2) and prevents rapid spread of influenza in the lungs.

Dendritic cells migrate to the local lymph node and present antigen to T cells. Under the influence of T helper type 1 (T_H1) cells, CTLs begin to appear after 2–3 days. These cells clear the residual infected cells and thus sterilizing immunity is achieved.

Influenza also elicits an antibody response and IgM antibodies begin to appear after about 5 days. These neutralizing antibodies bind to hemagglutinin and prevent virus from infecting cells. The antibody response against influenza develops too late to have a major role in helping to clear established infection and it is most important in preventing re-infection with an identical viral strain.

Influenza is a relatively unstable RNA virus and undergoes spontaneous mutation. Gradual mutations slowly change the viral genome and result in antigenic drift. More rapid, extensive mutations, or the possibility of recombinant genetic events with animal virus, dramatically change the viral genome and cause antigenic shift. Influenza uses **antigenic drift** and **antigenic shift** to overcome antibodies; drift causes annual mild epidemics and shift causes more severe epidemics every few years (Fig. 24.6).

Influenza vaccine is very successful at preventing infection in individuals at risk of severe complications (for example, patients with chronic chest problems). The vaccine uses killed influenza virus and to be effective it must contain the most up-to-date strains. Manufacturers must constantly update the vaccine using prevalent strains.

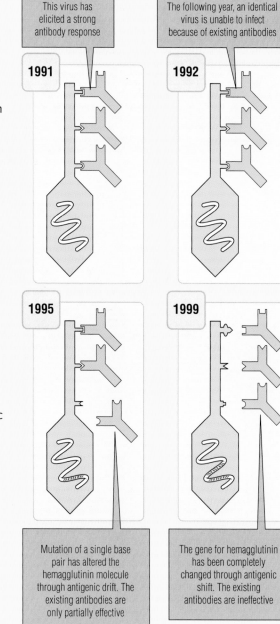

Fig. 24.6 Single base pair mutations causing drift are relatively frequent. Shift occurs much less often, probably when human influenza virus exchanges gene sequences with animal viruses (**recombination**). Such events overcome immunity on an enormous scale, triggering global epidemics.

Bone marrow   Thymus   Lymph node

Fig. 24.7
RNA and DNA viruses use different strategies to evade the immune system

	RNA viruses	DNA viruses
Examples	HIV, Influenza	Hepatitis B, Herpes virus family
How they evade the immune response	Small unstable genomes. Although RNA viruses may produce immunosuppressive proteins such as NEF (see Ch. 32), they rely on mutations to evade the immune response. The viral life cycle results in frequent mutations which allow the virus to evade the immune response, particularly CTL responses.	Large, stable genomes. Encode proteins which impair the immune response; for example, EBV produces a homolog to Bcl-2, which impairs apoptosis. CMV produces a protein which impairs antigen presentation. Mutations take place only gradually.
Vaccine issues	Mutations mean that influenza vaccines have to be revised each year. For HIV, vaccines will have to reflect the wide range of different strains that exist around the world.	Where they exist, current vaccines are successful, but the emergence of mutations may cause problems in the future.

CMV, cytomegalovirus; CTL, cytotoxic T cells; EBV, Epstein–Barr virus.

This polysaccharide is conjugated to a protein antigen, eliciting T cell help. Even young children respond to conjugate vaccines and there will be good affinity maturation

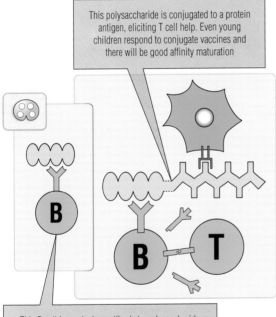

Fig. 24.8 Conjugated vaccines for meningococci *(Neisseria meningitidis)* and *Haemophilus* are already in use and a vaccine for pneumococci is being developed.

This B cell is producing antibody to polysaccharide independently of T cell help. This can not occur in young children and there is no affinity maturation

LEARNING POINTS

Can you now:

- Describe three different types of vaccine currently in use and how they vary in their safety and efficacy?
- Describe two different types of whooping cough vaccine and why they are used in different countries?
- Explain why influenza vaccine may need to be given every year?
- Describe two newer approaches to vaccination?

Hypersensitivity reactions

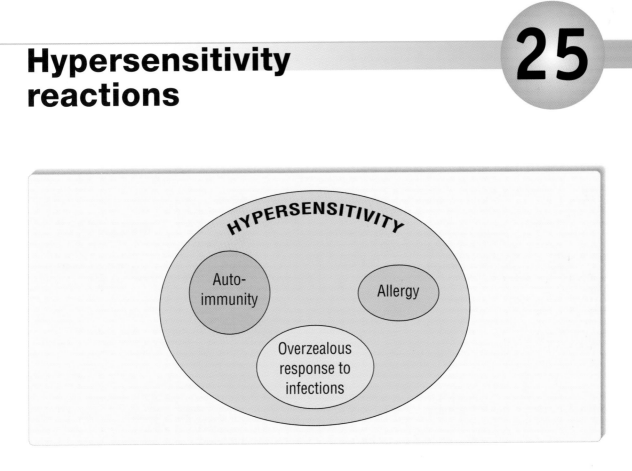

Excessive immune responses that cause damage are called **hypersensitivity reactions**. Hypersensivity reactions can occur in response to three different types of antigen:

- Infectious agents. We have already discussed how the immune system sometimes overreacts to infections and causes disease; when the immune response contributes to the symptoms of infection, the resultant disease is a type of hypersensitivity.
- Environmental substances. Hypersensitivity can occur in response to innocuous environmental antigens—one example of this is allergy. For example, in hay fever, grass pollens themselves are incapable of causing damage; it is the immune response to the pollen that causes harm.
- Self antigens. Normal host molecules can trigger immune responses, referred to as autoimmunity, and when these cause hypersensitivity **autoimmune disease** is the result.

Hypersensitivity reactions use four different mechanisms for causing disease; these are the topics of Chapters 25 to 30.

Types of triggers for hypersensitivity

Hypersensitivity to infectious agents

Not all infections are capable of causing hypersensitivity reactions. For example, although the common cold elicits a strong immune response, this never appears to cause harm.

Infections that are capable of eliciting hypersensitivity do not do so in every case. In Chapter 19 we discussed how hepatitis B virus infection can result in chronic hepatitis in some individuals. Another example is *Mycobacterium leprae*, which can elicit two types of response:

- In **lepromatous leprosy** there is a weak T helper (T_H) 1 response to mycobacteria, which continue to replicate. Although the mycobacteria spread throughout the body and the patient remains infectious to others, patients do not always develop severe symptoms.
- In **tuberculoid leprosy** there is a very strong T_H1 response, which leads to production of granulomata (Fig. 25.1). Mycobacteria are locked into the granulomata and the infection does not usually become widespread. The patient is not infectious to others. However, as a granuloma grows it can damage tissues, especially nerves. Tuberculoid leprosy is, therefore, a form of hypersensitivity.

Why different people develop either lepromatous or tuberculoid leprosy is probably genetically determined. It is likely that polymorphisms in immune response genes, such as the MHC (Ch. 8) or tumor necrosis factor (TNF) (Ch. 22), affect the outcome of *M. leprae*

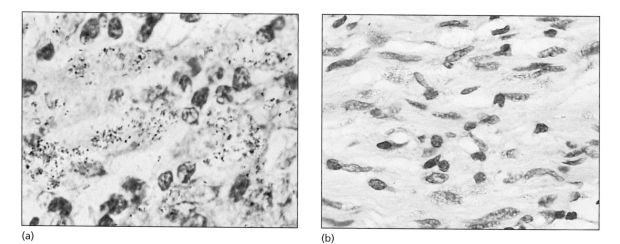

(a)　　　　　　　　　　　　　　(b)

Fig. 25.1 Leprosy. (a) A biopsy from a patient with lepromatous leprosy. There are many mycobacteria but very little immune reaction. (With permission from Cotran, R.S., Kumar, V. and Collins, T. 1998. *Pathologic basis of disease*, 6th edn. W.B. Saunders, St. Louis.) (b) In tuberculoid leprosy, there are far fewer mycobacteria but much more reaction in the form of macrophages and T cells. (Courtesy of Professor Umberto De Girolami, Brigham & Women's Hospital, Boston.) Compare this with Figure 22.3 showing *M. tuberculosis* infection.

infection. Drugs can further modify the outcome of *M. leprae* infection.

Another, very different, example of an infection causing hypersensitivity is immune complex disease caused by streptococci, which is discussed below.

Hypersensitivity to environmental substances

For environmental substances to trigger hypersensitivity reactions, they must be fairly small in order to gain access to the immune system. Dusts trigger off a range of responses because they are able to enter the lower extremities of the respiratory tract: an area that is rich in adaptive immune response cells. These dusts can mimic parasites and may stimulate an antibody response. If the dominant antibody is IgE, they may subsequently trigger immediate hypersensitivity, which is manifest as allergies such as **asthma** or **rhinitis**. If the dust stimulates IgG antibodies it may trigger off a different kind of hypersensitivity, for example, farmer's lung (Ch. 29).

Smaller molecules sometimes diffuse into the skin and these may act as haptens, triggering a delayed hypersensitivity reaction. This is the basis of contact dermatitis caused by nickel, discussed in Box 25.4.

Drugs administered orally, by injection or onto the surface of the body can elicit hypersensitivity reactions mediated by IgE or IgG antibodies or by T cells. Immunologically mediated hypersensitivity reactions to drugs are very common and even very tiny doses of drug can trigger life-threatening reactions. These are all classified as **idiosyncratic adverse drug reactions**. We return to this topic in Chapter 30.

A word of caution is needed here. Lay people, and many clinicians, refer to any hypersensitivity reaction to exogenous substances as **allergy** and the term originally meant any altered reaction to external substances. A related term, **atopy**, refers to immediate hypersensitivity mediated by IgE antibodies. In this book, this more restrictive definition is also used for allergy because it helps to explain the specific diagnosis and treatment of hypersensitivities mediated by IgE.

Hypersensitivity to self antigens

A degree of immune response to self antigens is normal and is present in most people. When these become exaggerated or when tolerance to further antigens breaks down, hypersensitivity reactions can occur. This is autoimmune disease and is discussed in Chapter 27.

Types of hypersensitivity reaction

The hypersensitivity classification system used here was first described by Coombs and Gell (Fig. 25.2). The system classifies the different types of hypersensitivity reaction by the types of immune response involved. Each type of hypersensitivity reaction produces characteristic clinical disease whether the trigger is an environmental, infectious or self antigen. For example, in type III hypersensitivity the clinical result is similar whether the antigen is streptococcus, a drug or an autoantigen such as DNA.

Hypersensitivity reactions are reliant on the adaptive immune system. Prior exposure to antigen is required to prime the adaptive immune response to produce IgE (type I), IgG (types II and III) or T cells (type IV). Because prior exposure is required, hypersensitivity reactions do not take place when an individual is first

Bone marrow　　　Thymus　　　Lymph node

Fig. 25.2
Coombs and Gell classification of hypersensitivity

	Type I: immediate hypersensitivity	Type II: cell-bound antigen	Type III: immune complex	Type IV: delayed hypersensitivity
Onset	Seconds—if IgE preformed	Seconds—if IgG preformed	Hours—if IgG preformed	2–3 days
Infectious trigger	Schistosomiasis	Immune hemolytic anemias	Poststreptococcal glomerulonephritis	Hepatitis B virus, tuberculoid leprosy
Environmental trigger	House dust mite, peanut, etc.	Immune hemolytic anemias	Farmer's lung	Contact dermatitis
Autoimmunity	Not applicable	Immune hemolytic anemias	Systemic lupus erythematosus	Insulin-dependent diabetes, celiac disease, multiple sclerosis, rheumatoid arthritis
Adaptive immune system mediators	IgE	IgG	IgG	T cells
Innate immune system effectors	Mast cells, eosinophils	Complement, phagocytes	Complement, neutrophils	Macrophages

exposed to antigen. In each type of hypersensitivity reaction the damage is caused by different adaptive and innate systems, each of which should now be familiar to you through discussion of their role in clearing infections.

Type I

Type I hypersensitivity is mediated through the degranulation of mast cells and eosinophils. The effects are felt with minutes of exposure (see Box 25.1) and this type of hypersensitivity is sometimes referred to as **immediate hypersensitivity** and is also known as allergy (Ch. 26).

Type II

Type II hypersensitivity is caused by IgG reacting with antigen present on the surface of cells. The bound immunoglobulin then interacts with complement or with Fc receptor on macrophages. These innate mechanisms then damage the target cells using processes that may take several hours, as in the case of drug-induced hemolysis (Box 25.2).

Type III

Immunoglobulin is also responsible for type III hypersensitivity. In this case immune complexes of antigen and antibody form and either cause damage at the site of production or circulate and cause damage elsewhere. Immune complexes take some time to form and to initiate tissue damage. Poststreptococcal glomerulonephritis is a good example of **immune complex disease** (Box 25.3 and Ch. 29).

BOX 25.1
Type I hypersensitivity: hay fever

A 16-year-old boy has had a runny nose and sore eyes since the beginning of July. His symptoms improve indoors, but they return within minutes of going outside. He has never been ill before, although his two sisters both have asthma. A skin prick test is performed (Fig. 25.3) and this shows allergy to some common grass pollens. It is almost impossible for him to avoid exposure to pollens, so for the rest of the pollen season he is treated with antihistamines.

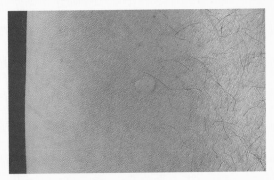

Fig. 25.3 Skin prick test. A pollen extract was dropped onto the patient's skin, which was then gently pricked. Within 10 minutes, the area became itchy and a wheal developed, surrounded by erythema. (With permission from the Department of Medical Illustration, St Bartholomew's Hospital, London.)

 Blood vessel   Gut   Peripheral tissue

BOX 25.2
Type II hypersensitivity: drug-induced hemolysis

A woman in her 30s presents with acute fatigue and breathlessness. Two days earlier, she was given penicillin antibiotic for a urinary tract infection. She has had the same antibiotic once before without problems. She is found to be pale and mildly jaundiced. The laboratory shows that her red cells are being destroyed in the circulation. Further testing shows that her serum contains antibodies that react with penicillin coating her red cells, confirming the diagnosis of penicillin-induced **immune hemolytic anemia**.

Penicillin is a low-molecular-weight compound that is unable to act as an antigen in its own right, but can act as a **hapten** (Fig. 25.4) (see also Box 5.1 and Fig. 5.3). In penicillin-induced hemolysis, prior exposure to penicillin induces IgG antibodies. On re-exposure, penicillin binds to red cells and it becomes a target for IgG. The IgG-coated red cells are taken up and destroyed by the spleen (Fig. 25.5).

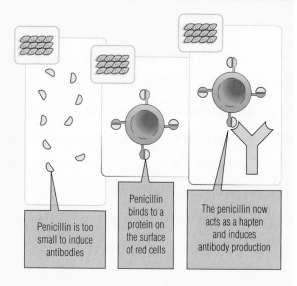

Penicillin is too small to induce antibodies

Penicillin binds to a protein on the surface of red cells

The penicillin now acts as a hapten and induces antibody production

Fig. 25.4 Haptens interact with normal proteins from a variety of host tissues.

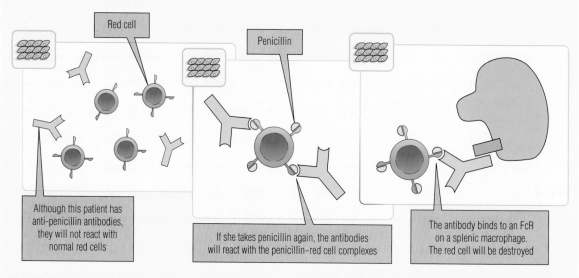

Red cell

Penicillin

Although this patient has anti-penicillin antibodies, they will not react with normal red cells

If she takes penicillin again, the antibodies will react with the penicillin–red cell complexes

The antibody binds to an FcR on a splenic macrophage. The red cell will be destroyed

Fig. 25.5 Penicillin-induced immune hemolysis. Destruction of red cells takes place within 24 hours of re-exposure to the antigen. FcR, Fc receptor.

Type IV
The slowest form of hypersensitivity is that mediated by T cells (type IV hypersensitivity). This can take 2–3 days to develop and is referred to as **delayed hypersensitivity**. (Box 25.4 and Ch. 30).

Diagnosis and treatment of hypersensitivity
There are major differences in how the types of hypersensitivity reaction are diagnosed and treated. For example, although skin tests are used to diagnose both type I and type IV hypersensitivity, the exact type

Bone marrow   Thymus   Lymph node

BOX 25.3
Type III hypersensitivity: poststreptococcal glomerulonephritis

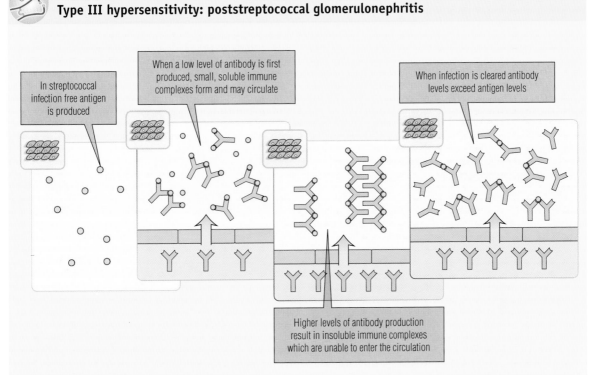

Fig. 25.6 Poststreptococcal glomerulonephritis. Acute infections such as streptococcus can trigger circulating immune complexes until the antigen is cleared.

An 11-year-old boy presents to his family physician with a 3 day history of swelling of the legs and scrotum. He complained of a sore throat about 2 weeks earlier. His urine contains blood and protein. Taken together, these are the findings of acute **glomerulonephritis**. A throat swab is taken and the bacterium β-hemolytic streptococcus is grown. He is started on antibiotics for the infection and over the next 3 weeks his edema improves. When he is reviewed at this stage his urine is normal.

This child had typical poststreptococcal glomerulonephritis. Streptococci induce a potent antibody response. These antibodies interact with antigen and small circulating immune complexes are produced as a result, especially when antigen is still in excess (Fig. 25.6). These complexes have a tendency to localize in the glomerulus and cause type III hypersensitivity, using mechanisms described in detail in Chapter 29.

Circulating immune complexes occur during other infections. Some individuals with hepatitis B virus infection are unable to control infection with adequate T cell responses (Ch. 22) and there is ongoing viral replication. Even though these individuals produce high levels of antibody, there may still be antigen excess and circulating immune complexes may form (Fig. 25.7).

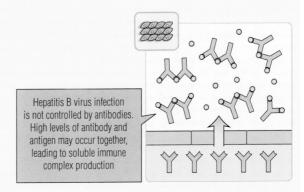

Fig. 25.7 Chronic infections such as hepatitis B virus cause more long-lasting immune complex disease.

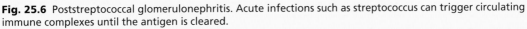

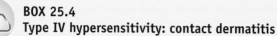

BOX 25.4
Type IV hypersensitivity: contact dermatitis

An 18-year-old construction worker developed an itchy rash on his face and hands. A dermatologist thinks this is contact dermatitis and organizes a patch test, including para-aminobenzoate (PAB, found in sun screens) and dichromate (DO3, found in cement). Patch testing (Fig. 25.8) confirms sensitivity to these chemicals and the rash improves on avoiding exposure.

Contact dermatitis is an example of type IV delayed hypersensitivity. The skin lesions consist of T cells and macrophages and develop 24–72 hours after exposure to the antigen. In this way, the lesions of contact dermatitis are very similar to those induced by a tuberculin skin test.

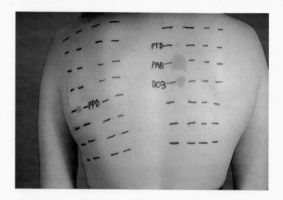

Fig. 25.8 In the patch test, the sensitizing antigen is placed on the skin under a dressing. This photograph shows a typical positive reaction at 48 hours. At the cellular level, the evolution of this test is very similar to a tuberculin skin test (Fig. 22.9). (With permission from the Department of Medical Illustration, St Bartholomew's Hospital, London.)

of testing depends on the type of disease suspected. Treatment for each type of hypersensitivity is also very different, as we shall explain in the following chapters.

A criticism of the Coombs and Gell classification system is that it is simplistic; many diseases are caused by an overlap of different types of hypersensitivity. However, some knowledge of the classification system makes it easier to understand how the different disorders come about and how they can be effectively diagnosed and treated.

In this book, we have not provided an exhaustive list of hypersensitivity disorders or worked through the different anatomical systems. This is because an understanding of the mechanisms of hypersensitivity enables students to apply this knowledge to other disease settings. There are many more hypersensitivity reactions than we have had an opportunity to discuss in detail.

LEARNING POINTS

Can you now:

- Explain the Coombs and Gell classification of hypersensitivity reactions?
- Give two examples of infection causing different types of hypersensitivity?
- Give three examples of how normally innocuous substances may cause hypersensitivity?
- Contrast the two different tests described in this chapter?

Bone marrow   Thymus   Lymph node

Immediate hypersensitivity (type I): allergy

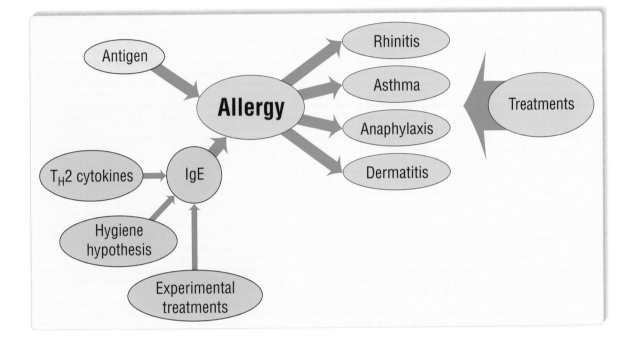

Definitions

The immunological definition of **atopy** is an immediate hypersensitivity reaction to environmental antigens, mediated by IgE. Such reactions tend to run in families and these families are said to have inherited the atopy trait. Although the term **allergy** was originally defined as altered reactivity to exogenous antigens, it is now often used synonymously with atopy. Allergic diseases include anaphylaxis, rhinitis, asthma, some types of dermatitis or eczema and food allergies. The distinction between true allergy and other reactions is important because some of the treatments for allergy would be inappropriate for other types of reaction.

Usually, allergies are very rapid reactions mediated by IgE. However, some allergic reactions continue for a long time (for example, when the environmental antigen cannot be easily avoided) and they develop into a late phase reaction characterized by T cell infiltrates. This is called the **late phase response** and is discussed below.

The types of allergy are shown in Figure 26.1.

Antigen

Antigens that trigger allergic reactions are referred to as **allergens**. Allergens are present in the environment as small particles or low-molecular-weight substances that penetrate the body after being inhaled, eaten or administered as drugs. Inhaled antigens include pollens, fungal spores and the feces of the house dust mite. Animal allergens include salivary proteins; these become airborne after the animal has licked itself and the saliva dries on the fur. Some insect venoms are allergens and these are injected directly into the skin.

For food allergens to cause symptoms they must either be absorbed through the mucosa of the mouth and lips (in which case they cause symptoms very rapidly) or be resistant to digestive enzymes and low pH (in which case absorption is delayed and symptoms occur later) (Box 26.1).

An important part of the treatment of allergy is identification and avoidance of allergens. Careful history taking facilitates identification of allergens. For example, a patient with a runny nose (rhinitis) is likely to be sensitive to aeroallergens. If symptoms occur predominantly in summer, grass pollens are the likely culprit. If symptoms occur all year round and mainly indoors, sensitivity to house dust mite feces is likely. House dust mite allergy occurs in areas where a cold climate dictates the need for central heating, heavy bedding and thick carpets—the habitat of this mite.

Fig. 26.1
Allergic diseases

Clinical disease	Symptoms	Characteristics
Asthma	Reversible airways obstruction in the bronchi	Infection, exercise and changes in temperature can also cause changes in air flow
Rhinitis	Discharge, sneezing and nasal obstruction	
Allergic conjunctivitis	Redness of conjunctiva and itchy eyelids	Often co-exists with rhinitis
Urticaria	Usually acute; itchy edema of the cutaneous tissues; the lesion is identical to that induced by skin prick testing	Allergy accounts for about two thirds of cases of urticaria
Angioedema	Usually acute; non-itchy edema of the subcutaneous tissues	Some forms, for example lip swelling, may be manifestations of food allergy
Atopic eczema	Usually chronic; itchy inflammation	A minority of cases are caused by food allergy
Anaphylaxis	Low blood pressure, angioedema and airways obstruction	

BOX 26.1
Food allergy

A 6-year-old boy has developed a number of skin problems. He has had a rash affecting his arms and legs since the age of 3. More recently he has developed a second itchy rash, lasting several minutes, which is associated with eating prawns. These symptoms are suggestive of urticaria (Fig. 26.2). On examination, all that can be seen are signs consistent with mild atopic eczema (Fig. 26.3).

Because his eczema is mild, it is possible to do skin prick testing, which confirms the allergy to prawns. He is also found to be allergic to egg yolk, which he has been eating regularly since he was a toddler.

His parents are advised that he should avoid egg and prawns. Over the next few weeks he has no more attacks of urticaria and his eczema improves. Because avoidance of egg yolks imposes severe dietary restrictions, a food challenge is undertaken. He is given very small doses of egg yolk and, 2 days

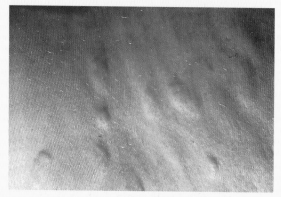

Fig. 26.2 Urticaria is an itchy rash caused largely by release of histamine leading to vasodilatation and increased capillary permeability. Acute urticaria is often allergic, while chronic urticaria often has other causes. (With permission from the Department of Medical Illustration, St Bartholomew's Hospital, London.)

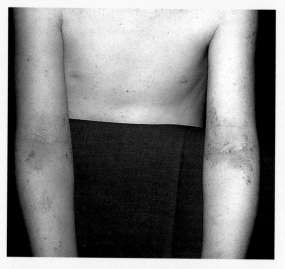

Fig. 26.3 Atopic eczema causes thickened, itchy weeping skin, especially affecting the flexures of the knees and elbows. (With permission from the Department of Medical Illustration, St Bartholomew's Hospital, London.)

Bone marrow   Thymus   Lymph node

BOX 26.1
Food allergy (*contd.*)

later, his eczema does flare up—confirming a diagnosis of egg yolk-induced atopic eczema.

Urticaria is often an acute manifestation of allergy in the skin while atopic eczema is a chronic response, characterized by infiltration of T cells and eosinophils in the skin. Atopic eczema is analogous to the delayed phase of asthma, but unlike asthma, eczema often improves spontaneously around adolescence.

It is not clear why allergy to foods is sometimes manifest in the skin. In many cases of urticaria and eczema, allergens are not identified and other mechanisms are probably responsible. Finding specific IgE against food allergens supports a diagnosis of food allergy. The gold standard test for confirming that allergy is responsible for symptoms is a food challenge, which can be done double blind so that neither the investigator nor patient know whether they have in fact been exposed to the food. When food allergy is investigated as a cause for more unusual symptoms in this way, a causal relationship is usually ruled out. Food allergy is often blamed for a wide variety of symptoms—including migraine, hyperactivity and chronic fatigue—but there is no evidence to support this.

Further clues to the identity of allergens can be provided by knowledge of cross-reacting allergens.

- In penicillin allergy the allergen is the β-lactam core of the penicillin molecule. Patients experience symptoms with different members of the penicillin family, for example amoxicillin and flucloxacillin. Patients with penicillin allergy can react to other families of antibiotics such as cephalosporins, which also contain β-lactam ring structures (see also Box 5.1).
- Some plant allergens are cross-reactive; for example patients who have both springtime rhinitis and allergy to foods may be sensitive to proteins present in birch pollen as well as hazelnut, apple, carrot and potato.
- Patients with rubber allergy are often sensitive to food allergens in banana, avocado, kiwi fruit and figs. These plants are related to the rubber plant.

Cells

The major cells involved in allergy, mast cells and eosinophils, have been described Chapter 21 where we explained how these cells evolved to have a role in killing parasites. Mast cells are resident in a wide number of tissues (rather like macrophages) while eosinophils migrate into tissues where type I hypersensitivity is taking place (rather like neutrophils attracted to sites of inflammation). These cells release the mediators that cause the symptoms of allergy.

Antibody

IgE is required for type I hypersensitivity reactions. B cells class switch to IgE production when they are co-stimulated by interleukin (IL) 4, secreted by T helper 2 (T_H2) cells. Once IgE is produced, it binds to the high-affinity receptor FcεRI, expressed on resting mast cells resident in tissues and eosinophils that have been activated and migrated into tissues. If antigen crosslinks the IgE bound to the FcεRI, these cells release the mediators of type I hypersensitivity. On stimulation, mast cells also release more IL-4. This provides a positive feedback system for the production of more IgE and T_H2 cells. Thus, once a T cell response to an antigen has deviated towards production of T_H2 cytokines, positive feedback sustains and enhances the response (Fig. 26.4). IgE production is inhibited by interferon γ (IFN-γ) secreted by T_H1 type T cells (see Box 26.2).

Very high levels of IgE are seen in patients infected with parasites, for example schistosomiasis. Levels of IgE may also be high in people who have inherited the atopy trait, although they can be normal. The presence of IgE against specific allergens is required for allergic reactions to that allergen, but this does not always predict clinical symptoms. Specific IgE can be measured using enzyme-linked immunosorbent assays (ELISA), although in diagnosing allergy, it is more often useful to do **skin prick testing**.

Skin prick testing is the preferred method for allergy testing. When the antigen crosslinks IgE on mast cell FcεRI, there is a rapid release of histamine, causing a local flare and wheal reaction. Skin prick tests give immediate results, which the patient can see, they are cheap and they may be more reliable than specific IgE testing. Skin prick testing is generally safe. Skin prick testing is not possible when patients have taken antihistamines or have extensive atopic dermatitis. Figure 26.6 shows skin prick testing in a patient with asthma.

Predisposition to allergy

Like all forms of hypersensitivity, predisposition to allergy is caused by environmental and genetic factors.

 Blood vessel Gut ⬛ Peripheral tissue

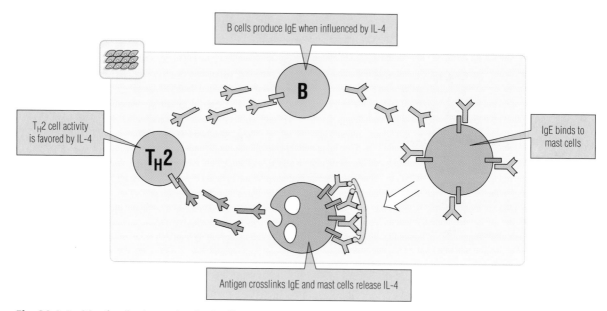

B cells produce IgE when influenced by IL-4

T$_H$2 cell activity is favored by IL-4

B

IgE binds to mast cells

T$_H$2

Antigen crosslinks IgE and mast cells release IL-4

Fig. 26.4 Positive feedback sustains the T cell response as long as antigen (allergen) is available and more IL-4 and more IgE are produced. The IL-4 produced may favor IL-4 production by T cells responding to other antigens.

The environmental component may be explained by the "hygiene hypothesis", and genetic factors by the atopy trait.

Atopy trait

In the West, up to 40% of the population have the atopy trait with exaggerated IgE responses to allergens. The risk of allergy tends to run in families; family members either have allergies themselves or are at risk of allergy because they have high levels of IgE against specific allergens. Affected family members may have different allergies, for example asthma, hay fever or eczema, in response to very different allergens. It is the risk of allergy that is inherited, not the specific allergy.

The genetics of allergy suggests that many genes are involved; inheritance is not usually Mendelian. For example, the genes for IL-4 and FcεRI are both polymorphic and have been associated with the risk of allergy. Interestingly, the FcεRI gene inherited from the mother appears to affect atopy more than the same gene inherited from the father. Other genes must also be involved, but unlike the other types of hypersensitivity, the MHC does not play a significant role.

Hygiene hypothesis

The incidence of allergies in the developed world is increasing. This is suggestive of the effects of a changing environmental factor. Several strands of evidence support the hygiene hypothesis: that exposure to bacteria in early life decreases the risk of allergy:

- children with asthma tend to live in cleaner houses than those without asthma
- growing up on farms and exposure to livestock decreases the risk of asthma
- asthma is rare in areas where tuberculosis is common.

At birth, most individuals have T cells with a bias towards T$_H$2-type cytokine production, possibly as a result of cytokines such as IL-4 and IL-10 secreted by the placenta (Ch. 32). The hygiene hypothesis suggests that exposure to organisms that promote a T$_H$1 response early in life deviates the immune response away from T$_H$2 responses. *Mycobacterium tuberculosis* and other bacterial infections stimulate T cells to secrete IFN-γ, which inhibits T$_H$2 responses (Fig. 26.7). These factors would be expected to work when immune responses to potential allergens are developing, and so they can only operate early in life.

The hygiene hypothesis may in future be translated into clinical benefits. For example, vaccination with *Mycobacterium vaccae*, a non-virulent mycobacterium, is being tested for benefits on the airways in patients with asthma. Studies are already underway with recombinant IL-12, which reduces the number of eosinophils in the airways of asthma patients. IL-12 treatment does not appear to improve asthma, however (Fig. 26.8).

In individuals who have already developed allergies, infection can make allergies worse. For example, respiratory viral infections can trigger attacks of asthma. In patients with established asthma, infection in the respiratory tract may trigger the secretion of chemokines and cytokines that attract and activate T$_H$2 cells and eosinophils, as bystanders.

BOX 26.2
Studies of T helper cells

In mice, it is possible to define two types of mature T helper cell. T_H1 cells secrete cytokines (for example IFN-γ) that promote killing of intracellular organisms through the actions of macrophages and natural killer cells. T_H2 cells respond to extracellular antigen and favor the production of IgE and type I hypersensitivity, by secreting cytokines such as IL-4 and IL-5.

Much of what is known about these polarized T cell populations has been derived from mice grown in extreme conditions that favor the production of only T_H1 or T_H2 cells. For example, mice exposed to parasites can produce almost exclusively T_H2 type cells. From this kind of experiment we know that T_H2 cells have a wide range of effects in developing allergy (Fig. 26.5).

T_H2 cells have a key role in establishing IgE-mediated responses and type I hypersensitivity. There is now considerable knowledge as to what favors the production of T_H2 cells over T_H1 cells at the very beginning of the immune response. In mice, T_H2 production is favored by the presence of IL-4 when naive T cells encounter antigen for the first time. Furthermore, a special population of mouse T cells must respond to antigen in order for IL-4 secretion to occur.

Research on mice has been useful in identifying the molecules and cells involved in allergy, but unfortunately, much less is known about how T_H2 responses develop in humans. In fact, very polarized T_H2 or T_H1 responses are only very rarely seen in humans. All we really know is that T_H2 responses are favored in humans when the individual has a family background of atopy and antigen is encountered at mucosal surfaces, such as the airway.

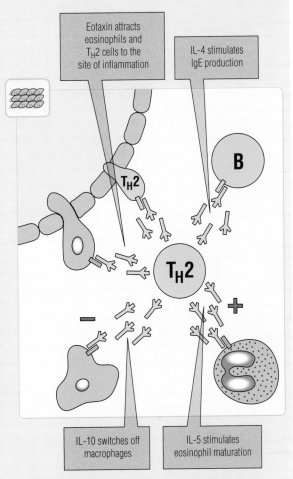

Fig. 26.5 Effects of T_H2 cytokines and chemokines in allergy. Interleukin (IL) 10 secreted by T_H2 cells switches off macrophages, reducing T_H1-induced inflammation. Interferon γ (IFN-γ) secreted by T_H1 cells inhibits T_H2 cells.

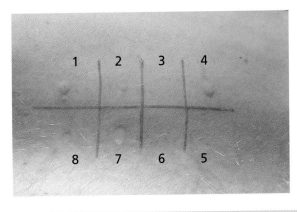

Fig. 26.6 Skin prick testing of aero-allergens in asthma. Clockwise from top left: 1, house dust mite; 2, grass pollen; 3, dog fur; 4, positive control (histamine); 5, vegetative control (saline); 6, cat fur; 7, tree pollen; 8, grass pollen. (With permission from the Department of Medical Illustration, St Bartholomew's Hospital, London.)

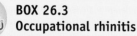

**BOX 26.3
Occupational rhinitis**

A 17-year-old student is working over the summer as a veterinary assistant. Each time he enters the clinic he suffers from bouts of sneezing and runny eyes. He has a history of pollen sensitivity and two of his sisters have asthma. Allergy to animal proteins is suspected and he is referred to an allergy clinic. Skin prick testing is done against a panel of possible allergens he encounters at his work.

The skin prick testing shows that he does not react to dog, cat or horse proteins, but he has a strong reaction to latex. Latex is used in the manufacture of clinical gloves. In clinical environments, microscopic latex particles become airborne and they can trigger attacks of rhinitis and conjunctivitis.

The clinic switches to plastic gloves for the duration of his summer job and his symptoms improve considerably. He is advised to avoid exposure to latex, for example to consider the use of latex-free, rather than rubber, condoms.

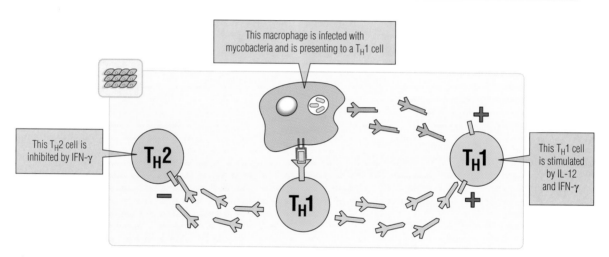

Fig. 26.7 T_H1 cytokines inhibit T_H2 cells. The hygiene hypothesis suggests allergy is suppressed by cytokines released during T_H1 responses. IFN-γ, interferon γ.

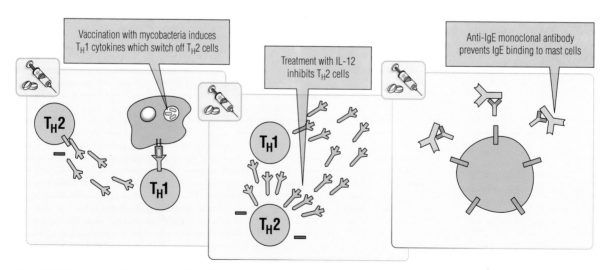

Fig. 26.8 Experimental treatments for allergy include vaccination, recombinant cytokines (e.g., interleukin 12, IL-12) and monoclonal antibodies.

Bone marrow   Thymus   Lymph node

Mediators of early phase

The early phase of allergy is caused by mediators released by mast cells when IgE bound to FcϵRI is crosslinked by allergen. Anaphylaxis is the most serious type of allergy and can occur when allergen enters the body from any route. Mast cells release preformed histamine and rapidly synthesize prostaglandins through the cyclo-oxygenase pathway (Ch. 20). These mediators cause vasodilatation and an increase in vascular permeability. Fluid shifts from the vascular to the extravascular space and there is a fall in vascular tone. The result of widespread mast cell activation is a dramatic fall in blood pressure, which is characteristic of anaphylactic shock.

In other forms of allergy, there are more localized changes in blood vessels, restricted to the site of allergen entry. For example, in allergic rhinitis, inhaled allergens stimulate mast cells in the nasal mucosa. There is then vasodilatation and edema in the nose, causing nasal stuffiness and sneezing. Leukotrienes, products of the lipo-oxygenase pathway (Ch. 20), increase mucus secretion, which causes the discharge characteristic of allergic rhinitis.

Increased mucus secretion in the bronchi also occurs in asthma and contributes to the airflow obstruction. However, in the lungs leukotrienes cause smooth muscle contraction and this has the most dramatic effects on airflow reduction (Fig. 26.9)

All of these effects can take place within minutes of exposure to allergen. Symptoms persist whilst exposure to allergen continues. Even if the patient is able to avoid the allergen, late-phase response may then occur (Box 26.4).

Mediators of late phase

Type I hypersensitivity reactions are generally characterized by immediate symptoms after exposure to allergens. For example, an asthmatic patient allergic to cats will develop airways obstruction, characterized by wheeze, seconds after exposure to cat fur. The symptoms improve after an hour or so as the immediate response dies down (Fig. 26.11).

Several hours after the acute episode, the airflow in the bronchi may deteriorate again, reflecting the migration of leukocytes, particularly eosinophils, into the bronchi in response to chemokines. The late phase may last several hours (Fig. 26.11).

In some individuals, this process becomes self perpetuating as T_H2 cells in the bronchial wall secrete cytokines such as IL-4 and more attractant chemokines (Fig. 26.12). The result is chronic allergic inflammation in the airways. Mediators released by eosinophils include peroxidase, eosinophil major basic protein and cationic protein, which all cause direct damage to bronchial tissue. As a result of the chronic allergic

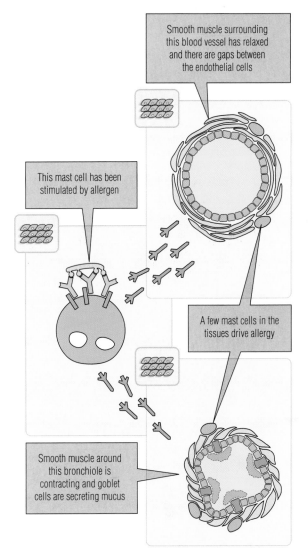

Smooth muscle surrounding this blood vessel has relaxed and there are gaps between the endothelial cells

This mast cell has been stimulated by allergen

A few mast cells in the tissues drive allergy

Smooth muscle around this bronchiole is contracting and goblet cells are secreting mucus

Fig. 26.9 Mediators of the early phase of allergy have different consequences depending on the target tissue.

inflammation, the bronchial smooth muscle is hypertrophic and mucus secretion is increased; airflow becomes persistently, rather than intermittently, reduced.

Infections exacerbate the inflammation and symptoms by attracting more inflammatory cells to the airway. Once the lining of the airway has become inflamed, it is susceptible to any irritant, for example cigarette smoke, and changes in endogenous steroid secretion (Box 26.4).

Treatment

General measures in the treatment of allergy include identifying and avoiding possible allergens. This is not

BOX 26.4
Asthma

A 13-year-old girl presents to the pediatricians with impaired exercise tolerance. She was diagnosed with asthma 4 years ago. She has previously always had episodic disease, typically after exposure to cats, and always responded to inhaled β_2-adrenergic agonists. For the last few months her symptoms have been constant rather than intermittent and she has been performing poorly in sports at school. She has a personal history of atopic eczema and a family history of asthma.

The pediatricians find that she is wheezy and that her **peak flow**, a measure of airways obstruction, is reduced. Her parents are given a meter and record peak flow at home for 5 days. These recordings show she has unstable airways obstruction, but that her airflow is never normal (Fig. 26.10). This is characteristic of poorly controlled asthma. Her asthma is present even when she is not exposed to cats and is causing striking airways instability. She is started on an inhaled corticosteroid twice a day and her symptoms improve considerably.

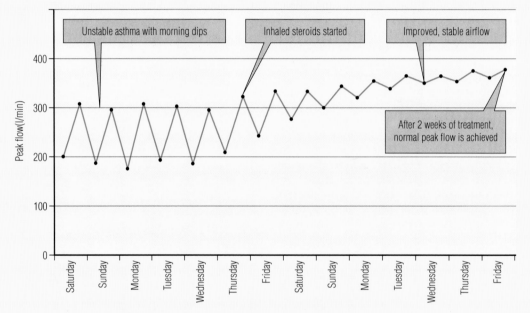

Unstable asthma with morning dips

Inhaled steroids started

Improved, stable airflow

After 2 weeks of treatment, normal peak flow is achieved

Fig. 26.10 When peak flow is measured twice a day, it is shown to be lower in the morning in unstable asthma. These morning dips correspond to troughs in endogenous corticosteroid secretion.

always possible when the allergen is widespread in the environment, for example grass pollen. Other treatments involve the use of drugs or desensitization.

Drug treatments

Some drugs block the end effects of mediator release; for example β_2-adrenergic agonists, such as salbutamol, mimic the effects of the sympathetic nervous system and work mainly by preventing smooth bronchial muscle contraction in asthma (Fig. 26.13). Epinephrine (adrenaline) is an important drug used in the treatment of anaphylaxis. In anaphylaxis, the blood pressure falls dramatically because fluid shifts out of blood vessels and into the tissues when vessel permeability increases. Epinephrine (adrenaline) can increase the blood pres-

sure and reverse airways obstruction and be life saving in anaphylaxis (Box 26.5).

Corticosteroids are widely used in the prevention of symptoms in patients with allergy and these are discussed in detail in Chapter 30. Corticosteroids can prevent the immediate hypersensitivity reaction, the late phase and chronic allergic inflammation. To avoid side-effects, corticosteroids are often given topically in allergies, for example inhaled steroids are used in asthma.

Sodium cromoglicate has some effects in preventing allergy attacks. It is thought to work by stabilizing mast cells and reducing degranulation.

Specific receptor antagonists block the effects of leukotrienes. Montelukast, for example, reduces the amount of airways inflammation in asthma.

Bone marrow   Thymus   Lymph node

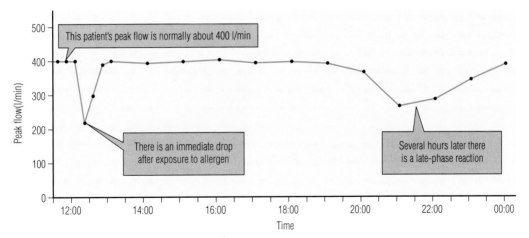

Fig. 26.11 Following exposure to cat fur, this patient has severe asthma symptoms that return after an interval of several hours.

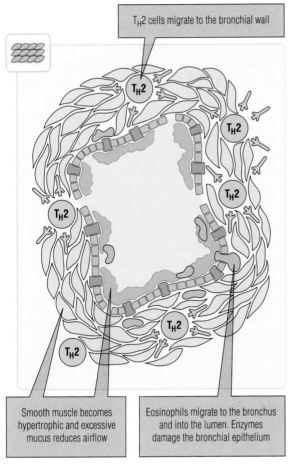

Fig. 26.12 Chronic allergic inflammation: compare this with the changes of acute asthma in the bronchus in Figure 26.9.

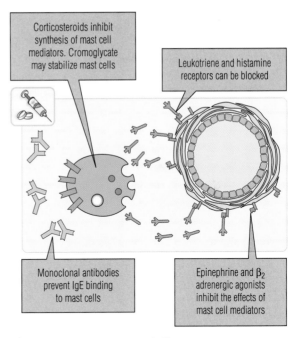

Fig. 26.13 Drug treatment of allergy.

Antihistamines block specific histamine receptors. Antihistamines are not very useful in asthma, because this mediator is not released by lung mast cells, but they have an important role in allergies affecting the skin and nose.

Newer drugs that block the effects of the T_H2 type cytokines, IL-3, IL-4 and IL-5, have not been shown to improve symptoms in allergy.

Omalizumab is a monoclonal antibody that binds to IgE and prevents it binding to the FcεR. Omalizumab

BOX 26.5
Bee sting anaphylaxis

A 6-year-old boy has been brought into the emergency room in an unconscious state. He was at a picnic when he suddenly developed swelling of the face and tongue, complained of feeling nauseous and then collapsed. His mother thinks he may have been stung by a bee. There is no personal or family history of allergy and he has been previously stung by bees with no ill effects.

On arrival at the emergency room he has angioedema of the face and tongue (Fig. 26.14). There is a bee sting on his left forearm, which is also swollen. His blood pressure is low and his heart rate is fast. A diagnosis of **anaphylaxis** is made.

He is immediately treated with intramuscular epinephrine (adrenaline) and recovers promptly. Although he is kept in hospital for 24 hours, his condition improves steadily and he requires no further treatment.

Two weeks later he attends the allergy clinic. A skin prick test using bee venom is very carefully carried out and it is strongly positive. Because he lives in the country, avoidance of bees is impractical.

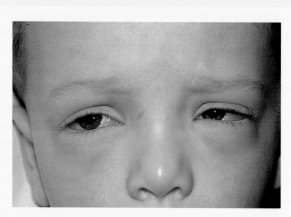

Fig. 26.14 Angioedema can be seen as an isolated feature of allergy or as a part of anaphylaxis. (With permission from the Department of Medical Illustration, St Bartholomew's Hospital, London.)

His parents are advised about the nature of anaphylaxis and they are issued with an epinephrine (adrenaline) injection to use if he is stung again and develops symptoms. He is also started on a course of desensitization.

---

reduces the number of circulating and airway eosinophils and prevents both the immediate and late phases of asthma after exposure to house dust mite. Omalizumab is a humanized chimeric antibody (see Box 9.1) and it is, therefore, thus less likely to provoke anti-mouse antibodies.

To date, there are no drugs available to clinicians to block specifically the effects of chemokines, enzymes such as mast cell tryptase or toxic proteins such as eosinophil major basic protein.

Desensitization

Desensitization or immunotherapy is a well-established technique that aims to improve allergy symptoms caused by specific allergens. It is most useful when single allergens are involved in symptoms and it often used to prevent anaphylaxis resulting from insect stings. Insect venom is injected intradermally in escalating doses. Although treatment starts with very small doses of venom, there is a risk of precipitating a full-blown anaphylactic attack. Therefore, desensitization must be carried out by trained staff with access to resuscitation equipment. Over time, the patient is given injections with increasing quantities of venom, eventually corresponding to the amount of venom in an insect sting. At this point, over 90% of patients will not develop anaphylaxis if they are stung again.

Desensitization works by inducing T_H1 cells, which then drive production of IgG against the allergen. After an insect sting, the venom will rapidly be bound by IgG and so it will no longer be available to crosslink IgE on mast cells (Fig. 26.15). Desensitization illustrates how a different route of administration induces different T cell populations: T_H1 in the case of intramuscular administration, T_H2 in the case of a sting into the skin.

Bone marrow   Thymus   Lymph node

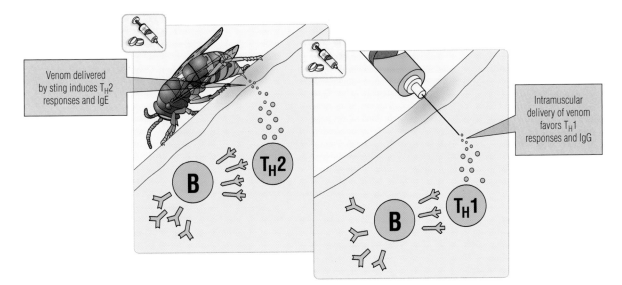

Fig. 26.15 Desensitization induces IgG anti-venom antibodies.

LEARNING POINTS

Can you now:

- Describe the mechanisms of the early and late phases of allergy?
- Describe the techniques used to identify allergens involved in immediate hypersensitivity?
- Contrast T_H1 and T_H2 cells?
- Understand the genetic and environmental factors that predispose to allergy and how these operate at an immunological level?
- Describe anaphylaxis and its immediate treatment?
- Outline the types of drugs used to treat allergy?

Autoimmunity

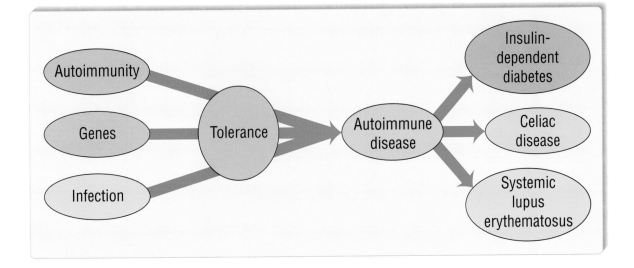

Some autoimmunity is normal

Autoimmune responses include antibodies and T cells with specificity for self antigens and are common in healthy individuals.

Autoantibodies are antibodies directed at normal cellular components, referred to as autoantigens. Most healthy individuals produce some autoantibodies, although these are usually very low level and require sensitive tests for their detection. Higher affinity autoantibodies, detectable with routine clinical tests (Box 27.1), are found in some normal people, especially women and the elderly. For example, low levels of antinuclear antibodies are seen in 20% of elderly patients.

It may seem strange that despite so many checkpoints in B cell ontogeny (Ch. 14) autoimmune responses still occur. Many of these autoantibodies are **natural antibodies**. Natural antibodies are immunoglobulins secreted by a special subset of B cells (B-1, which express CD5, see Fig. 14.11) regardless of whether or not exposure to the relevant antigen has taken place. The background to natural antibodies is discussed in Chapter 14. These B cells start life in the peritoneum and migrate to the gut and break some of the rules that normally apply to B cells: their immunoglobulin genes do not undergo gene rearrangement, they only secrete IgM, and they are able to secrete immunoglobulin without T cell help. Because B-1 cells do not alter their immunoglobulin genes in response to antigen exposure, the

immunoglobulin never improves its fit to specific antigen. This means that, although natural antibodies bind a wide number of antigens with low affinity, they never have high affinity binding to a small number of specific antigens.

Natural antibodies secreted by B-1 cells have a number of different activities (Fig. 27.2).

- Natural antibodies bind with low affinity to antigens present on a large number of bacteria. This activates complement and their physiological role is to help to clear invading bacteria rapidly. Thus, natural antibodies are acting like molecules of the innate immune system: they do not rely on genetic recombination and they are present before an infection starts.
- Natural antibodies cross-react with the inherited A and B antigens of red cells. Unless they have inherited either A or B antigens, individuals make anti-A and anti-B even if they have never been exposed to red cells from another person (Ch. 28). Humans also have natural antibodies against sugars expressed on cells of other animal species. These xenogeneic natural antibodies are discussed further in Chapter 33.
- Another consequence of their low specificity is that natural antibodies can also bind to a series of normal cellular constituents, for example nuclear proteins and DNA. This explains why some normal people have anti-nuclear antibodies. The

BOX 27.1
Tests for autoantibodies

Immunofluorescence is widely used in the diagnosis of autoimmune disease (see Ch. 5 for techniques). Direct immunofluorescence is used to detect proteins (for example IgG or complement components) that have been deposited in the tissues during a disease process. The biopsy tissue is incubated with sheep antibodies against the appropriate protein (Fig. 27.1a). The sheep antibody is conjugated to a fluorescent label, which will emit visible light when exposed to ultraviolet light under a microscope (for example, Fig. 27.13). Direct immunofluorescence is an inconvenient test because it requires the patient to have a biopsy.

Indirect immunofluorescence tests for antibodies in the serum and it does not require a biopsy. In many cases it is the preferred method of diagnosing autoimmunity. Indirect immunofluorescence uses tissue obtained from animals, such as mice, to which human autoantibodies will bind. A section of the tissue is incubated with patient's serum. Bound immunoglobulin is then detected with a sheep

continued

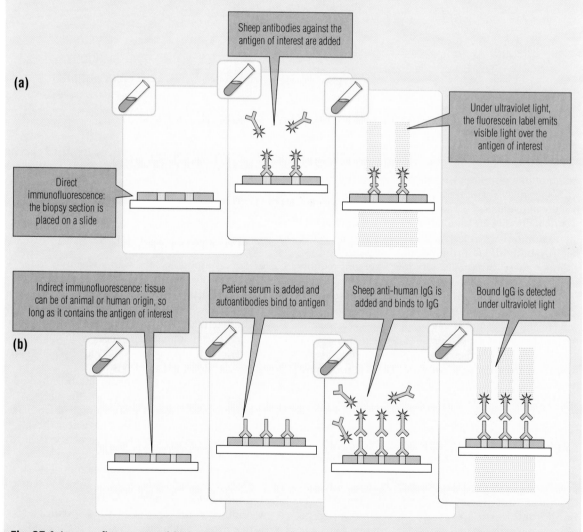

Fig. 27.1 Immunofluorescence. (a) Direct immunofluorescence looks for antigens in tissue. (b) Indirect immunofluorescence looks for antibodies in serum.

Bone marrow   Thymus   Lymph node

BOX 27.1
Tests for autoantibodies (*contd.*)

antibody conjugated to a fluorescent label (Fig. 27.1b). Islet cell (Fig. 27.7) and endomysial antibodies (Fig. 27.8) are illustrations of indirect immunofluoresence in this chapter. This technique is cheap and can often give very specific information about the specificities of autoantibodies: for example, specific types of anti-nuclear antibody (Ch. 29).

Autoantibodies can also be detected with enzyme-linked immunosorbent assays (ELISA), which use the principles described in Chapter 5. Purified antigen is required for ELISA tests. The autoantigen is linked to a solid support, usually plastic wells. The ELISA

detects the amount of patient antibody that has bound to the fixed antigen.

ELISA tests are routinely used to supplement indirect immunofluorescence testing for many diseases; for example, gliadin antibodies, detected by ELISA, are used to supplement testing for endomysial antibodies. However, not all autoantigens have been purified in sufficient quantities for ELISA testing and, although relying on older technologies, indirect immunofluorescence is likely to remain the technique of choice for diagnosing autoimmune disease.

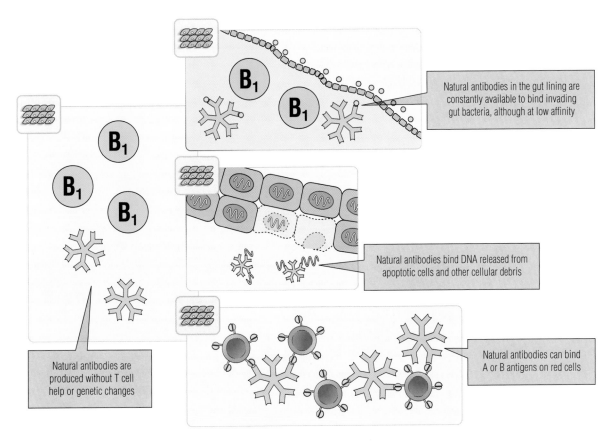

Fig. 27.2 Natural antibodies bind a range of antigens with low affinity. Natural antibodies are usually IgM pentamers.

autoantigen binding ability of natural antibodies may be an accidental consequence of cross-reactivity, but these antibodies may have a role in, for example, clearing up cellular debris.

There are also T cells which break the normal immuno-logical rules. These autoreactive T cells are able to recognize and secrete cytokines in response to autoantigens, such as MHC, and they are present in most normal individuals in very small numbers. Little is known about these T cells and there is no clear evidence for a physiological role. Autoreactive T cells must be closely regulated normally through peripheral tolerance (Ch. 14) because, even though most people have them, autoimmune disease only occurs in a minority of people.

Autoimmunity versus autoimmune disease

Autoimmune disease occurs when autoreactive T cells or autoantibodies cause tissue damage through hypersensitivity reaction types II to IV, discussed in Chapter 25. When autoantibodies cause tissue damage, they are described as being pathogenic. Unlike infectious antigens, autoantigens are almost impossible to clear, despite the immune system's best efforts; consequently, once initiated, autoimmune diseases tend to be active for a long time. Autoimmune diseases are very common and tend to cause chronic diseases. They can affect any organ system and occur at any age. Understanding how autoimmune diseases arise helps us to diagnose, treat and even prevent these problems.

One possibility is that the natural autoantibodies mentioned above cause autoimmune disease. However, there is evidence that T cells initiate autoimmune disease as follows:

- even autoimmune diseases caused by IgG-mediated mechanisms (hypersensitivity types II

and III) require T cell help in order for affinity maturation to produce pathogenic antibodies
- transfer of T cells from an animal with autoimmune disease to a healthy animal can transfer disease
- autoimmune diseases are often linked to specific MHC genes, which, of course, regulate T cells but not B cells.

There is little evidence that the B-1 cells, which secrete harmless natural antibodies, can also produce the high-affinity, specific antibodies that can cause autoimmune disease without T cell help.

For T cells to mediate autoimmune disease, they need to overcome tolerance mechanisms. Before we describe how they may do this, we offer a brief reminder about how T cells are tolerized to autoantigen.

A reminder about T cell tolerance

Tolerance prevents the immune system responding to specific antigens and has been described in Chapters 14 and 15. T cells are initially tolerized to autoantigens in the thymus; this is central tolerance. Any T cell that binds at high affinity to self peptide in the thymus will be deleted by apoptosis: **negative selection** (Fig. 27.3).

However, it is not possible for every self peptide to be expressed in the thymus, so some autoreactive T cells may escape negative selection. For example, it is unlikely that every possible peptide from a remote, complex organ like the brain is expressed in the thymus and so some brain-specific T cells may reach the periphery.

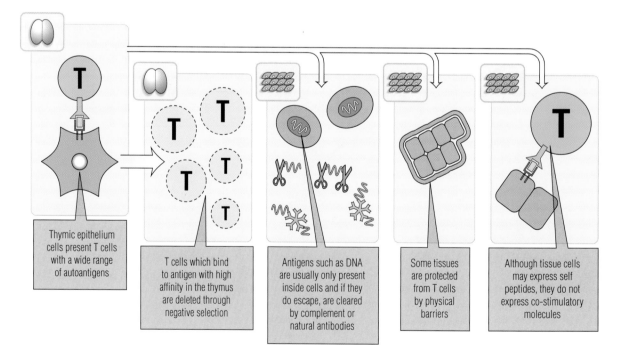

Thymic epithelium cells present T cells with a wide range of autoantigens

T cells which bind to antigen with high affinity in the thymus are deleted through negative selection

Antigens such as DNA are usually only present inside cells and if they do escape, are cleared by complement or natural antibodies

Some tissues are protected from T cells by physical barriers

Although tissue cells may express self peptides, they do not express co-stimulatory molecules

Fig. 27.3 T cell tolerance. The majority of autoreactive T cells are killed in the thymus. Peripheral tolerance and sequestration of antigens prevent T cells reacting with autoantigens in the periphery.

Bone marrow   Thymus   Lymph node

In the normal course of events, autoreactive T cells may never encounter specific antigen if it is locked away in an **immunologically privileged site**. Immunological privilege can be brought about by physical barriers that prevent entry of lymphocytes or antibody. For example, the blood–brain barrier makes the brain a "no go" area for the immune system. Alternatively there may be molecular devices that prevent immune surveillance of some tissues; testicular cells express Fas, which induces apoptosis in any T cells that manage to enter the testis.

Other autoreactive T cells may enter tissues that express specific antigen and **peripheral tolerance** normally prevents these T cells from responding. Tissue cells express MHC class I at all times and they can be induced to express MHC class II. However, autoreactive T cells emerging from the thymus also require expression of co-stimulatory molecules such as CD80 (B7) or CD40. Rather than become stimulated, naive T cells will undergo apoptosis or become anergic when they recognize antigen on non-professional antigen-presenting cells. Anergic cells remain alive, but are prevented from responding to antigen.

The breakdown of T cell tolerance

Tolerance can break down centrally or peripherally. Most evidence suggests that peripheral events are most important in humans.

Breakdown of central tolerance

Self peptides are expressed at variable levels in the thymus. For example, insulin is expressed in the normal thymus, where it tolerizes T cells through negative selection. The level of insulin expression in the thymus is genetically determined. Some individuals express low levels of thymic insulin and they are less likely to delete insulin-reactive T cells (Fig. 27.3). These individuals produce peripheral T cells that can respond to insulin and they are at higher risk of the autoimmune disease insulin-dependent diabetes (see below). Inheritance of certain MHC alleles also affects the risk of type I diabetes.

Breakdown of peripheral tolerance

Some of these breakdown mechanisms occur as a result of genetic differences, others occur as a result of environmental factors such as infections (Fig. 27.4).

Tissue cells acquire the ability to present self peptides

Professional antigen-presenting cells, such as monocytes and macrophages, are recruited to sites of infection. These cells express co-stimulatory molecules and cytokines that enable naive T cells to respond to self peptides expressed by tissue cells. In this mechanism, an appropriate inflammatory response to infection spreads to include inappropriate responses to self antigens.

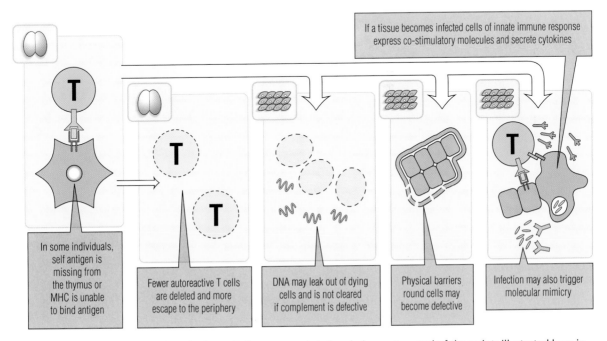

If a tissue becomes infected cells of innate immune response express co-stimulatory molecules and secrete cytokines

In some individuals, self antigen is missing from the thymus or MHC is unable to bind antigen

Fewer autoreactive T cells are deleted and more escape to the periphery

DNA may leak out of dying cells and is not cleared if complement is defective

Physical barriers round cells may become defective

Infection may also trigger molecular mimicry

Fig. 27.4 How T cell tolerance breaks down. Tolerance needs to break down at several of the points illustrated here in order for autoimmune disease to develop.

 Blood vessel   Gut   Peripheral tissue

Molecular mimicry

Molecular mimicry is used to describe a situation in which an immune response to an infection elicits antibodies or T cells that cross-react with host tissues. An example of this is acute rheumatic fever, which can occur rarely following infection with the bacterium β-hemolytic streptococcus. Patients develop a complex of symptoms including rash, heart and nervous system involvement. In these individuals, streptococcal infection induces antibodies that cross-react with heart tissue and trigger type II hypersensitivity. In this instance, streptococcal antigens mimic heart antigen. The infection is able to overcome the tolerance mechanisms that normally prevent the production of autoreactive antibodies because streptococcus activates the innate immune response, through its pattern-recognition molecules. Rheumatic fever is a transient illness and does not cause the chronic disease that is typical of most autoimmune disease. Similar bacteria can cause poststreptococcal glomerulonephritis (Ch. 25) through a very different mechanism.

Molecular mimicry has been cited as a mechanism for many other autoimmune diseases. For example, ankylosing spondylitis is a rheumatological disease that tends to occur in individuals who inherit HLA-B27. It was initially proposed that infectious agents expressed antigens that cross-reacted with HLA-B27 and that ankylosing spondylitis was caused by T cells reacting to HLA-B27. However, when researchers looked for T cells that reacted to HLA-B27 in ankylosing spondylitis patients, they were no more common than in healthy controls. Molecular mimicry is probably not solely responsible for many autoimmune diseases.

Cryptic antigens become exposed

Some molecules are normally rapidly removed from the extracellular environment. For example, DNA released by dying cells is removed by binding molecules such as mannan-binding lectin and complement component C1. The enzyme clears any residual DNA. If DNA cannot be removed by these mechanisms, it may provoke an immune response, which may be the first step in development of the autoimmune disease systemic lupus erythematosus (see Box 27.4, below).

Some antigens are normally kept physically separated from the immune system. The testis is an example of a tissue that is not usually patrolled by T cells. Following vasectomy, sperm antigens leak out of the genital system. These antigens cause the production of autoantibodies against sperm in some patients. Such patients remain infertile, even if the vasectomy is reversed, because of the anti-sperm antibodies.

Some autoimmune diseases

Insulin-dependent diabetes mellitus

Insulin-dependent diabetes mellitus (IDDM) is an example of type IV hypersensitivity. T cells invade the pancreatic islets and specifically destroy the insulin-secreting beta cells. Antibodies against beta cells and their components are produced at the beginning of the disease and these are sometimes useful in diagnosis.

If an identical twin develops IDDM, there is a 35% chance his or her twin will also do so; this is called the **concordance rate**. In Caucasians, IDDM occurs frequently in people who inherit the HLA allele *DQ2*. In most *HLA-DQ* alleles, position 57 in the HLA-DQ β-chain is occupied by an aspartic acid residue. With HLA-DQ2, this position is replaced by another amino acid residue. Figure 27.5 shows how this single amino acid residue change in the β-chain of HLA-DQ2 affects the risk of developing IDDM.

Other genes also affect the risk of diabetes. Polymorphisms affecting the expression of insulin in the thymus affect the risk of diabetes, because low expression allows insulin-reactive T cells to reach the periphery.

Even in identical twins the risk of concordance for diabetes is only 35%, so environmental factors must be very important. The likely environmental culprit is infection, which may cause low-grade inflammation in the pancreatic islets. The inflammatory signals attract innate immune system cells, which express co-stimulatory molecules and secrete cytokines. These allow antigens to be presented to autoreactive T cells (Fig. 27.6 and Box 27.2).

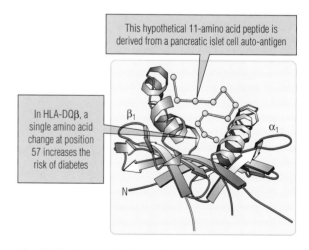

Fig. 27.5 Current thinking is that HLA-DQ2 has reduced binding for a pancreatic islet cell antigen. Autoreactive T cells cannot be deleted in the thymus and the potential for autoimmunity to increased.

Bone marrow   Thymus   Lymph node

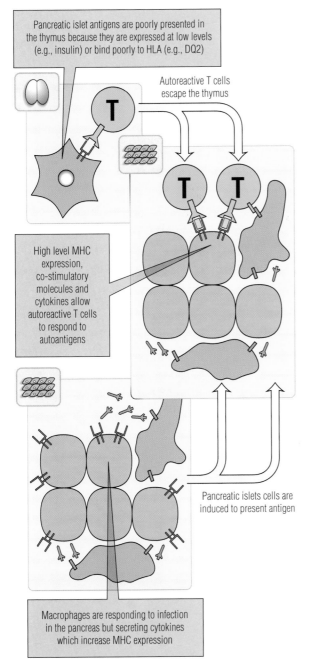

Pancreatic islet antigens are poorly presented in the thymus because they are expressed at low levels (e.g., insulin) or bind poorly to HLA (e.g., DQ2)

Autoreactive T cells escape the thymus

High level MHC expression, co-stimulatory molecules and cytokines allow autoreactive T cells to respond to autoantigens

Pancreatic islets cells are induced to present antigen

Macrophages are responding to infection in the pancreas but secreting cytokines which increase MHC expression

Fig. 27.6 Pathogenesis of insulin-dependent diabetes. In people who have inherited HLA alleles that increase the number of circulating autoreactive T cells, infection may trigger a full-scale attack on islet cells.

Celiac disease

Celiac disease is an autoimmune disease in which lymphocytes and macrophages infiltrate the jejunum. Celiac disease is, therefore, a type IV delayed hypersen-

BOX 27.2
Insulin-dependent diabetes mellitus

An 8-year-old boy has been performing poorly at school for several weeks. He is drinking large amounts of water. His mother is concerned because his older sister was diagnosed as having diabetes after having the same symptoms.

The boy has a moderately raised fasting glucose but there are no ketones in his urine; these findings are not diagnostic of diabetes. His serum is tested by indirect immunofluorescence for autoantibodies and it is shown to contain islet cell antibodies (Fig. 27.7), which are very suggestive of insulin-dependent diabetes (IDDM). He starts taking insulin and, 5 years later, has had no complications of diabetes.

The autoantibodies seen in IDDM are generally not required for the diagnosis in individuals who have high blood glucose and ketones in the urine. Their presence may help to make the diagnosis in patients with less clear features, as in this case.

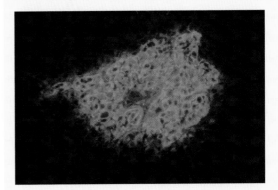

Fig. 27.7 This slide shows antibodies against pancreatic islet beta cells. Exocrine cells outside the islet do not fluoresce. Indirect immunofluorescence was used with patient's serum and normal pancreatic tissues. The other autoantibodies seen in IDDM (anti-glutamic decarboxylase and anti-insulin) are detected using enzyme-linked immunosorbent assay (ELISA). These antibodies are present in 90% of new diabetics and in high-risk relatives who go on to develop diabetes.

sitivity reaction against an exogenous antigen, gliadin, and an autoantigen, tissue transglutaminase.

- Wheat, rye and barley contain a protein called gluten, which in turn contains a polypeptide, gliadin. When gliadin is removed from the diet, the symptoms of celiac disease and jejunal histology improve.

- Tissue transglutaminase is an enzyme that converts the amino acid glutamine to glutamic acid. It can irreversibly bind to substrate peptides. Endomysial antibodies are an indirect way of detecting antibodies to tissue transglutaminase (Box 27.3).

Identical twins have a high concordance rate (75%) for celiac disease. The majority of patients with this disease have inherited the *HLA-DQ2* allele. In celiac disease, jejunal T cells recognize gliadin peptides bound to HLA-DQ2. However, pockets on the side of the peptide-binding groove on HLA-DQ2 only bind charged amino acids; gliadin will not bind unless glutamine residues have been converted to glutamic acid by tissue transglutaminase (Fig. 27.9). As a result of binding to gliadin, tissue transglutaminase itself becomes a target of autoantibodies (Fig. 27.10).

Members of the same family will often develop IDDM and celiac disease (Box 27.4). Family members may also be at higher risk of developing autoimmune thyroid or adrenal disease or gastritis. These diseases frequently co-exist in the same individuals and they are termed organ-specific autoimmune diseases.

Systemic lupus erythematosus

Systemic lupus erythematosus (SLE) is an autoimmune disease mediated by immune complexes, i.e., type III hypersensitivity. The hypersensitivity reaction in SLE is mediated by antibodies against DNA and other nuclear components such as ribonucleoproteins (Fig. 27.11).

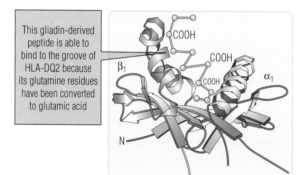

This gliadin-derived peptide is able to bind to the groove of HLA-DQ2 because its glutamine residues have been converted to glutamic acid

Fig. 27.9 Gliadin peptides bound to HLA-DQ2.

BOX 27.4
Organ-specific autoimmune disease

The HLA genes are all closely situated on chromosome 6 and they tend to be inherited as a block, called a haplotype. One relatively common haplotype consists of HLA alleles *B8, DR3* and *DQ2*. It is the inheritance of this haplotype that explains why a range of autoimmune disease occur in families. The *HLA-DQ2* allele increases the risk of IDDM and celiac disease. It is not clear which genes in the MHC are associated with the organ-specific autoimmune diseases and there are many possible candidate genes (see Figs 8.2 and 8.10).

BOX 27.3
Celiac disease

The younger sister of the diabetic patient discussed in Box 27.2 develops diarrhea and weight loss. She is shown to have mild malabsorption. Her serum is tested by indirect immunofluorescence and is found to contain IgA autoantibodies against endomysium (Fig. 27.8). ELISA testing shows that she has antibodies against gliadin. These findings are suggestive of celiac disease, and a jejunal biopsy shows she has atrophy of the villi, also consistent with this. The patient is started on a gluten-free diet and her symptoms improve dramatically. The endomysial antibodies are no longer present 6 months later.

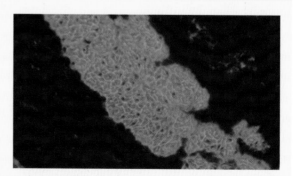

Fig. 27.8 Patients with celiac disease have autoantibodies against endomysium, connective tissue surrounding bundles of smooth muscle fibers. In the test illustrated here, the smooth muscle fibers lie in the wall of the esophagus. Endomysium is a good source of tissue transglutaminase, the autoantigen in celiac disease.

Bone marrow   Thymus   Lymph node

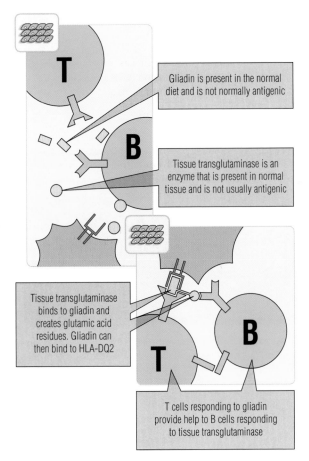

Gliadin is present in the normal diet and is not normally antigenic

Tissue transglutaminase is an enzyme that is present in normal tissue and is not usually antigenic

Tissue transglutaminase binds to gliadin and creates glutamic acid residues. Gliadin can then bind to HLA-DQ2

T cells responding to gliadin provide help to B cells responding to tissue transglutaminase

Fig. 27.10 The pathogenesis of celiac disease. Jejunal damage in celiac disease is mediated by T cells responding to deamidated gliadin, bound to HLA-DQ2. These T cells produce cytokines, such as interferon γ, which may damage villi. The pathogenic role of the antibodies produced against gliadin and tissue transglutaminase is unclear, although both antibodies are useful diagnostically.

There is a detailed description of how SLE causes disease in Chapter 29. In this chapter we are concerned with how antibodies against DNA are generated. Genes play an important role in the pathogenesis of SLE; the concordance rate for SLE in identical twins is about 60%. Two sets of genes appear to be important in the pathogenesis of SLE in humans.

Gender. In general, autoimmune diseases are more common in women, although SLE is an extreme example, affecting women 20 times more frequently than men. The higher incidence of autoimmunity in women is probably related to higher levels of the sex hormone estrogen. SLE can sometimes develop shortly after starting estrogen-containing contraceptive pills and it often gets worse during pregnancy, when estrogen levels are high. Estrogen has the physiological effect of

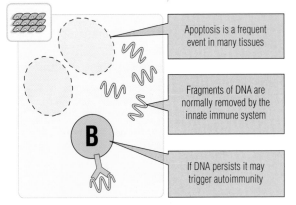

Apoptosis is a frequent event in many tissues

Fragments of DNA are normally removed by the innate immune system

If DNA persists it may trigger autoimmunity

Fig. 27.11 The pathogenesis of systemic lupus erythematosus (SLE). The role of estrogens and drugs in causing SLE is not clear.

increasing antibody production and it may thus increase autoantibody secretion. Some autoimmune diseases (for example, IDDM) affect men and women equally (see Ch. 35).

Debris clearing proteins. Some proteins of the innate immune system are involved in clearing up cellular debris. For example, MBL and C1 protein can recognize and bind fragments of DNA. These fragments are then cleared, perhaps through phagocytosis. DNA may also be cleared by an enzyme normally present in the blood: DNAse. Patients with low levels of C1q, MBL or DNAse are at higher risk of SLE, presumably because DNA produced as a result of cell death is able to trigger production of anti-DNA antibodies.

Overview of autoimmune disease

In this chapter, we have illustrated the pathogenesis of autoimmune disease. The risk of autoimmune disease is conferred by inheritance of one or more genes that impair tolerance mechanisms. Infection is probably the most important environmental factor trigger. Understanding how these factors interact helps us to develop strategies for improved diagnosis, treatment and prevention of autoimmune disease.

Diagnosis

Although many autoantibodies do not cause damage, they are a useful diagnostic tool for autoimmune disease. When the molecular basis for autoimmunity is known, very specific tests may be developed. For example, the autoantibodies in celiac disease were originally described as binding to endomysium. We now know that these antibodies react with tissue transglutaminase. New ELISAs, using tissue transglutaminase as an antigen, are being evaluated for diagnosing celiac disease.

BOX 27.5
Systemic lupus erythematosus

A 34-year-old woman develops painful swollen wrist joints and a rash on her face (Fig. 27.12). A skin biopsy is taken for direct immunofluorescence. It is shown to contain IgG and complement deposits (Fig. 27.13). These findings are diagnostic of systemic lupus erythematosus. This case history is continued in Chapter 29.

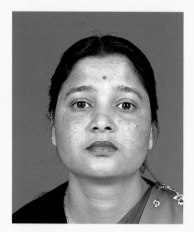

Fig. 27.12 The butterfly rash is characteristic of systemic lupus erythematosus. (Courtesy of Dr R. Cerio, Royal London Hospital, UK.)

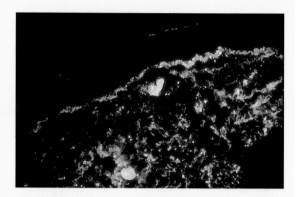

Fig. 27.13 Direct immunofluorescence can be useful in the diagnosis of systemic lupus erythematosus because it can show deposits of IgG and complement in the skin. Just how these deposits are formed is discussed in Chapter 29. (Courtesy of Dr R. Cerio, Royal London Hospital, UK.)

Treatment

Now that we know the amino acid sequences of the peptides that bind to HLA-DQ2 in celiac disease, we may be able to develop therapies based on blocking peptides (Fig. 27.14). Such peptides are being investigated in celiac disease.

Prevention

Members of the family of a patient with IDDM are at risk of diabetes themselves, especially if they have anti-islet cells or anti-glutamic acid decarboxylase antibodies. Because these high-risk individuals can now be identified with some certainty, various studies have investigated ways of preventing the onset of clinical diabetes. Strategies such as immunosuppressive drugs can delay the onset of diabetes, but soon after the drugs are stopped (they are too toxic to be used for long periods of time) the disease becomes apparent.

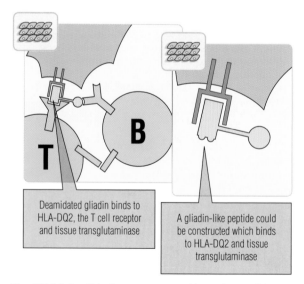

Deamidated gliadin binds to HLA-DQ2, the T cell receptor and tissue transglutaminase

A gliadin-like peptide could be constructed which binds to HLA-DQ2 and tissue transglutaminase

Fig. 27.14 Peptide therapy may enable patients with celiac disease to have normal diets. Note that the constructed peptide binds HLA-DQ2 but is not recognized by the T cell receptors.

Bone marrow   Thymus   Lymph node

LEARNING POINTS

Can you now:

- List what evidence there is for autoimmunity in normal, healthy individuals?
- Describe the origin and function of natural antibodies?
- Describe how the immune system tolerates most autoantigens and how tolerance can break down?
- Using the examples of insulin-dependent diabetes, celiac disease and systemic lupus erythematosus, describe how genes and environmental factors work together to cause autoimmune disease?
- Describe how immunofluorescence tests and ELISAs are used to detect autoantibodies?
- Contrast direct and indirect immunofluorescence?

 Blood vessel   Gut   Peripheral tissue

Antibody-mediated hypersensitivity (type II)

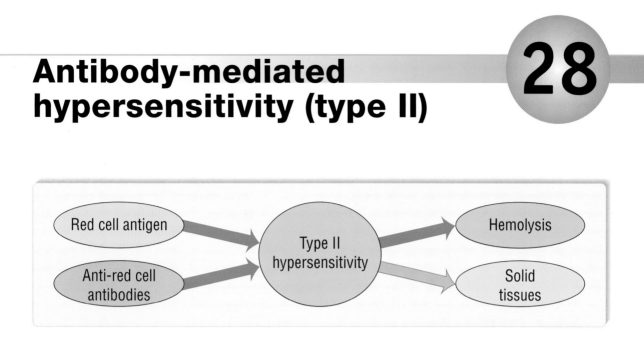

Type II hypersensitivity reactions are a consequence of IgG or IgM binding to the surface of cells. Antibody binding frequently damages red blood cells, either through activation of complement or because the antibodies opsonize the target erythrocytes. This is referred to as immune-mediated hemolysis. Antibody binding may also damage solid tissues. The antigen may then be cellular or part of the extracellular matrix (for example, basement membrane). Less often, antibodies may modify the function of cells by binding onto receptors for hormones, which we illustrate with autoimmune thyroid disease and Wegener's granulomatosis. Hyperacute graft rejection is also a version of type II hypersensitivity and this is discussed in Chapter 33.

IMMUNE-MEDIATED HEMOLYSIS

Causes

Red cell antigens

Red cells express a variety of antigens some of which are alleles inherited in a Mendelian fashion (Fig. 28.1).

The rhesus blood group system consists of three loci, C, D and E, of which D is the most important. Most individuals express a D locus antigen and so they are **rhesus positive**. About one in six people are homozygous for a null D allele; they express no D antigen and so they are **rhesus negative**. D is a conventional protein antigen and rhesus negative individuals make IgG anti-D after exposure to the antigen.

The A and B blood group antigens are sugar molecules inherited in a co-dominant fashion: an individual can inherit the A antigen (blood group A), the B antigen (blood group B), both A and B (blood group AB) or a null allele (blood group O). The A and B antigens are similar to sugars expressed on bacteria. Anti-A

and anti-B are natural antibodies (Ch. 27), physiologically produced as a defense against bacteria and capable of cross-reacting with A or B red cell antigens. Hence individuals who are blood group O, and have inherited neither A nor B antigen, will produce IgM against A and B, whether or not they have been exposed to these antigens.

Other antigens are non-allelic—the same molecule is expressed by everyone. For example the I antigen is expressed by adults on the surface of red cells. I behaves as a regular self antigen and should not normally elicit anti-I antibodies.

Antigens of the ABO and rhesus systems are alloantigens: they differ from person to person. The antibodies produced against these antigens can cause type II hypersensitivity when cells are transferred from one individual to another, for example in blood transfusion or during pregnancy.

Antigens of the rhesus and I systems can act as autoantigens. They can cause type II hypersensitivity when they become targets of autoimmunity.

Anti-red cell antibodies

IgM antibodies against red cell antigens are produced as natural antibodies against A and B or as auto antibodies against I in some types of autoimmune hemolytic anemia (AIHA; see below). IgM antibodies are very effective at activating complement, causing damage through activation of the membrane attack complex (Fig. 28.2).

IgG antibodies are produced against rhesus antigens, either as a response to allogeneic stimulation (Box 28.1) or in some types of AIHA (see below). IgG is not very effective in activating complement and does not cause haemolysis in the circulation. Instead, IgG-coated red cells are recognized by Fc receptors on resident macrophages in the liver and spleen. These macrophages

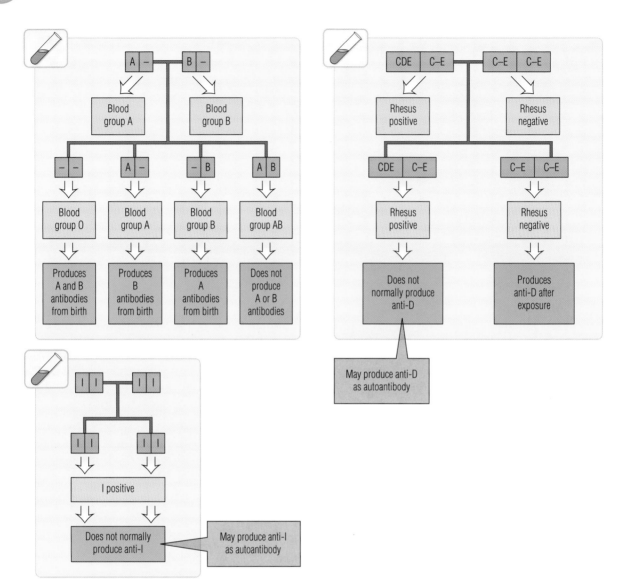

Fig. 28.1 Genes (orange), antigens (yellow) and antibodies (blue) involved in the blood group systems. Alloantibodies are produced spontaneously against A and B, and after exposure to D. D and I may become targets for autoantigens.

are stimulated by bound cells to phagocytose fragments of the red cells, which are damaged in the process.

Types of immune-mediated hemolysis

Alloimmune hemolysis

The rhesus antigens behave like a conventional antigen: exposure is required in order to produce IgG antibody. This most frequently occurs in pregnancy when rhesus antibodies cross the placenta and cause hemolytic disease of the newborn (Box 28.1).

Incompatibility in the ABO system is the commonest cause of serious blood transfusion reactions. For example, an A-positive individual requiring a transfusion will possess natural antibodies against B-positive cells. If B-positive cells are inadvertently transfused, they will be rapidly hemolysed in the circulation. The hypersensitivity reaction can take place within seconds of the donor cells entering the recipient.

Units of blood for transfusion contain mainly red cells and very little antibody-containing plasma. The recipient's antibodies and the donor's red cell antigens must be checked for compatibility prior to transfusion. A Coombs' test (Box 28.2) is used to check that the recipient does not have antibodies that may bind donor cells. In emergencies, when the laboratory does not have time to determine the recipient's blood group, O cells, which have neither A nor B antigens, can be used for transfusion into any type of recipient.

Bone marrow   Thymus   Lymph node

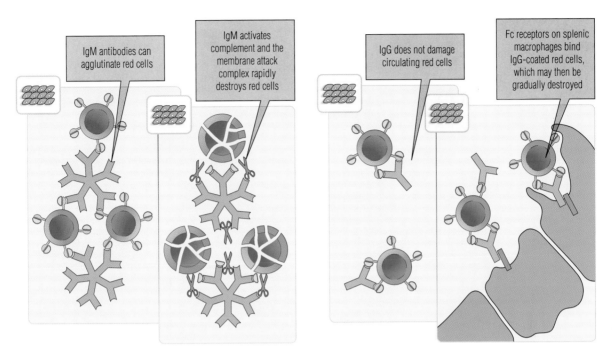

Fig. 28.2 Mechanisms of immune hemolysis. IgM antibodies are more dangerous than IgG antibodies in immune hemolysis.

BOX 28.1
Hemolytic disease of the newborn

A woman presents to the antenatal clinic at 28 weeks of pregnancy. She is a refugee from a developing country. In the past she has had two miscarriages in midpregnancy. Over the next few weeks the pregnancy runs smoothly, but the woman is found to be rhesus blood group negative. Further tests show that she has antibodies to the rhesus D antigen. At 34 weeks of pregnancy an ultrasound scan shows signs of fetal distress. Labor is induced and a baby girl is born. She is profoundly anemic. A Coombs' test on the baby's blood is positive, confirming the diagnosis of hemolytic disease of the newborn.

If a rhesus-negative woman carries a rhesus-positive fetus, she will produce antibodies if fetal cells leak into the maternal circulation. This can occur during pregnancy and following miscarriage. In our patient, the previous miscarriages were not the result of rhesus incompatibility, but they sensitized the mother to produce antibodies (Fig. 28.3). The IgG antibodies produced crossed the placenta and bound fetal red cells, which were then destroyed in the fetal spleen and liver.

The treatment for hemolytic disease of the newborn is exchange transfusion, a technique that replaces fetal red cells with donor rhesus-negative cells.

Hemolytic disease of the newborn is entirely preventable through the use of anti-D injections (Fig. 28.4).

Anti-A or anti-B antibodies only very rarely cause hemolytic disease of the newborn, because IgM natural antibodies are not actively transported across the placenta.

continued

 Blood vessel | Gut | Peripheral tissue

BOX 28.1
Hemolytic disease of the newborn (*contd.*)

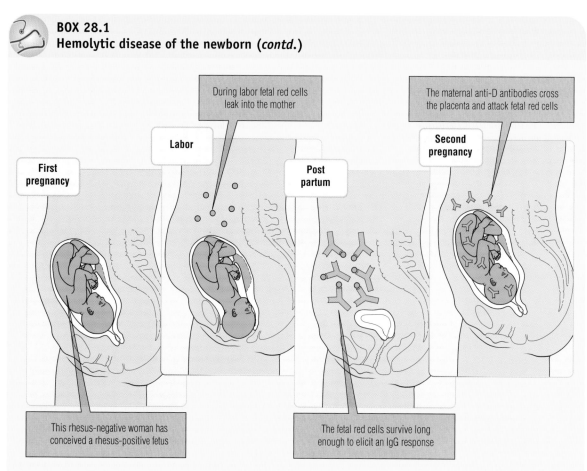

During labor fetal red cells leak into the mother

The maternal anti-D antibodies cross the placenta and attack fetal red cells

Labor

Second pregnancy

First pregnancy

Post partum

This rhesus-negative woman has conceived a rhesus-positive fetus

The fetal red cells survive long enough to elicit an IgG response

Fig. 28.3 Hemolytic disease of the newborn.

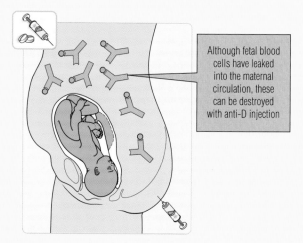

Although fetal blood cells have leaked into the maternal circulation, these can be destroyed with anti-D injection

Fig. 28.4 Anti-D antibody should be given to rhesus-negative women after the birth of a rhesus-positive child or following a miscarriage. Anti-D destroys rhesus-positive fetal cells in the maternal bloodstream before she has an opportunity to make her own anti-D, which can affect the next pregnancy. Anti-D is a type of passive immunotherapy and it can prevent hemolytic disease of the newborn when used appropriately.

Bone marrow   Thymus   Lymph node

BOX 28.2
Coombs' test

Coombs' test is used to determine when cells are coated with antibody (direct Coombs' test) or to identify when there are antibodies capable of binding red cells (indirect Coombs' test).

The direct test is used, for example, to test whether red cells are coated with alloantibodies in a child affected by hemolytic disease of the newborn. The red cells are incubated with an anti-human IgG. If the red cells are coated with immunoglobulin the red cells will be agglutinated by the animal antibody (Fig. 28.5). The indirect Coombs' test can be used to check whether a blood transfusion recipient has pre-existing antibodies that may bind donor cells. This is the basis of cross-matching for blood transfusion.

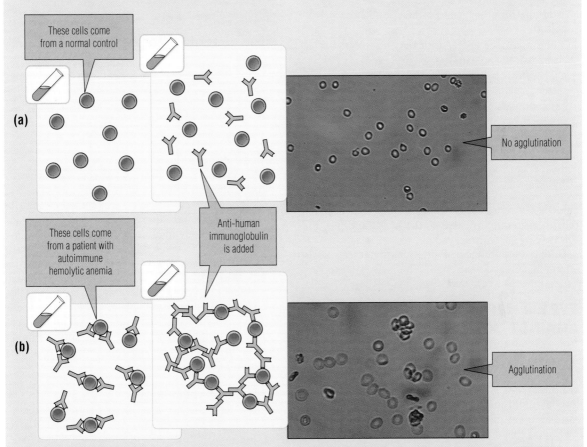

These cells come from a normal control

(a)

No agglutination

These cells come from a patient with autoimmune hemolytic anemia

Anti-human immunoglobulin is added

(b)

Agglutination

Fig. 28.5 The Coombs' test. (a) The direct test detects cells coated with IgG in vivo. (b) The indirect test detects antibodies that could bind cells.

Autoimmune hemolysis

Autoimmune hemolytic anemia (AIHA) can be triggered by infections or drugs (see Box 25.2) or it can be part of generalized autoimmune diseases such as systemic lupus erythematosus (see Ch. 29). Autoantibodies can also be produced by malignant clones of B cells in diseases such as chronic lymphatic leukemia or lymphoma. However, most cases of AIHA are not explained. Red cell antigens can become targets for IgG and IgM autoantibodies.

The commonest type of AIHA is caused by IgG autoantibodies against rhesus antigens. The antibody-coated red cells are only slowly removed by the spleen and the onset of anemia is gradual (Box 28.3).

The I antigen is generally the target when IgM antibodies cause AIHA. Much more rapid and dangerous intravascular hemolysis occurs as a result of complement activation. Another feature of IgM antibodies is that they often bind red cells best at temperatures

BOX 28.3
Autoimmune hemolytic anemia

A 45-year-old woman has developed increasing fatigue over 3 weeks. She is jaundiced and the spleen is enlarged. A blood count shows features of hemolysis. A direct Coombs' test shows her red cells are coated with IgG.

There is no evidence of underlying disease or infection and the patient has received no drugs, so the cause remains unexplained: this is referred to as **idiopathic** autoimmune hemolytic anemia (AIHA).

She is initially treated with corticosteroids. These function in AIHA by inhibiting the phagocytosis by macrophages in the liver and spleen. After 6 weeks on steroids, her condition has continued to deteriorate. She undergoes a splenectomy, after which her hemoglobin returns to normal.

The hazards of splenectomy are discussed in Box 13.1.

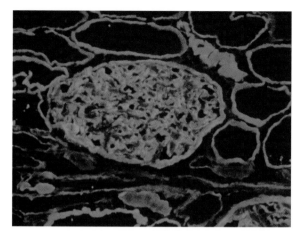

Fig. 28.6 Indirect immunofluoresence has been used to detect autoantibodies in this patient with Goodpasture's syndrome. Kidney tissue is used as the target antigen for this test. There is linear staining along the glomerular basement membrane.

below 37°C. These cold hemagglutinins can cause red cells to aggregate in vessels in the hands and feet and this may cause ischemic damage.

Similar alloimmune and autoimmune processes can affect platelets and neutrophils.

TYPE II HYPERSENSITIVITY AGAINST SOLID TISSUES

Autoantibodies can also attack and damage components of solid tissues. For example, in Goodpasture's syndrome, IgG autoantibodies bind a glycoprotein in the basement membrane of the lung and glomeruli. Antibasement membrane antibody activates complement and this can trigger an inflammatory response. Goodpasture's sydrome damages the basement membrane, leading to bleeding in the lungs (hemoptysis) and glomeruli (hematuria) and acute renal failure. Anti-basement membrane antibody can be detected by indirect immunofluorescence (Fig. 28.6) and can be removed by plasmapheresis (see below).

TYPE II HYPERSENSITIVITY AND STIMULATORY ANTIBODIES

In other situations, antibodies bind to cells and stimulate their activity. We illustrate this with Graves' disease and Wegener's granulomatosis.

Graves' disease

Graves' disease is the commonest cause of hyperthyroidism, often affecting young women (Box 28.4) with a family history. Graves' disease is linked to the HLA allele *DR3*. In Graves' disease, the thyroid is stimulated by an autoantibody that binds onto the thyroid-stimulating hormone receptor (Fig. 28.8). Graves' disease is thus a special type of type II hypersensitivity. In pregnant women with Graves' disease, IgG thyroid-stimulating antibody can cross the placenta and causes transient neonatal hyperthyroidism. Graves' disease is associated with exophthalmos (protruding eyes) resulting from T cells infiltrating the orbit of the eye. Exophthalmos is thought to be caused by an orbital antigen that cross-reacts with a thyroid antigen (Box 28.4).

Wegener's granulomatosis

A much rarer disease is Wegener's granulomatosis, a type of blood vessel inflammation (**vasculitis**) affecting the nose, lungs and glomeruli. Patients with Wegener's granulomatosis have autoantibodies that react with proteinase 3, a proteolytic enzyme present in neutrophils (Box 28.5). These autoantibodies are referred to as classical anti-neutrophil cytoplasmic antibodies (cANCA) and they produce a typical indirect immunofluorescence pattern (Fig. 28.9a). Proteinase 3 is normally present in the cytoplasm, but when neutrophils are activated, for example by cytokines released during infections, it is expressed on the cell surface. Proteinase 3 then becomes accessible to cANCA antibodies, which bind neutrophils, inhibit migration and stimulate the oxidative burst, cytokine and enzyme release. Neutrophils damage vessels in Wegener's granulomatosis by being immobilized in

 Bone marrow   Thymus   Lymph node

BOX 28.4
Graves' disease

A 62-year-old woman complains of increasing anxiety and restlessness. Her doctor notices that she has an enlarged thyroid gland and fast pulse: both signs of hyperthyroidism. In addition she has exophthalmos (Fig 28.7). Blood tests show that her thyroid gland is overactive and she has autoantibodies to thyroid peroxidase and the thyroid-stimulating hormone receptor. These are diagnostic of Graves' disease.

She is treated with anti-thyroid drugs and her symptoms improve.

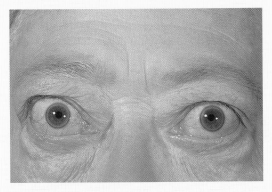

Fig. 28.7 This woman with Graves' disease has exophthalmos (protruding eyes) because of swelling of the orbital soft tissue. (With permission from the Department of Medical Illustration, St Bartholomew's Hospital, London.)

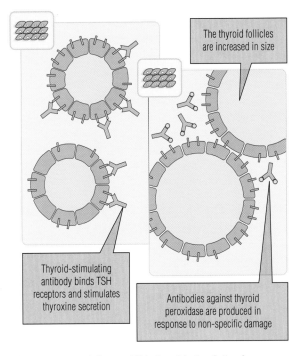

The thyroid follicles are increased in size

Thyroid-stimulating antibody binds TSH receptors and stimulates thyroxine secretion

Antibodies against thyroid peroxidase are produced in response to non-specific damage

Fig. 28.8 Graves' disease. TSH, thyroid-stimulating hormone.

vessel walls and then triggering inflammation. Why the nose, lungs and glomeruli are particularly affected is not clear.

A second set of anti-neutrophil cytoplasmic antibodies (ANCA) produce a perinuclear pattern on immunofluorescence (pANCA) and tend to react with a second neutrophil enzyme, myeloperoxidase (MPO). These pANCA/MPO antibodies are also associated with vasculitis, which tends to affect the glomeruli and not other organs (Fig. 28.9b).

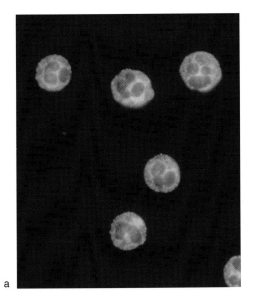

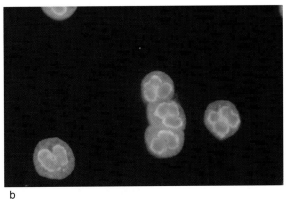

Fig. 28.9 Anti-neutrophil cytoplasmic antibodies (cANCA). These images show indirect immunofluorescence using patient serum on normal neutrophils. (a) cANCA (anti-proteinase 3) seen in Wegener's granulomatosis. (b) pANCA (anti-myeloperoxidase) seen in patients with other forms of vasculitis.

 Blood vessel Gut Peripheral tissue

BOX 28.5
Wegener's granulomatosis

A 40-year-old lady presents in acute renal failure. She has a history of nasal stuffiness and nose bleeds. Ulcerated lesions are present in the nose. Renal biopsy shows glomerulonephritis. A serum sample reacts with neutrophil cytoplasm on indirect immunofluorescence (Fig. 28.9a). Further ELISA testing shows the patient's serum reacts with proteinase 3. These abnormalities are consistent with a multiorgan vasculitis called Wegener's granulomatosis, and the patient's kidney function improved with plasmapheresis. At the same time, the autoantibodies disappeared from her blood.

PREVENTION AND TREATMENT OF TYPE II HYPERSENSITIVITY

Allogeneic hemolytic reactions are preventable. Transfusion reactions can be prevented by carefully checking the donor and recipient are compatible and that the recipient has no antibodies that could react with donor red cells (cross-matching). Hemolytic disease of the newborn is preventable by ensuring that rhesus-negative women receive anti-D after miscarriage or labor.

When type II hypersensitivity is mediated by IgM, such as during an ABO-incompatible blood transfusion, it is very hard to block the effector mechanism. This is because complement activation takes place very rapidly and there are no safe, effective complement-blocking drugs.

Treatment of IgG-mediated type II hypersensitivity aims to reduce autoantibody levels or prevent effector cells from causing damage.

Although some immunosuppressive drugs can reduce B cell autoantibody secretion, this approach is not particularly successful in type II hypersensitivity. Plasmapheresis (Fig. 28.10) reduces autoantibody levels, but is uncomfortable and time consuming for patients and is reserved for situations where antibody needs to be rapidly removed, such as Wegener's granulomatosis and Goodpasture's syndrome.

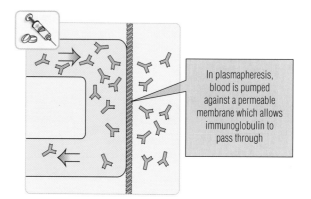

In plasmapheresis, blood is pumped against a permeable membrane which allows immunoglobulin to pass through

Fig. 28.10 Treatment of type II hypersensitivity by plasmapheresis.

LEARNING POINTS

Can you now:

- List the antigens involved in auto- and allo-immune hemolysis?
- Explain how IgG and IgM antibodies can cause hemolysis?
- Describe how autoantibodies cause hyperthyroidism?
- Explain how autoantibodies cause the symptoms of Wegener's granulomatosis?
- List which tests are used to diagnose these autoimmune diseases?
- List preventive actions and treatments for type II hypersensitivity diseases?

Bone marrow   Thymus   Lymph node

Immune complex disease (type III hypersensitivity)

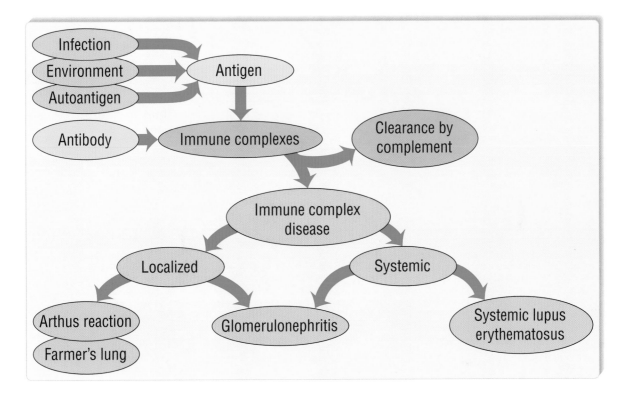

Immune complexes are lattices of antigen and antibody; they may be localized to the site of antigen production or circulate in the blood. They are produced as part of the normal immune response and are usually cleared by mechanisms involving complement, as described below. Immune complexes cause disease in a number of situations.

Antigens in immune complexes

For immune complexes to develop, antigen must be present for long enough to elicit an antibody response. Immune complexes usually form when antigen is in excess of antibody (Fig. 29.1). Immune complexes may form when antigen is produced from one of three sources:

- infectious antigens
- innocuous environmental antigens
- autoantigens.

Infectious antigens

Most infections are short lived and controlled by the immune response. Even in such rapidly controlled

infections, immune complexes may cause hypersensitivity, for example after streptococcal infection (see Ch. 25). Infections such as hepatitis B are not always controlled and can cause sustained high levels of antigen in blood (**antigenemia**), resulting in more chronic disease.

Innocuous environmental antigens

Harmless environmental antigens can elicit an IgG response if they are small enough to enter the tissues. A good example is fungal spores, which cause the localized immune complex disease farmer's lung (Box 29.1). Drugs are also environmental antigens and sometimes cause localized immune complexes, for example the **Arthus reaction** (Box 29.2).

Drugs can also cause circulating immune complexes. This leads to a disorder referred to as **serum sickness**. The name was coined in the period before antibiotics were available, when patients with infections were given immune horse serum. Nowadays, serum sickness most often happens as a result of the occasional use of mouse monoclonal antibodies to treat cancer or autoimmune

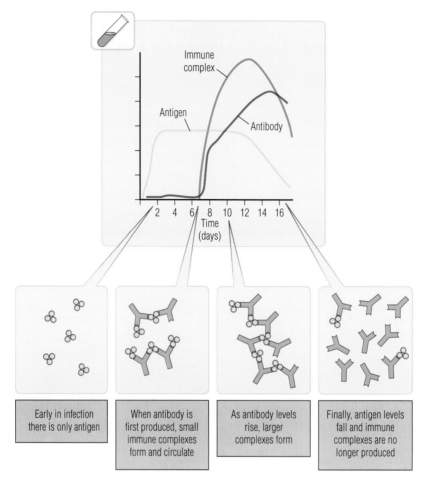

Fig. 29.1 Small immune complexes form when antigen is in excess and more likely to enter the circulation.

disease (Ch. 30). Repeated exposure leads to production of anti-mouse antibodies and circulating immune complexes. Serum sickness then causes fever, rash and joint pains. This problem can be overcome by genetically manipulating the mouse antibodies in order to humanize them.

Autoantigens

Autoantigens can only cause immune complex disease in the presence of autoantibodies. DNA is an antigen in systemic lupus erythematosus (SLE; Box 29.3). DNA is released into the circulation when cells die, especially if innate immune system mechanisms usually responsible for clearing DNA are defective (see Ch. 27). DNA that is not rapidly cleared is able to elicit an antibody response.

Antibodies in immune complexes

IgG in immune complexes activates effectors such as complement as well as macrophages and neutrophils,

through their Fc receptors. IgG antibodies capable of forming immune complexes can be detected in precipitin assays. In these tests, immune complexes form between the test antigen and antibodies from patient's serum (Fig. 29.6).

Clearance of immune complexes

Immune complexes form in normal individuals when antibodies are produced at high levels during infections. The immune complexes must be cleared or they will cause disease through the mechanisms described below. Two mechanisms involving complement clear immune complexes (also see Ch. 19).

Complement breaks down large soluble complexes

Immune complexes of antigen and immunoglobulin contain high numbers of immunoglobulin Fc in close proximity, which activates complement through the

Bone marrow   Thymus   Lymph node

BOX 29.1
Farmer's lung

A 23-year-old farmer complains of breathlessness, cough, malaise and fever on several occasions after feeding his cattle. The symptoms develop several hours after exposure to hay and last about 2 days. A blood sample shows he has precipitating IgG antibodies against mold extract (Fig. 29.6). In addition, his symptoms are reproduced 5 hours after deliberate challenge with mold spores in hospital, confirming a diagnosis of farmer's lung. He is instructed to breathe through a filter mask when handling hay and his symptoms do not recur.

Patients with farmer's lung produce IgG antibodies against proteins in mold spores. Immune complexes form in the lungs after exposure to spores. Over several hours these immune complexes trigger inflammation in the alveoli. (Fig. 29.2). The process is very different from IgE-mediated hypersensitivity, which produces immediate symptoms on exposure to antigen and does produce fever or symptoms outside the lungs.

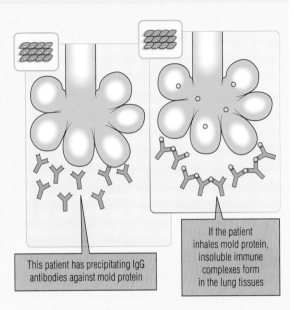

This patient has precipitating IgG antibodies against mold protein

If the patient inhales mold protein, insoluble immune complexes form in the lung tissues

Fig. 29.2 Farmer's lung.

BOX 29.2
The Arthus reaction

A drunk medical student has lacerated his leg and he is in the emergency room to have the wound sutured. His last tetanus vaccine was just over 5 years earlier. In accordance with hospital policy, a booster tetanus vaccination is given, although, in the resulting struggle, this is inadvertently given intradermally. Twelve hours later, a painful lesion at the site of the vaccination wakes him from his sleep (Fig. 29.3). This is an Arthus reaction.

Vaccines are usually given intramuscularly in order for the antigen to diffuse into the lymphoid system. Antigens injected intradermally cannot diffuse out rapidly. The purpose of tetanus booster vaccination is to maintain high antibody levels in individuals who repeatedly injure themselves. Our medical student, therefore, had a local depot of antigen and pre-existing antibodies. Immune complexes formed in situ and activated complement, mast cells and neutrophils, triggering a very localized type III hypersensitivity reaction.

The Arthus reaction develops more slowly than the immediate type I hypersensitivity reaction, but faster than the delayed type IV hypersensitivity reaction.

Thus, the delay in onset of a skin reaction to exogenous antigens gives important clues to the nature of the mediators. IgE-mediated reactions occur within 5 minutes, immune complexes cause symptoms after 12 hours or so and T cell lesions develop 2 to 3 days after exposure.

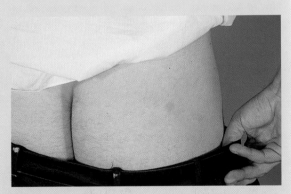

Fig. 29.3 The Arthus reaction takes 12 hours to develop because immune complexes must form in situ and then activate mast cells and neutrophils. (With permission from the Department of Medical Illustration, St Bartholomew's Hospital, London.)

 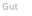

BOX 29.3
Systemic lupus erythematosus

A 34-year-old woman with joint pains and a rash has been diagnosed with systemic lupus erythematosus (SLE; see Box 27.5). Indirect immunofluorescence shows her blood contains an anti-nuclear antibody (Fig. 29.4) and ELISA (enzyme-linked immunosorbent assay) testing shows she has a high level of antibodies against DNA. Her joint pains initially respond well to non-steroidal anti-inflammatory drugs and her rash improves when she avoids strong sunlight.

One year later, at the rheumatology clinic, she mentions that her joint pain is now much worse. Routine urine testing shows a high level of protein and her renal function is deteriorating. Because SLE can cause a range of different renal problems, a

biopsy is carried out. Direct immunofluorescence shows deposits of complement and IgG in the glomeruli, consistent with immune complex disease (Fig. 29.5). The findings are similar to those from the skin biopsy carried out earlier (Fig. 27.13). Conventional microscopy shows that she has a cellular inflammatory infiltrate in the glomerulus. The prognosis for this kind of renal disease in SLE is poor. The patient was treated with several intravenous courses of the immunosuppressive drug cyclophosphamide and her renal function and joint problems improved considerably.

The joint, skin and kidney involvement are very typical of circulating immune complex disease. In addition to joint, skin and kidney involvement, SLE can affect the central nervous system and placenta, the latter causing miscarriage.

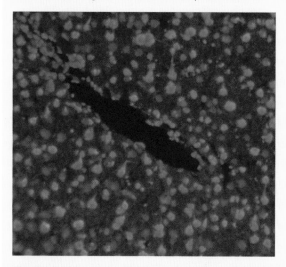

Fig. 29.4 This is an indirect immunofluorescence slide showing anti-nuclear antibody. The patient's serum is reacted with rat liver in this test.

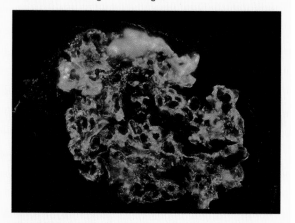

Fig. 29.5 This is a direct immunofluorescence slide showing IgG deposited in the kidney of a patient with systemic lupus erythematosus. For direct immunofluorescence, tissue from the patient is required.

classical pathway (Fig. 29.7). Small molecular components, especially activated C3, are produced through activation of the complement pathway. These molecules insert themselves into, and break up, the lattice of the immune complex.

Complement receptor 1 transfers complexes to phagocytes

Red cells transfer circulating immune complexes from tissues and blood to the phagocytes of the liver and spleen. Red cells express complement receptor 1 (CR1), the receptor for activated C3. Immune complexes bind to the complement receptor CR1 on red cells, which then circulate through the liver and

spleen. In the liver and spleen, receptors take up the immune complexes and, in doing so, stimulate the macrophages to phagocytose them (Fig. 29.7). This mechanism is very efficient and can entirely remove immune complexes from the circulation in a few minutes. Furthermore, because the spleen is home to a large population of B cells, antigens originally present in the periphery are rapidly presented to B cells to boost antibody production.

Failure of clearance

These immune complex clearance mechanisms can be saturated in situations where there is excessive, ongoing production of immune complexes, for

 Bone marrow   Thymus   Lymph node

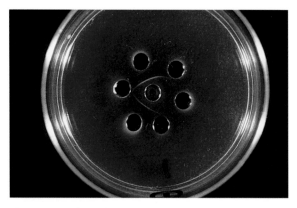

Fig. 29.6 In this gel precipitation assay, patient's serum is placed in the central well and mold (*Micropolysporum faeni*) spore protein in a peripheral well. The contents of the wells diffuse towards one another. If there are precipitating IgG antibodies against the mold proteins, a precipitin line will form. This is also exactly what happens in the alveoli of patients with farmer's lung.

example in antigenemia resulting from chronic infection. Some individuals lack complement and, because the mechanisms described cannot function, they are predisposed to immune complex disease (Box 19.4).

Mechanisms of inflammation

Immune complexes not cleared rapidly cause damage by activating components of the innate immune system (Fig. 29.8).

- Complement is activated by immune complexes. Although this process helps to clear complexes, low-molecular-weight anaphylatoxins are produced, which increase permeability of blood vessels and are chemotactic for leukocytes.
- Complexes bind onto, and activate, cells such as neutrophils, mast cells and platelets. Neutrophils and mast cells release proteolytic enzymes, which damage blood vessels and initiate inflammation. Activated platelets bind to the endothelium and form thrombi.

If antigen is present predominantly at one site, immune complexes cause localized damage, for example the Arthus reaction (Box 29.2) and farmer's lung (Box 29.1). Small complexes, produced when antigen is in excess, enter the circulation and form circulating immune complexes. Circulating complexes cause damage to blood vessels, ranging from inflammation of the vessel walls to occlusion of the vessel and ischemic damage. Immune complex disease is one cause of vessel inflammation (**vasculitis**). Circulating immune complexes cause damage at specific sites, especially the kidney, skin and joints.

Immune complex disease in the kidney

Involvement of the kidney in type III hypersensitivity is a common cause of renal failure. The kidney is often affected because blood pressure in the glomerulus is four times higher than that in the systemic circulation. High blood pressure increases immune complex

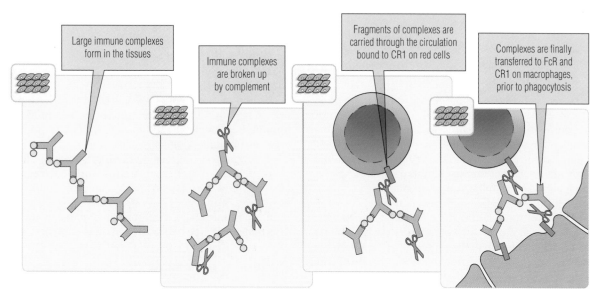

Large immune complexes form in the tissues

Immune complexes are broken up by complement

Fragments of complexes are carried through the circulation bound to CR1 on red cells

Complexes are finally transferred to FcR and CR1 on macrophages, prior to phagocytosis

Fig. 29.7 Clearance of immune complexes. Red cells are not damaged when immune complexes are transferred to macrophages. CR1, complement receptor 1; FcR, Fc receptor.

Blood vessel   Gut   Peripheral tissue

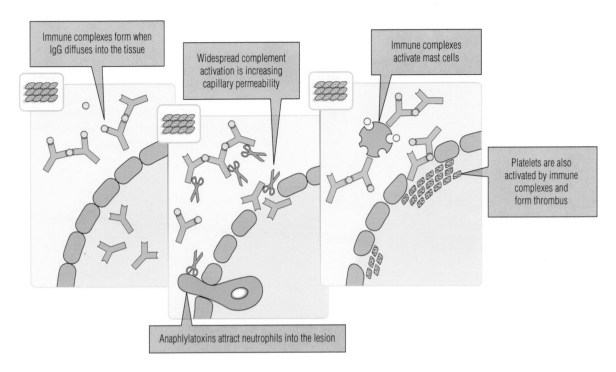

Immune complexes form when IgG diffuses into the tissue

Widespread complement activation is increasing capillary permeability

Immune complexes activate mast cells

Platelets are also activated by immune complexes and form thrombus

Anaphlylatoxins attract neutrophils into the lesion

Fig. 29.8 Immune complexes cause damage by activating the innate immune system.

deposition in vessel walls. Glomerular cells express the complement receptor CR1, which may predispose to immune complex deposition at this site. Synovial cells also express CR1, which may explain why joints are also often involved in circulating immune complex disease.

Immune complex disease in the kidney can result in two clinically defined syndromes:

- **nephrotic syndrome**, in which protein leaks into the urine and there is gradual onset renal failure
- **nephritis**, in which there is rapid-onset renal failure, blood and protein in the urine and hypertension.

Both types of disease are produced by inflammation in the glomeruli (**glomerulonephritis**). In the nephrotic syndrome, immune complexes are deposited in the glomerular basement membrane where they activate complement (Fig. 29.9). This usually causes subtle damage to the basement membrane, which allows proteins to leak into the urine. In nephritis, by comparison, there is a cellular infiltrate in addition to complement activation. Neutrophils are attracted into the glomeruli and the resulting inflammation causes blood and protein to leak into the urine, impairing the ability of the kidney to excrete toxic metabolites. Which type of glomerular lesion is produced depends on several factors, including the size of immune complexes, the rate at which they are produced and the duration of immune complex production.

In poststreptococcal glomerulonephritis, the renal disease is dramatic but short lived because infection is brought under control by the immune response. When drugs cause immune complex-mediated kidney disease, stopping the drug improves kidney function. In SLE, the immune complexes contain autoantigens and so the renal disease has gradual onset but is not self-limiting (Box 29.3).

Immune complexes are not the only immunological cause of glomerulonephritis. Renal damage can also occur in Wegener's granulomatosis and Goodpasture's syndrome (Ch. 28) and when immunoglobulin light chains damage the kidney in multiple myeloma (Ch. 34).

The immunology work-up is crucial in the investigation of nephritis and the nephrotic syndrome. Indirect immunofluoresence is used to find antibodies implicated in immune complex disease (for example anti-DNA antibodies) or other types of autoantibody, for example anti-neutrophil cytoplasmic antibody (cANCA) and anti-glomerular basement membrane antibody. Sometimes it is necessary to do direct immunofluorescence on a renal biopsy specimen to determine what type of process is causing damage.

Treatment of immune complex disease

Antigen avoidance is possible in some cases of type III hypersensitivity, for example, farmer's lung or some drugs and vaccines. In the case of autoantigens, however (for example, DNA), avoidance is clearly not possible.

In autoimmune causes of immune complex disease, corticosteroids block some of the damage caused by effector cells, for example neutrophils. Cyclophosphamide is an alkylating agent that impairs DNA synthesis and prevents rapid proliferation of cells such as lymphocytes. Although cyclophosphamide has some effects on T cells, its main benefit is in reducing B cell proliferation and hence autoantibody levels. Cyclophosphamide is often used in severe SLE.

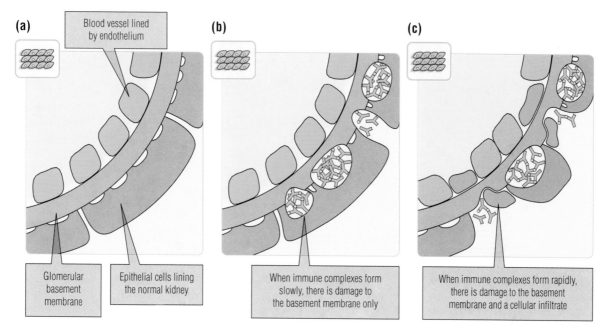

(a)
Blood vessel lined by endothelium

Glomerular basement membrane

Epithelial cells lining the normal kidney

(b)
When immune complexes form slowly, there is damage to the basement membrane only

(c)
When immune complexes form rapidly, there is damage to the basement membrane and a cellular infiltrate

Fig. 29.9 Nephrotic syndrome. (a) A normal glomerulus. (b) Slow complex formation, for example in hepatitis B virus infection. (c) Rapid complex formation, for example following streptococcal infection.

LEARNING POINTS

Can you now:

- Describe the antigens and antibodies that cause immune complexes?
- Explain how immune complexes are normally cleared?
- Describe the pathogenesis of farmer's lung, as an example of local immune complex disease?

- Describe the pathogenesis of SLE as an example of systemic autoimmune disease?
- Contrast direct and indirect immunofluorescence in the diagnosis of SLE?
- Explain why the kidney is frequently involved in immune complex disease?
- Describe two clinical outcomes of immune complex disease in the kidney?

Blood vessel　　　Gut　　　Peripheral tissue

Delayed hypersensitivity (type IV)

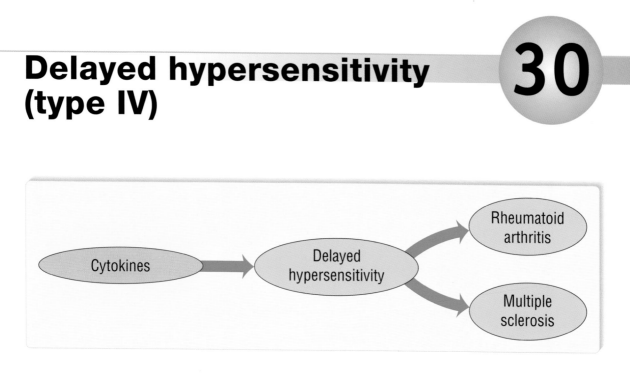

Delayed hypersensitivity was originally defined as reactions taking place 2–3 days after exposure to antigen, for example tuberculin skin testing (Box 22.4). We now know that delayed hypersensitivity is characterized by T helper 1 (T_H1) cells driving inflammatory responses mediated by macrophages.

Delayed hypersensitivity can be a physiological reaction to pathogens that are hard to clear, for example, hepatitis B virus and *Mycobacterium tuberculosis*. Mycobacterial infections trigger the most extreme delayed hypersensitivity reactions, which are characterized by granuloma formation, extensive cell death and the appearance of caseous necrosis (Ch. 22).

Delayed hypersensitivity can also occur in response to innocuous environmental antigens such as nickel in some cases of contact dermatitis. These antigens must have a low molecular weight in order to enter the body. The very small size of these substances means that they must act as **haptens** in order to become antigenic. Contact dermatitis occurs as a result of exposure to a wide range of other chemicals including cosmetics and, normally harmless, plant extracts (for example, poison ivy).

Delayed hypersensitivity reactions also take place against autoantigens. For example, in insulin-dependent diabetes (Ch. 27) T cells respond to pancreatic islet cell antigens, damaging the islets and eventually preventing insulin secretion.

Delayed hypersensitivity reactions are driven by T_H1 cells

In Chapter 20 we described how delayed hypersensitivity reactions are initiated when tissue macrophages recognize the presence of danger signals and initiate the inflammatory response. Dendritic cells, loaded with antigen, migrate to local lymph nodes where they present antigen to T cells. Specific T cell clones proliferate in response to antigens and these migrate to the site of inflammation. T cells and macrophages stimulate one another through the cytokine network (Ch. 22). Tumor necrosis factor (TNF) is secreted by both macrophages and T cells and stimulates much of the damage in delayed hypersensitivity (Fig. 30.1).

Because of the need for antigen presentation by T cells, delayed hypersensitivity reactions are often associated with very specific HLA alleles, as in insulin-dependent diabetes and celiac disease (Ch. 27).

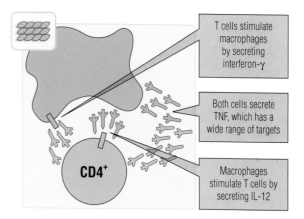

Fig. 30.1 Tumor necrosis factor (TNF) mediates many of the clinical features of delayed hypersensitivity reactions, for example rheumatoid arthritis. IL, interleukin.

Type IV hypersensitivity disease

In this chapter, we discuss two other common auto-immune diseases caused by delayed hypersensitivity: rheumatoid arthritis (RA) and multiple sclerosis (MS). Celiac disease and insulin-dependent diabetes were discussed in Chapter 27.

Rheumatoid arthritis

RA is a common disabling condition. In RA, the synovial membrane lining both joints and tendon sheaths is swollen up to 100 times its normal size. The synovium is infiltrated by chronic inflammatory cells including T cells and macrophages (Box 30.1). The inflammatory process is driven by the T cells, although it is not yet proven what antigen these are responding to. There is some evidence that the synovial T cells are responding to **heat shock proteins** (HSP). HSPs were first discovered in bacteria, where they are produced in response to heat and other stress. Very similar bacterial HSPs are found in human cells, and it is possible that infection triggers a response against bacterial HSP which then directs T cells against human HSP. This mechanism would represent a type of molecular mimicry (Ch. 27).

Cytokines secreted by T cells and macrophages in the synovium cause the majority of symptoms in RA (Fig. 30.4). Although RA is predominantly a delayed hypersensitivity reaction, T cell cytokines stimulate B cells in the synovium to produce rheumatoid factor. This autoantibody is a natural antibody: it can be produced without any T cell help. Rheumatoid factor is frequently produced during chronic infections, presumably as a bystander effect of T cell cytokines. Hence rheumatoid factor is not specific for RA. In RA, rheumatoid factor may produce immune complexes within the joint, adding to the inflammation.

Multiple sclerosis

MS is a severe disease; 50% of patients will be disabled within 15 years of onset. Early in MS, there are recurrent bouts of inflammation affecting different parts of the central nervous system (CNS). Later in MS, there is progressive disease and the myelin sheath, which surrounds and insulates neurons, is destroyed.

BOX 30.1
Rheumatoid arthritis

A 50-year-old man complains of a 6 month history of pain in his hands, wrists and feet. The pain is worse in the morning, when his joints are stiff for an hour or so. The small joints in his hand are swollen and tender (Fig. 30.2). He is making an acute phase response with an elevated sedimentation rate and C reactive protein. A radiograph of his hands shows erosions (Fig. 30.3), typical of rheumatoid arthritis. His blood also contains rheumatoid factor: IgM anti-IgG autoantibodies. These are not diagnostic of rheumatoid arthritis but they do indicate a poor prognosis.

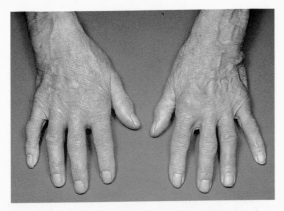

Fig. 30.2 Swelling of the metacarpophalangeal and proximal interphalangeal joints is characteristic of rheumatoid arthritis. (With permission from the Department of Medical Illustration, St Bartholomew's Hospital, London.)

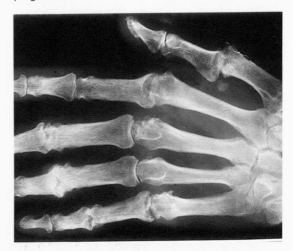

Fig. 30.3 This radiograph shows erosions—areas of "bitten out" bone along the joint margins of the metacarpophalangeal joints—in rheumatoid arthritis. (With permission from the Department of Medical Illustration, St Bartholomew's Hospital, London.)

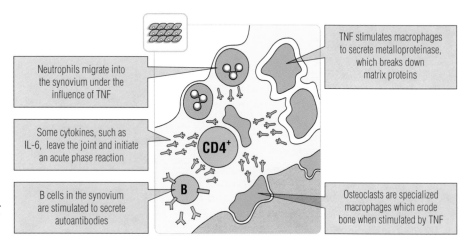

Fig. 30.4 Most of the features of rheumatoid arthritis are attributable to the effects of cytokines. IL, interleukin; TNF, tumor necrosis factor.

Labels in figure:
- Neutrophils migrate into the synovium under the influence of TNF
- Some cytokines, such as IL-6, leave the joint and initiate an acute phase reaction
- B cells in the synovium are stimulated to secrete autoantibodies
- TNF stimulates macrophages to secrete metalloproteinase, which breaks down matrix proteins
- Osteoclasts are specialized macrophages which erode bone when stimulated by TNF
- CD4⁺
- B

MS affects about 1 per 1000 people in Northern Europe and central North America. In more tropical areas, the prevalence is much lower. Individuals that move from lower to higher risk areas have an increased risk of developing MS, suggesting that environmental factors are more important than genes for the geographical variation in prevalence. Two strands of evidence support infections as being the environmental trigger for MS:

- demyelination is very occasionally seen following documented infections, such as measles
- in patients with MS, infections can precipitate exacerbations of symptoms.

Genes are involved to a lesser extent in MS; the concordance rate amongst identical twins is only 30%.

Initially in MS there are acute attacks of inflammatory lesions consisting of T cells and macrophages in the affected nervous tissue. The inflammatory lesions cause the reversible, relapsing disability typical of early MS (Fig. 30.5 and Box 30.2).

The chronic disability in MS is the result of another process—demyelination. Demyelinated nerve cells are no longer able to conduct impulses and they cannot always recover.

There are also B cells in the CNS that secrete antibodies against myelin basic protein. In equivocal cases, the demonstration of antibody production in the CNS can help to make a diagnosis of MS. Between attacks, there is usually recovery of function, at least early in the disease.

(b)

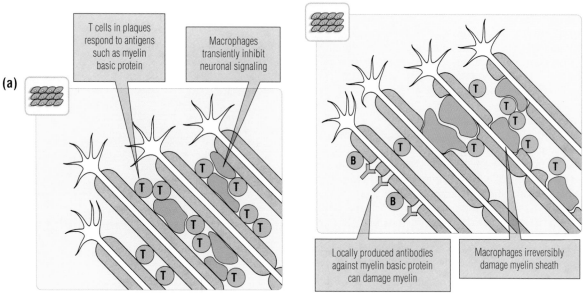

(a)

Labels in figure:
- T cells in plaques respond to antigens such as myelin basic protein
- Macrophages transiently inhibit neuronal signaling
- Locally produced antibodies against myelin basic protein can damage myelin
- Macrophages irreversibly damage myelin sheath

Fig. 30.5 Multiple sclerosis. The lesions in acute relapsing (a) and chronic progressive (b) multiple sclerosis are different.

BOX 30.2
Multiple sclerosis

A 22-year-old woman complains of visual impairment in her left eye. Six months earlier she had noticed numbness and tingling in both legs for approximately 3 weeks. A magnetic resonance imaging (MRI) brain scan is performed and this shows many lesions in the white matter (Fig. 30.6). The diffuse, asymmetrical lesions are consistent with the patchy inflammation that is seen in MS, and a diagnosis of probable MS is made. Over the next few weeks her vision improves, but after 18 months she develops leg weakness. An MRI scan at this time reveals new white matter lesions. The findings of patchy neurological disease affecting different parts of the nervous system at different times is very suggestive of MS.

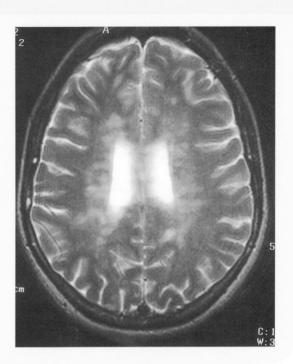

Fig. 30.6 This magnetic resonance brain scan shows plaques of demyelination. (Courtesy of Dr J. Evanson, Royal London Hospital, UK.)

Treatment

In delayed hypersensitivity it is sometimes possible to avoid environmental antigens, for example, some types of contact dermatitis are improved by avoiding exposure to nickel. In celiac disease, avoiding dietary gluten improves symptoms and reduces levels of anti-endomysium antibodies. In these examples, an exogenous antigen is driving an autoimmune disease. Where the cause is an endogenous antigen, treatment is more complex. Options currently used are anti-inflammatory and immunosuppressive drugs.

Anti-inflammatory drugs

Anti-inflammatory drugs work by cutting down the mediators released during inflammation, usually by cells of the innate system (Fig. 30.7). For example nonsteroidal anti-inflammatory drugs (such as indometacin) inhibit arachidonic acid metabolism (Ch. 21).

Corticosteroids have some effects in MS, but only at high, intravenous doses. Corticosteroids probably work in MS by reducing the actions of macrophages (Box 30.3). Corticosteroids are of some value in RA but are too toxic for long-term use.

All these drugs have serious side-effects and, furthermore, they do not alter the immune response to environmental or autoantigens.

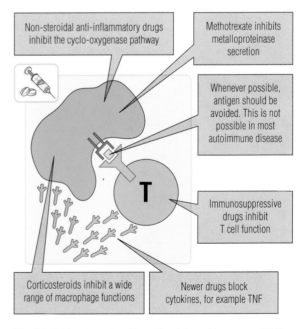

Non-steroidal anti-inflammatory drugs inhibit the cyclo-oxygenase pathway

Methotrexate inhibits metalloproteinase secretion

Whenever possible, antigen should be avoided. This is not possible in most autoimmune disease

Immunosuppressive drugs inhibit T cell function

Corticosteroids inhibit a wide range of macrophage functions

Newer drugs block cytokines, for example TNF

Fig. 30.7 Treatment options for delayed hypersensitivity.

BOX 30.3
The therapeutic role of corticosteroids

Endogenous corticosteroids suppress the immune response during physiological stress. Corticosteroids are often used as immunosuppressive drugs during the treatment of autoimmunity, allergy and following transplantation. Their effects are mediated by affecting gene transcription when used at low to moderate doses. Corticosteroids bind specific receptors, which transport them to the nucleus and are responsible for binding to regulatory gene sequences. At higher doses they affect cell signaling directly.

Although corticosteroids are thought to affect the transcription of 1% of all genes in a wide range of cells, their dominant therapeutic effects are on phagocytes. Effects on lymphocytes may largely be a result of poor antigen processing and co-stimulation provided by phagocytes.

The side-effects of corticosteroids are well known. From the immunological point of view, immunosuppression is a particular concern and it may result in reactivation of infections normally controlled by macrophages, for example, tuberculosis.

BOX 30.4
Blocking the effects of tumor necrosis factor

TNF is a key cytokine in delayed hypersensitivity reactions, for example RA. Three strategies have been developed to prevent TNF binding to receptors on cells involved in the inflammatory response (Fig. 30.8).

- Mouse monoclonal antibodies can prevent TNF binding to its receptor. However, patients produce antibodies against the mouse-specific epitopes on the immunoglobulin. These neutralizing antibodies prevent the anti-TNF from working and this can cause serum sickness-like reactions (see Ch. 29).
- Chimeric antibodies are engineered to combine mouse and human fragments; chimeric anti-TNF antibodies are very effective—up to 80% of patients with RA have clinical improvements. Although the risks of anti-mouse antibodies are reduced with chimeric antibodies, this monoclonal

continued

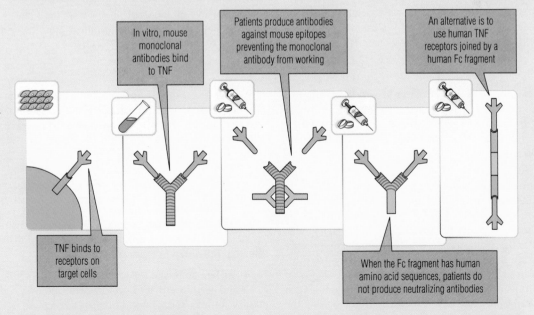

> In vitro, mouse monoclonal antibodies bind to TNF

> Patients produce antibodies against mouse epitopes preventing the monoclonal antibody from working

> An alternative is to use human TNF receptors joined by a human Fc fragment

> TNF binds to receptors on target cells

> When the Fc fragment has human amino acid sequences, patients do not produce neutralizing antibodies

Fig. 30.8 Monoclonal antibodies can block the effects of tumor necrosis factor (TNF) in rheumatoid arthritis; for example, the formation of new erosions is prevented.

 Blood vessel   Gut   Peripheral tissue

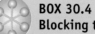

BOX 30.4
Blocking the effects of tumor necrosis factor (*contd.*)

antibody is recommended for use in combination with methotrexate, an immunosuppresive drug.

- A different strategy has been to make recombinant TNF receptor/Fc molecules, to mop up TNF. These are constructed using human protein sequences to overcome problems with neutralizing antibodies. These molecules are also effective in RA.

TNF has a physiological role in combating infections. One concern over drugs that block the effects of TNF is that they may predispose to infections. Some patients have developed tuberculosis following TNF-blocking drugs. These drugs are also very expensive, and, unfortunately, are not available for many patients with RA.

BOX 30.5
Supplementing the effects of a beneficial mediator: interferon-β

Recombinant IFN-β has benefits in some patients with MS and delays the development of acute attacks of nervous system inflammation. There is still not enough experience to say whether IFN-β has long-term benefits and can prevent the chronic disability associated with demyelination.

You will remember from Chapter 19 that the type I interferons (IFN-α and IFN-β) have potent antiviral effects and weaker immunostimulatory effects (increasing antigen presentation and activating natural killer cells). It is not clear exactly how IFN-β works in MS, but there are two possible explanations:

- reduction of TNF secretion: this is an unexpected finding since IFN-β only weakly interacts with components of the immune system and other TNF-blocking strategies can worsen MS

- prevention of viral infections that could trigger off episodes of MS.

No matter how it works, there are some important drawbacks with IFN-β treatment for MS. Firstly, IFN-β activates the acute phase response and patients often complain of fever. Second, if patients produce anti-IFN-β antibodies, treatment stops being effective. IFN-β is produced using recombinant technology in non-human cells; because these cells do not add sugar molecules to the IFN-β molecule in the same way as human cells, recombinant IFN-β is antigenic. When technology is used to make the recombinant IFN-β molecule resemble the human molecule, the risk of developing neutralizing antibodies is reduced by 50%. Finally, like most recombinant proteins, IFN-β is very expensive.

New approaches are looking at specific mediators in the immune process and attempting either to block harmful effects (e.g., those of TNF (Box 30.4)) or to mimic useful effects (e.g., interferon-β (IFN-β; Box 30.5)).

Immunosuppressive drugs

Immunosuppressive drugs inhibit the specific immune response that drives delayed hypersensitivity and are most relevant in autoimmune delayed hypersensitivity, when antigen cannot be avoided. Immunosuppressive drugs are dealt with in Chapter 33 as they are most often used in transplant recipients. The benefits of immunosuppressive drugs must be balanced against their dangerous side-effects, particularly increasing the risk of infection. For example, in insulin-dependent diabetes, pancreatic islet cell function can be maintained while patients receive immunosuppresive drugs.

However, the drugs would have to be given for life and the side-effects are unacceptable; insulin replacement is a safer option. Immunosuppressive drugs have not been widely tested in MS.

Some hypersensitivity reactions are driven by mixed mechanisms

The Gell and Coombs classification of hypersensitivity (Ch. 25) is an oversimplification and many diseases overlap the different types. For example:

- the late phases of the type I reactions in asthma and atopic dermatitis are characterized by T cell infiltrates, more typical of type IV reactions
- although MS and RA are both type IV reactions, autoantibodies (anti-myelin basic protein and rheumatoid factor) play an important role.

 Bone marrow   Thymus   Lymph node

Other diseases mix hypersensitivity to environmental antigens and autoantigens:

- in celiac disease, there is a hypersensitivity reaction to an environmental antigen but also features of autoimmunity, such as antibodies to tissue transglutaminase.

Understanding the different types of hypersensitivity gives clues to the diagnosis and treatment of these important conditions. For example, diagnosis by finding autoantibodies and therapeutic use of plasmapheresis are appropriate in Wegener's granulomatosis, but not in RA.

Immunologically mediated drug reactions

Drug reactions are common, affecting up to 15% of hospital patients. The majority of reactions are predictable and directly related to the pharmacological effects of the drug. For example, if a patient is given an incorrectly high dose of a sedative drug, they will sleep for longer than expected. Other side-effects are less predictable and these are described as being **idiosyncratic**. Some of these reactions may occur when a patient lacks an enzyme responsible for metabolizing a drug. For example, a patient that has low levels of the appropriate metabolizing enzyme will experience excessive sleepiness even after the correct dose of sedative.

Idiosyncratic drug reactions also commonly have an immunological basis. Some of these effects are mediated by the innate immune system, for example, morphine can stimulate mast cell degranulation, leading to histamine release and the development of the itchy rash urticaria. Reactions can also involve the adaptive system and they can cause any type of hypersensitivity (Fig. 30.9). These reactions only occur after a patient has previously been exposed to a drug so that antibodies or reactive T cells can develop.

It is important to diagnose the cause of these reactions, because repeat exposure can lead to life-threatening reactions. Laboratory tests can provide indirect evidence of immunological hypersensitivity. For example, elevated blood mast cell tryptase levels suggest mast cell involvements through innate mechanisms or type I hypersensitivity. Direct tests such as specific IgE testing (Ch. 26) are not often helpful, because the patient may be reacting to one of several metabolites, rather than the drug itself.

Fig. 30.9
Immunologically mediated drug reactions

Hypersensitivity type	Reaction	Useful test
I	Anaphylaxis to penicillin	Specific IgE test (Ch. 27)
		Skin prick testing (with caution!)
II	Drug-induced hemolysis	Coombs' test (Ch. 28)
III: localized	Arthus reaction to vaccines	Antibody levels (Ch. 29)
III: circulating complexes	Serum sickness with monoclonal antibodies	
IV	Contact dermatitis to antibiotic-containing cream	Patch testing (Ch. 25)

LEARNING POINTS

Can you now:

- Recall how delayed hypersensitivity reactions rely on the cytokine network?
- Describe the pathogenesis, diagnosis and treatment of the common disorders multiple sclerosis and rheumatoid arthritis?
- Describe the benefits and problems of recombinant proteins, such as interferon-β and anti-tumor necrosis factor monoclonal antibodies, being used in delayed hypersensitivity?
- Describe the benefits and limitations of corticosteroids in delayed hypersensitivity?
- Describe how the Gell and Coombs classification of hypersensitivity is used to diagnose and treat a wide range of disorders?

 Blood vessel Gut ▦ Peripheral tissue

Primary immunodeficiency

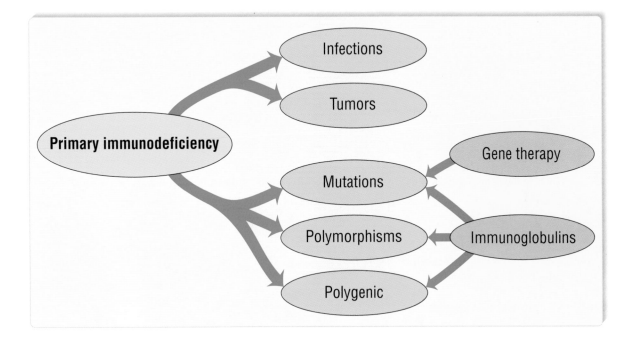

Significance of immunodeficiency

Immunodeficiency results in an increased risk of opportunist infections and tumors. Two types are recognized:

1. *Primary immunodeficiencies* have a genetic basis and are relatively rare
2. *Secondary immunodeficiency* is more common and is caused by lesions outside the immune system; in these cases, treating the external problem, for example chronic lymphocytic leukemia, will improve the immune response.

Infections provide clues to the type of immunodeficiency

Repeated or unusual infection is an important sign of immunodeficiency. The type of infection gives clues to the cause and degree of immunodeficiency (Fig. 31.1).

Repeated bacterial infection is a sign of defective antibody production, as antibody is a key player in the eradication of extracellular organisms. A typical example is recurrent respiratory infection caused by *Pneumococcus* or *Haemophilus* spp., which leads to irre-

versible damage to the bronchi: bronchiectasis. Infections with staphylococci, Gram-negative organisms and fungi are characteristic of a reduced number or abnormal function of phagocytes. For unknown reasons, some complement defects predispose to meningococcal meningitis (Ch. 19).

Defective T cells or macrophages tend to predispose to infection with intracellular organisms such as protozoa, viruses and intracellular bacteria, including mycobacteria and salmonella (Fig. 31.1). Reactivation of latent herpesvirus infection is particularly linked to T cell immunodeficiency. Recurrent attacks of cold sores or shingles may suggest mild immunodeficiency. Herpesvirus-induced tumors, notably Kaposi's sarcoma (human herpes virus 8) and non-Hodgkin's lymphoma (Epstein–Barr virus), are characteristic of T cell dysfunction and these are discussed further in Chapter 34.

The degree of T cell immunodeficiency is also reflected in patterns of mycobacterial infection (Fig. 31.1). *Mycobacterium tuberculosis* is a virulent organism causing lung infection in immunocompetent people. In mild T cell immunodeficiency, the same organism spreads outside the lungs. More severe immunodeficiency will predispose to widespread infection with

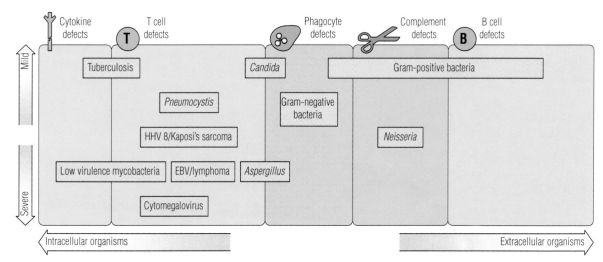

Fig. 31.1 Repeated or unusual infection suggests the presence of immunodeficiency. The type of opportunist infection also gives clues to the degree and cause of immunodeficiency. EBV, Epstein–Barr virus; HHV, human herpesvirus.

mycobacteria of low virulence normally found in the environment (for example, *Mycobacterium avium intracellulare* complex) or in vaccines (e.g., BCG).

Causes of primary immunodeficiency

The causes of primary immunodeficiencies can be classified as:

- mutations: rare, affect any part of the immune system and cause severe disease
- polymorphisms: very common traits, affect any part of the immune system and cause a moderate increased risk of infection
- polygenic disorders: relatively common, affect mainly antibodies and cause severe disease.

Mutations and immunodeficiency

There are approximately 12 important mutations in genes for the innate and adaptive immune systems that cause immunodeficiency (Figs 31.2 and 31.3). Many mutations result in **severe combined immunodeficiency** (SCID), which refers to a group of disorders affecting both T and B cells. Some of these disorders are autosomally inherited (e.g., RAG deficiency; see Box 7.1) and there may be a family history of consanguinity (marriage of related individuals). Others are X-linked (e.g., γ-chain deficiency (Box 12.3) and the hyper-IgM syndrome (Box 16.3)) and there may be a history of early deaths in maternal uncles (Box 31.1). The Di George syndrome (Fig. 31.3; see also Box 15.1) is caused by a large part of chromosome 22 being translocated to other chromosomes and is not usually inherited.

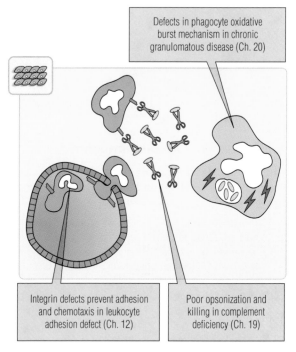

Defects in phagocyte oxidative burst mechanism in chronic granulomatous disease (Ch. 20)

Integrin defects prevent adhesion and chemotaxis in leukocyte adhesion defect (Ch. 12)

Poor opsonization and killing in complement deficiency (Ch. 19)

Fig. 31.2 Defects in the innate immune system are characterized by infections with extracellular pathogens.

Polymorphisms and immunodeficiency

Genetic polymorphisms are alleles (different forms) of the same gene occurring at a single locus in at least 1% of the population. Eye color is a good example of genetic polymorphism. HLA alleles are polymorphic

Bone marrow   Thymus   Lymph node

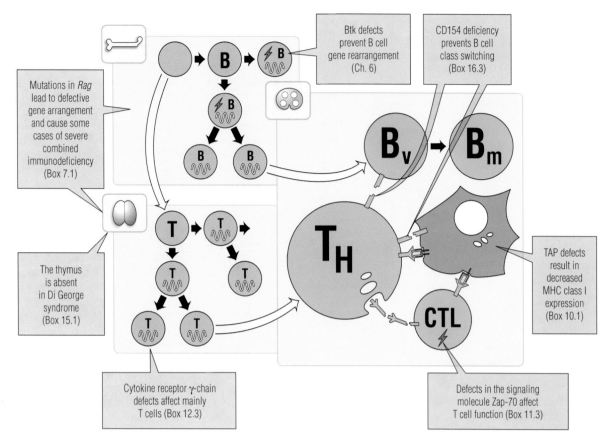

Fig. 31.3 Disorders with mainly T cell defects, for example, Di George syndrome and Zap-70 and Jak defects, present soon after birth with infections with intracellular pathogens. B cell disorders, for example, X-linked agammaglobulinemia, present around 6 months, when maternal antibody levels have fallen. Btk, Bruton's tyrosine kinase; CTL, cytotoxic T lymphocytes, TAP, transporter associated with antigen presentation.

and do affect the outcome of infections including hepatitis B, hepatitis C and human immunodeficiency virus (HIV) (Box 3.1). Individuals with HLA alleles that are unable to bind viral peptides have a worse outcome. Polymorphisms of the promoter for tumor necrosis factor (TNF) genes (associated with risk of cerebral malaria and septic shock; Ch. 22) and chemokines and their receptors (associated with risk of HIV; Ch. 32) are discussed elsewhere.

Mannan-binding lectin (MBL) is a collagen-like protein that binds sugars in bacterial cell walls and activates the classical complement pathway (Ch. 19). Polymorphisms in MBL and complement affect the risk of infections (Fig. 31.4). The effects of polymorphisms on individuals are small and may only be discovered in studies on populations.

Polymorphisms persist in different frequencies in different populations, affected by prevalent infections. The best known example lies outside the immune system. The hemoglobin S polymorphism (sickle cell anemia) protects against malaria and is more common in populations living in, or with origin in, malarious zones.

Polygenic disorders

Polygenic disorders are caused by the interaction of several genes, with a contribution from environmental factors. **Common variable immunodeficiency** (CVID) and deficiencies of IgA and IgG subclasses are common polygenic disorders affecting mainly antibody production. **IgA deficiency** affects about 1 in 600 people, although why infections are only seen in about one third of patients is unclear. Celiac disease (Ch. 27) is more common in patients with IgA deficiency.

CVID occurs in about 1 in 20 000 young people, affecting men and women equally. CVID is the commonest immunodeficiency requiring treatment. Patients have low levels of total IgG, although other findings (for example, levels of IgA, IgM, numbers of B and T cells) are variable. CVID is a convenient label for what will probably emerge as a heterogeneous group of diseases. CVID causes recurrent bouts of infection of the respiratory tract, starting in early adult life. Infections involving the gut, skin and nervous system are also common (Box 31.2). Autoimmunity is

BOX 31.1
Clinical challenges in severe combined immunodeficiency

The critical challenge in severe combined immunodeficiency (SCID) is recognition of the signs of immunodeficiency early enough to prevent life-threatening infections. A diagnosis of SCID should be considered if a patient has:

- unusual or recurrent infection
- failure to thrive and diarrhea
- unusual rashes
- a family history of neonatal death or of consanguinity
- a very low total lymphocyte count (below $1 \times 10^9/l$ ($10^3/\mu l$)).

If SCID is suspected and HIV infection has been excluded, the infant should be referred to a specialist center where the diagnosis will be confirmed and definitive treatment given (often bone marrow transplant). Until this can be done, the following simple steps are taken to avoid serious infection:

- avoid live vaccines, including BCG, measles, mumps, rubella and polio
- use prophylaxis against opportunist infections, for example, *Pneumocystis carinii* pneumonia.

common in CVID and frequently includes pernicious anemia and thyroid disease, arthritis and immune thrombocytopenia.

The genetic loci in IgA deficiency and CVID are not known but they may include the HLA genes. Although 25% of patients have a family history of either CVID or IgA deficiency, environmental factors are also important. Anti-rheumatic and anti-convulsant drugs have been implicated in precipitating both IgA deficiency and CVID.

Two types of related but milder primary immunodeficiency exist in patients with a tendency to develop recurrent infections with *Pneumococcus* or *Haemophilus* spp. despite normal total IgG. These patients may have a **deficiency of IgG2**, a subclass of IgG produced in response to polysaccharide antigens by B cells in the spleen (B-1 cells) without T cell help. In other patients, levels of IgG2 are normal but there is a failure to respond to polysaccharide antigens, with poor titers of antibodies to pneumococcal antigens, even after vaccination. **Specific antibody deficiency** is also seen transiently during infancy and following splenectomy (Box 13.1).

Diagnosis

The commonest indication for testing for primary immunodeficiency is chronic or recurrent bacterial respiratory infection at any age. IgG, IgA and IgM should be measured (see Box 31.3). In patients with low levels of immunoglobulins, causes of secondary immunodeficiency such as protein loss from the gut or kidneys should be excluded. If total immunoglobulins are normal, IgG subclasses and specific antibodies against *Haemophilus* and *Pneumococcus* spp. should be measured. If these tests are all normal, it is important to check that there are no problems with complement or neutrophil function (for example, chronic granulomatous disease, Ch. 20) before concluding that there is no immunodeficiency.

In more unusual patients with atypical viral, protozoal or mycobacterial infections, T cell immunodeficiency should be ruled out. HIV infection can be excluded by careful history taking and appropriate testing. In patients with suspected cellular immunodeficiency, lymphocyte numbers should be measured by flow cytometry (see Chs 5 and 32).

Genetic testing. Polymorphisms are believed to confer an evolutionary advantage to carriers and they are passed on to a relatively large proportion of any given population. This means that there are relatively few, discrete alleles for any given gene. It is relatively simple to detect these by simple tests, such as the polymerase chain reaction, although the value of such testing is unclear.

Testing for mutations is difficult because each affected family can carry a unique sequence. For example, there are several hundred mutations identified in the gene *btk* in families affected by X-linked agammaglobulinemia.

However, once a preliminary diagnosis of a disease caused by mutation is made, it can be confirmed by genetic testing. Genetic testing also determines whether family members are carriers and it can be used to carry out antenatal diagnosis in subsequent pregnancies.

Treatment

The aim of treatment is to prevent infection. In cases of mild immunodeficiency, such as IgG2 deficiency, prophylactic antibiotics may be adequate.

In more severe antibody deficiency, immunoglobulin replacement therapy is required (Fig. 31.9). Administration of immunoglobulin is a type of *passive immunotherapy* (Ch. 4, Box 4.2). Antibodies against a wide range of pathogens are needed, so immunoglobulin pooled from several thousand normal donors is used. Immunoglobulin replacement can be given intravenously or subcutaneously. Replacement therapy is very different from high-dose immunoglobulin replacement therapy, which is immunosuppressive.

Plasma donors are screened for HIV and hepatitis B and C antibodies. Manufacturing processes to purify

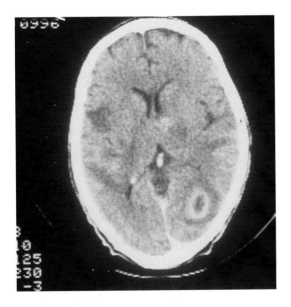

IgG will destroy many pathogens, but further steps are usually taken to reduce risk of hepatitis C carriage, for

Fig. 31.4 This patient has been unlucky enough to inherit polymorphisms in the genes encoding complement C2 and C4 and mannan-binding lectin. A computed tomographic brain scan shows fungal abscesses. Occurring singly, these polymorphisms are common and not strongly associated with infection. (With permission from the Department of Medical Illustration, St Bartholomew's Hospital, London.)

example, pasteurization (heating to 56°C) or adding detergents. None of these steps is guaranteed to remove **prions**, the agents responsible for "mad cow disease" and variant Creutzfeldt–Jakob disease. At the time of writing, plasma from the UK is not used in immunoglobulin manufacture because of the theoretical risk of transmission of prions.

In T cell deficiency, bone marrow transplant (BMT) may be required. BMT is discussed more fully in Chapter 33. When BMT is not an option (usually because no suitable donors are available), gene therapy may be attempted in patients with T cell defects.

BOX 31.2
A delayed diagnosis

A 28-year-old woman has been referred with daily sputum production and worsening shortness of breath. She had recurrent chest infections whilst a college student and she was unable to complete her degree. Over the past 7 years, her chest symptoms have become continuous. She has chronic sinusitis and has had three (unsuccessful) sinus drainage operations. She is non-smoker with an unremarkable family history.

On examination she has clinical signs of bronchiectasis, which is confirmed on computed tomography of her lungs (Fig. 31.5). Bronchiectasis is irreversible damage to the airways caused by repeated bouts of infection. *Haemophilus* bacteria are present in her sputum.

Her immunological investigations are shown in Figure 31.6.

Causes of secondary immunodeficiency were excluded and the diagnosis of common variable immunodeficiency was made. Her symptoms improved on intravenous immunoglobulin and she has completed her degree as a mature student.

continued

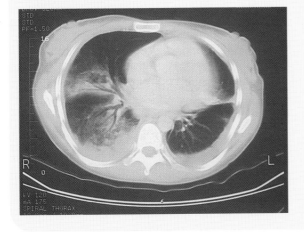

Fig. 31.5 This lung scan shows bronchiectasis in a woman with common variable immunodeficiency. Repeated bouts of infection damage the lining of the airways. Bronchiectasis is characterized by ragged dilatation of the bronchi. Although it is irreversible, bronchiectasis will stop progressing on immunoglobulin treatment. (With permission from the Department of Medical Illustration, St Bartholomew's Hospital, London.)

BOX 31.2
A delayed diagnosis (*contd.*)

Fig. 31.6
Immunological investigations in common variable immunodeficiency

Component	Patient values	Normal range
IgG (g/l)	2.2	7.0–18.0
IgA (g/l)	0.4	0.8–4.0
IgM (g/l)	0.4	0.4–2.5
CD3+ T cells (cells/μl)	420	820–2100
CD19+ T cells (cells/μl)	230	760–4200

BOX 31.3
Measuring immunological proteins

Many proteins can be measured using techniques reliant on immune complex formation. When antibodies are added to antigen, immune complexes will form. The physical nature of the immune complex will depend on the ratio of antigen to antibody. When these are present in equivalent molar quantities, large immune complexes form which precipitate out of solution. Immune complex formation (Fig. 31.7) is used in nephelometry to detect high concentration proteins (for example, IgG) and in single radial immunodiffusion for low concentrations of protein (for example, IgG subclasses; Fig. 31.8).

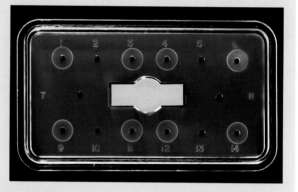

Fig. 31.8 Single radial immune diffusion is a sensitive assay used to measure low concentration proteins. The detecting antibody is dissolved in solid phase agarose. The patient sample is then added to a well in the agarose. A ring of precipitation will then form, the radius of which is related to the antigen concentration. Samples 2, 5, 7, 8, 10 and 13 have low levels of protein in this test. (With permission from The Binding Site Ltd, UK.)

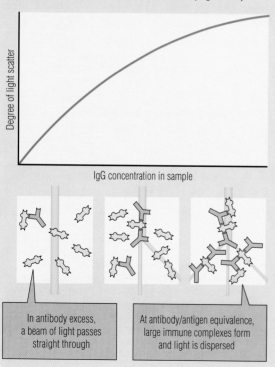

In antibody excess, a beam of light passes straight through

At antibody/antigen equivalence, large immune complexes form and light is dispersed

Degree of light scatter

IgG concentration in sample

Fig. 31.7 In nephelometry, insoluble immune complexes will scatter light that is transmitted through a solution, depending on the quantity of antigen or antibody. In this example, IgG is acting as the antigen. The antibody is usually produced in mice.

Bone marrow   Thymus   Lymph node

Fig. 31.9
Immunoglobulin products for replacement therapy

Product	Source	Indications
Immunoglobulin replacement therapy	Pooled from normal humans	Primary immunodeficiency
High-dose immunoglobulin	Pooled from normal humans	Immunosuppressive effects used in autoimmunity (Ch. 27)
Anti-D	Pooled from women with high levels of anti-D	Prevention of hemolytic disease of the newborn (Ch. 28)
Hyperimmune immunoglobulin	Pooled from humans with high titers of antibodies	Prevention of tetanus, rabies, varicella zoster and hepatitis B
Anti-venom	Plasma from immune horses	Treatment of snake bites
Monoclonal antibodies	Raised against specific human cells in mouse hybridomas	Used as immunosuppressants and in cancer treatment (Chs 9 and 34)

Gene therapy

Gene therapy uses recombinant technology to correct the genetic defect in stem cells, which can then reconstitute the immune system.

For gene therapy to be successful, several criteria must be met.

- The genetic mutation for each patient must be identified and there must be evidence that correcting the mutation will improve their condition. Insertion of normal genes may not correct a dominant mutation.
- The inserted gene must be regulated appropriately. For example, some of the kinase genes mentioned (*jak*, *btk*, Box 11.3) could cause inappropriate cell activation if they were constitutively active in recipient cells.
- The gene must be delivered to the cell safely. Viral constructs are often used to deliver the normal gene. Healthy humans contain many harmless retroviruses that may recombine genetic sequences with the viral vector. The new viruses produced may be able to cause disease.
- Gene therapy must not cause malignancy. If a gene with an active promoter is inserted next to an oncogene, the latter may become constitutively active and cause cancer. This is known as **insertional mutagenesis** and it remains a major cause for concern.

Gene therapy has been used successfully in a handful of patients with γ-chain deficiency, a type of X-linked SCID (Box 12.3). Stem cells are transfected with the γ-chain gene and give rise to large numbers of normal daughter cells. These cells proliferate and replace the abnormal cells because the transfected γ-chain gene allows them to proliferate in response to cytokines; these cells have a strong **survival advantage**. In the future, gene therapy is likely to be applied to other types of primary immunodeficiency caused by mutations.

LEARNING POINTS

Can you now:
- List the clinical features which would make you suspect primary immunodeficiency?
- List the primary immunodeficiencies caused by mutations, polymorphisms and polygenic factors?
- Outline the tests used to measure lymphocyte subsets and immunoglobulins?
- Construct a list of immunodeficiencies caused by the mutations mentioned in Figure 31.3? Refer to boxes in earlier chapters to describe the cellular and molecular defects.
- Write short notes on immunoglobulin replacement and gene therapy?

 Blood vessel Gut Peripheral tissue

Secondary immunodeficiency

32

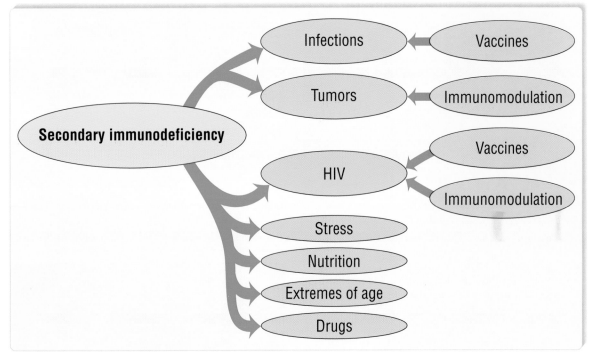

Secondary immunodeficiencies can be severe, for example, during human immunodeficiency virus (HIV) infection, myeloma and some drug treatments. Newer more sophisticated treatments such as transplants often require the use of immunosuppressant drugs to prevent rejection; this creates a group of immunodeficient individuals with special medical problems. Extremes of age and poor nutrition tend to cause milder, but significant, secondary immunodeficiency.

HIV INFECTION

Natural history

HIV infection is the most important cause of secondary immunodeficiency, affecting over 30 million people worldwide.

The HIV envelope, made up of gp120 molecules, binds CD4 in order to enter target cells, including CD4+ T cells, monocytes and dendritic cells. Gp120 also binds chemokine receptors, which increases the efficiency of viral entry. Following sexual exposure to HIV, the virus uses the CCR5 chemokine receptor on macrophages and dendritic cells to gain entry at mucosal sites (Fig. 32.1a).

Following non-sexual HIV transmission, for example sharing needles during intravenous drug use, these chemokine receptors are not as important.

Subsequently, there is active HIV replication in lymph nodes, with destruction of CD4+ T cells (Fig. 32.1b). Some newly infected patients develop rashes, feel unwell and have a fever. This stage may be referred to as **HIV seroconversion illness**, because it occurs at about the time antibodies to HIV appear.

Over the next few weeks, viral replication is reduced by specific cytotoxic T lymphocytes (CTL; Fig. 32.1c). A lower level of viral replication then continues in lymph nodes, and a steady state of virus production is matched by equivalent rate of clearance of virus and T cell death. This steady state may persist for several years. In some macrophages and T cells HIV integrates into the genome but does not replicate. These **latently infected** cells provide a reservoir of infection, because in the absence of replication, they are never recognized by the immune system. Signals from cytokines or the T cell receptor will increase transcription, enabling HIV replication any time the immune system responds to infection.

Reverse transcriptase is an HIV enzyme that transcribes viral RNA into DNA. Up to 1 in 10 000 bases

Blood vessel   Gut   Peripheral tissue

277

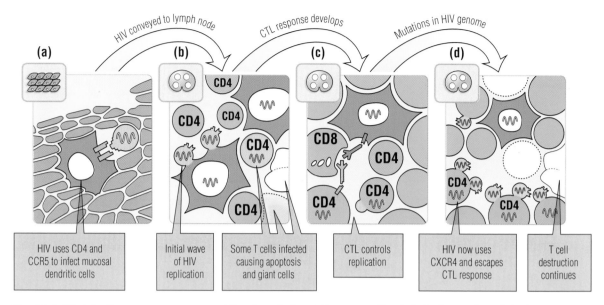

Fig. 32.1 HIV infection progresses more rapidly when viral mutations occur that help in the evasion of the immune response, e.g., switching CXCR chemokine receptor usage.

may be mutated during reverse transcription. These mutations affect the delicate balance between HIV and the host immune system. The altered immunogenicity of newer mutated strains enables HIV to evade the immune response. Mutated peptides may not bind to MHC or may not be recognized by T cell receptors, favoring outgrowth of these viruses and their progeny. Mutation may also enable HIV to bind the CXCR4 chemokine receptor on T cells (32.1d). These strains are more effective at infecting CD4⁺ T cells.

Concomitant with declining CD4 numbers, there is an increase in viral replication and measurable viremia. Up to 10^9 virions may be produced each day, many of which will contain mutated antigenic peptides.

Most patients with early HIV infection are symptom free. As the number of T cells declines, symptomatic infection with virulent organisms such as *Candida albicans* (Fig. 32.2) and *Mycobacterium tuberculosis* may occur. *Pneumocystis carinii* pneumonia (PCP) reflects more severe immunodeficiency and finally, when little residual immune response remains, low-virulence organisms such as atypical mycobacteria and cytomegalovirus (CMV) cause infections.

Tumors such as non-Hodgkin's lymphoma and Kaposi's sarcoma (Fig. 32.3) also occur and patients may develop dementia, caused by HIV infection of glial cells derived from monocytes.

Monitoring infection

Patients with HIV infection require immunological (CD4 cell counts) and virological (viral load) monitor-

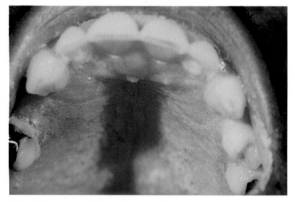

Fig. 32.2 The white lesions on this man's palate are oral candidiasis, which is a marker of mild immunodeficiency and it is often the first opportunist infection in patients with HIV. Oral candidiasis is often seen in other mild secondary immunodeficiencies. (With permission from the Department of Medical Illustration, St Bartholomew's Hospital, London.)

ing. The CD4 cell count is the number of blood lymphocytes expressing CD4, and different levels are associated with the risk of developing specific opportunist infections. CD4 cell levels form part of assessment schemes for progression of HIV infection (e.g., the Centers for Disease Control and Prevention (CDC) scheme). For example, patients with CD4 counts below $200/\mu l$ have a high risk of PCP and should receive prophylaxis. Prophylaxis against CMV and atypical mycobacteria should be considered if the CD4 count has fallen below $100/\mu l$.

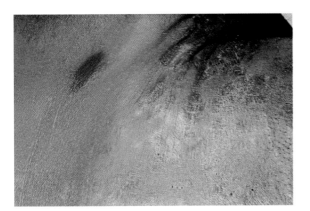

Fig. 32.3 Kaposi's sarcoma (KS) is a marker of moderate immunodeficiency and it is seen most frequently in HIV patients. In HIV infection, KS affects only some patient groups, for example gay men, probably because of the requirements for a second coinfection with human herpes virus 8. (With permission from the Department of Medical Illustration, St Bartholomew's Hospital, London.)

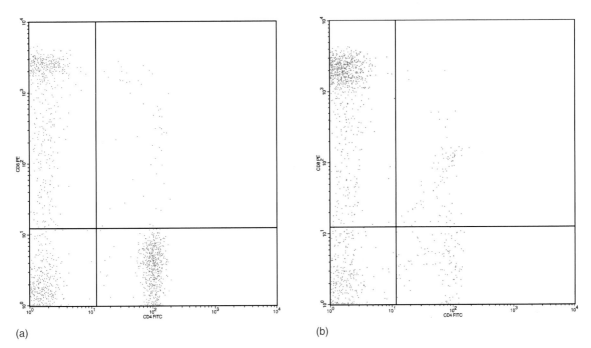

(a)   (b)

Fig. 32.4 In this test, lymphocytes are counted on the basis of CD4 (X axis) and CD8 (Y axis) expression. This is the same principle as that used in the test shown in Fig. 5.7. (a) Normal donor; there are plentiful CD4⁺ and CD8⁺ lymphocytes. (b) Patient with HIV infection; CD8 numbers are unchanged, but there are fewer CD4⁺ cells.

CD4 cell counts are done by flow cytometry, which gives reliable results, although a range of factors can affect them considerably (Figs 32.4 and 32.5).

Viral load tests measure HIV viremia and reflect long-term risk of disease progression. Viral load is used with CD4 cell counts to determine the use of anti-retroviral treatment which is combinations of inhibitors of the reverse transcriptase or the HIV protease (Box 32.1).

Factors affecting outcome of infection

Viral and host factors that affect the outcome of HIV infection provide clues to improvements in vaccines and treatments.

The HIV gene *nef* codes for a protein that inhibits the immune system by reducing the expression of MHC class I. This prevents recognition of infected cells by CTL. HIV strains with mutations in *nef* are poorly virulent and they have been considered in HIV vaccine development (Box 32.2). The most important variable host factor affecting HIV infection is chemokine receptor polymorphism. HIV infects cells at mucosal surfaces expressing the CCR5 family of chemokine receptors. Individuals homozygous for a polymorphism in the CCR5 receptor have a decreased risk of becoming infected with HIV after sexual exposure. There is some evidence that polymorphisms in CCR5 affect other viral infections, such as chickenpox, and

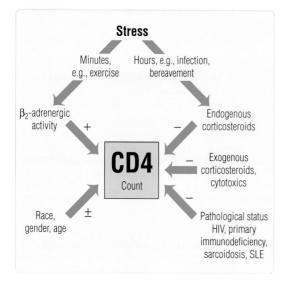

Fig. 32.5 Many factors affect CD4 cell counts, notably the effects of endogenous corticiosteroids. This has practical implications, for example, CD4 cell counts should be done at the same time each day and they should be avoided when patients are acutely ill.

BOX 32.1
Typical HIV history

A patient presented with rashes and fevers soon after an episode of unprotected sex. Figure 32.6 shows his CD4 cell counts. His initial HIV antibody test was negative, but he subsequently seroconverted. For 4 years he had no further problems, but when his long asymptomatic phase of infection ended he developed oral candidiasis. Effective antiretroviral treatment became available several years later and this improved his clinical and immunological state. Drug resistance developed 2 years later and cytomegalovirus infection was a consequence of his deteriorating immune function.

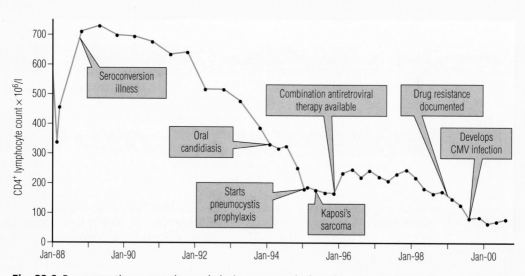

Fig. 32.6 Pneumocystis pneumonia prophylaxis was started when this patient's CD4 cell count fell below $200 \times 10^6/l$ ($200/\mu l$). This effectively prevented this life-threatening infection. CMV, cytomegalovirus.

Bone marrow   Thymus   Lymph node

BOX 32.2
nef mutations and low virulence

In the early 1980s, eight patients in Sydney were infected with HIV from contaminated blood products from a single donor. Five of these patients are alive over 14 years later; in three, CD4 cell counts remain high and viral load is undetectable. The viral strain in the blood donor and recipients was found to have a deletion in the *nef* gene.

Although *nef* mutations only rarely account for long-term survival in HIV infection, the discovery is of interest because it could be used to make attenuated HIV vaccines.

may improve outcomes after kidney transplantation. Polymorphisms in CCR5 do not yet appear to cause any harmful effects on the immune system and give some clues to new HIV treatments.

CTL responses to HIV vary between patients. For example, enhanced CTL responses protect some female sex workers against HIV, despite repeated unprotected intercourse, for up to 12 years. Some of these women have been exposed to HIV but have managed to establish **sterilizing immunity**. "Long-term non-progressors" are patients remaining well at least 10 years after HIV infection and they also have stronger than usual CTL activity against HIV.

CTL responses may remain strong if the virus does not mutate and evade the immune response. Alternatively, some individuals may have genetically determined enhanced ability to respond to HIV peptides. HLA polymorphisms may be important in determining the ability to make CTL in two different ways. Firstly, individuals may have inherited specific HLA alleles that are able to bind HIV peptides and present them to CTL. Secondly, individuals who are homozygous for all HLA alleles effectively have half as many different HLA molecules available for HIV peptide presentation as individuals who are heterozygous at all alleles. People who are heterozygous at all HLA alleles tend to have better outcomes after HIV infection, illustrating the importance of the generation of diversity (Box 3.1).

Vaccines

Figure 32.7 gives a summary of the current candidate vaccines for HIV. Antibodies alone do not guarantee protection from infection or disease progression; even patients dying of AIDS are able to mount strong antibody responses, as shown by persistently positive HIV ELISA (enzyme-linked immunosorbent assay) tests. Strong CTL responses are more important in protecting from HIV infection, as discussed above.

Fig. 32.7
Candidate HIV vaccines. No single candidate vaccine is yet proven to meet all the challenges produced by HIV

	Vaccine type				
	Intramuscular peptide	**Mucosal peptide**	**Recombinant virus**	**Attenuated virus**	**DNA vaccine**
Example	gp120	gp120	Canary pox–gp120	*nef* deleted	*gp120*
Effective against a range of HIV strains?	No	Unknown	Unknown	Unclear (see Box 32.2)	Unknown
Type of response	Long-lasting antibody; not CTL	Mucosal antibody and CTL	Weak antibody; strong CTL	Strong CTL	CTL; mucosal antibody if given intranasally
Safe?	Yes	Unknown	Risk of viral recombination	Risk of viral recombination	Unknown
Practical?	Yes	Yes	Requires special storage	Requires special storage	Yes

CTL, cytotoxic T lymphocyte.

Blood vessel   Gut   Peripheral tissue

HIV rapidly mutates, and viral samples obtained from different geographical sites show marked antigenic variations. Vaccines need to be effective against a range of mutations.

Finally HIV vaccines must be safe and practical for use in the developing world, where most new HIV infections take place.

Immunomodulation

What can be done to boost the immune response in HIV infection?

Administration of interleukin 2 (IL-2) on its own increases HIV replication because infected cells upregulate viral transcription along with host T cell genes. Antiretroviral therapy (ART) given alone cannot eradicate HIV integrated into the genome of resting cells, which will remain as a reservoir of virus. Administration of *both* IL-2 and antiretroviral drugs induces greater improvements in CD4 cell counts than drug therapy alone, and there is no increase in viral replication.

IL-2 activates HIV gene transcription and peptide expression and may facilitate killing of these cells, whilst antiretroviral therapy prevents HIV infecting new cells. The combined strategies reduce the number of latently infected T cells, as well as reducing HIV RNA levels. IL-2 can have side-effects, such as influenza-like symptoms, and its use in HIV will probably not be licensed unless clinical improvements can be documented in trials.

OTHER SECONDARY IMMUNODEFICIENCIES

Nutrition

Deficiency of zinc and magnesium impairs cell-mediated immunity, particularly T_H1-pattern cytokine secretion. This type of deficiency in micronutrients occurs in a wide range of situations, for example, in postoperative patients. Although vitamins, especially vitamins A and E, are required by the immune system their role is less significant than mineral nutrients.

Continued poor nutrition leads to a loss of fat cells. Fat cells normally secrete the hormone **leptin**, which has stimulatory effects on the immune system. Loss of fatty tissue may, therefore, cause mild immunodeficiency, mediated by low levels of leptin (Ch. 35).

Physiological stress

Acute or chronic stress has variable effects on the immune system, discussed in Chapter 35.

The immune system in the first year of life

Throughout the first year of life, the specific immune system remains immature. Although neonates have high numbers of T cells, these are all naive and so do not respond well to antigen (see Chs 14 and 17).

Fetal antibody synthesis begins at 20 weeks, but adult levels of IgG are not reached until about 5 years. For the first few months of life, infants are reliant on maternal IgG. Pregnant women produce increased immunoglobulins under the effects of estrogens. IgG is transported across the placenta by specialized Fc receptors in the last 10 weeks of pregnancy. Breast milk is an additional source of protection in early life and protects against lung and gastrointestinal infection. Bottle-fed infants are 60 times more likely to develop pneumonia in the first 3 months of life.

Premature babies face the greatest problems with infection because they have had less time to receive maternal immunoglobulin during the late stages of pregnancy. Immaturity of innate mechanisms such as lung surfactant (Ch. 19) can increase the risk of respiratory infection.

Many infants develop low levels of antibody during the first year of life. **Transient hypogammaglobulinemia of infancy** is caused by a delay in maturation of immunoglobulin synthesis, especially IgG2, at a time when maternal antibody levels are falling.

The aging immune system

The elderly suffer more infections than younger patients. This is in part because thymic function declines early in adult life. Fewer T cells emerge from the thymus and proliferation of T cells in the periphery is mainly responsible for maintaining adequate cell numbers.

Additionally, a biological clock is particularly important in T cells. Each time a cell divides, there is a stepwise shortening of telomeric DNA. When telomere length is considerably shortened cells can no longer divide. This **replicative senescence** affects T cells after about 40 divisions.

Aged B cells may show signs of a lifetime's exposure to microorganisms. Immunoglobulin synthesis is increased and outgrowth of B cell clones may lead to benign paraproteins or B cell malignancy (Ch. 34). This process is driven by Epstein–Barr virus (EBV). Autoantibodies are also commoner in the elderly but are not usually associated with disease.

Miscellaneous factors

B cell malignancy
Myeloma and chronic lymphocytic leukemia are malignancies of B cells (Ch. 34). Although both may produce large amounts of monoclonal immunoglobu-

 Bone marrow   Thymus   Lymph node

lin (paraprotein), they are associated with low levels of antibody against pathogens. Myeloma and chronic lymphocytic leukemia are very common causes of secondary immunodeficiency in the elderly. Thymoma is a rare tumor that can cause immunodeficiency in addition to autoimmune disorders such as myasthenia gravis.

Drugs

Drugs are common cause of secondary immunodeficiency and eliminating the offending drug will usually improve the immune response.

Immunosuppression is an expected side-effect of steroids and cytotoxic drugs and of the immunosuppressive regimens used in autoimmune disease and transplant rejection prophylaxis. Before starting such treatments, it is good practice to ensure the patient has no hidden infections (such as tuberculosis). Certain drugs can cause antibody deficiency as an unexpected side-effect. Among the most notorious are anticonvulsants, used to treat epilepsy.

Kidney disease

In nephrotic syndrome (Ch. 28), there may be significant renal protein loss and a reduction in blood levels of IgG and IgA with normal IgM.

Immunoglobulins can also be lost via the gut in severe diarrheal diseases. Renal failure and diabetes also cause secondary phagocyte defects, although the mechanism is not known.

BOX 32.3
Secondary immunodeficiency in acute illness

A previously healthy 30-year-old man was admitted following a car crash. He is unconscious and he has signs of cerebral edema. The patient has a tube inserted into his trachea, and a central venous line and urinary catheter are inserted. He is given high-dose corticosteroids in an attempt to reduce cerebral edema. After a series of convulsions, the anticonvulsant phenytoin is given intravenously (Fig. 32.8).

Two weeks later he is recovering from his neurological episode when he develops pneumonia (Fig. 32.9). In addition to physiological stress and poor nutrition, this patient has his innate barriers penetrated at three different sites and is then exposed to two drugs that impair the immune system. It is no surprise his defenses against infection are impaired!

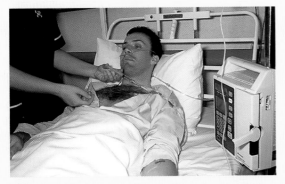

Fig. 32.8 In acutely ill patients admitted to hospital, many factors interact to cause immunodeficiency. This is made worse when physical barriers are breeched by cannulae and intravenous lines and because of the wide range of pathogens found inside hospitals. (With permission from the Department of Medical Illustration, St Bartholomew's Hospital, London.)

Fig. 32.9 The patient's chest radiograph shows abscesses typical of staphylococcal pneumonia. This avoidable, life-threatening infection is a consequence of multiple factors in this patient. (With permission from the Department of Medical Illustration, St Bartholomew's Hospital, London.)

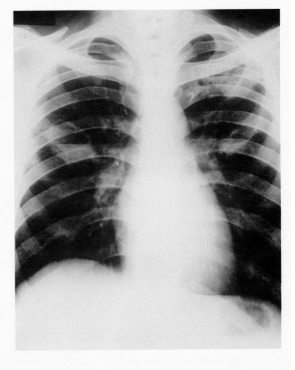

Blood vessel   Gut   Peripheral tissue

Infections

Infections can also cause immunodeficiency. Malaria and congenital rubella may cause antibody deficiency. Measles is well known for causing defects in cell-mediated immunity—sometimes enough to reactivate tuberculosis.

Many of these factors operate together in acutely ill patients (Box 32.3).

LEARNING POINTS

Can you now:

- Write short notes on the cells affected by HIV infection?
- Describe how you would monitor a patient with HIV infection?
- List host and virus factors which affect the course of HIV infection?
- Make a list of the challenges to be overcome by effective HIV infection?
- Explain which factors interact to predispose hospital patients to infection?

Bone marrow   Thymus   Lymph node

Transclamtation

33

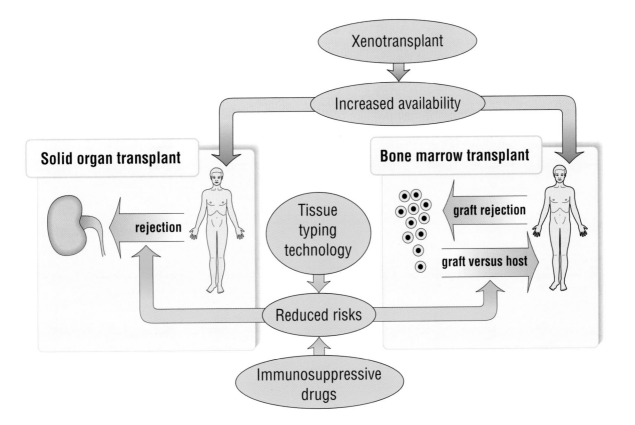

Transplantation terminology

Rejection refers to damage done by the immune system to a transplanted organ.

Autologous transplant refers to tissue returning to the same individual after a period outside the body—usually in a frozen state.

Syngeneic transplant refers to transplant between identical twins; there is usually no problem with graft rejection.

Allogeneic transplant takes place between genetically non-identical members of the same species; there is always a risk of rejection.

Xenogeneic transplant takes place between different species and this carries the highest risk of rejection.

SOLID ORGAN TRANSPLANTATION

When transplantation is indicated

Transplantation may be an option when the organs

shown in Figure 33.1 stop functioning. Several criteria must be met before transplantation:

- there must be good evidence that the damage is irreversible or that alternative treatments are not applicable
- the disease must not recur; for example, renal transplant is contraindicated in patients with Goodpasture's syndrome, who have anti-glomerular basement membrane antibodies (Ch. 28)
- the chances of rejection must be minimized
  — the donor and recipient must be ABO compatible
  — the donor must not have anti-donor HLA antibodies
  — the donor should be selected with a close as possible HLA type to the recipient: this is most important for kidney and stem cell transplant; it improves the outcome for cardiac transplant, but very often the urgency for a transplant, in a patient with severe cardiac failure, means that a mismatched heart is acceptable.

Fig. 33.1
Transplantation of a variety of tissues is now possible

Organ	Characteristics	Graft survival (%)
Cornea	No immunosuppression required because cornea does not become vascularized	Over 90
Kidney	Live related kidney donation often used; graft survival optimized by HLA match; immunosuppression required	Over 80
Pancreas	Usually transplanted along with kidneys in diabetics with renal failure; separated islet cells have also been infused into the vena cava	About 50
Heart	Used for coronary artery disease, cardiomyopathy and some congenital heart disease; immunosuppression required	Over 80
Liver	Used for alcoholic liver disease, primary biliary cirrhosis and virus-induced cirrhosis	Over 60: outcome not affected by degree of HLA matching
Stem cells	Used in malignancy, hematological conditions and some primary immunodeficiency; best results when there is a match of HLA *A, B, C* and *DR*	Up to 80

These conditions are not important for corneal grafts, because usually corneal transplants are not vascularized and so they do not become exposed to the recipient's immune system. Tissue typing techniques enable donor/recipient matching to be assessed (Box 33.1).

Mechanisms of rejection

Hyperacute rejection
Hyperacute rejection takes place within hours of transplantation and is caused by preformed antibodies binding to either ABO blood group or HLA class I antigens on the graft (Fig. 33.3). The recipient may have formed anti-HLA Class I antibodies following exposure to allogeneic lymphocytes during pregnancy, blood transfusion or a previous transplant. Antibody binding triggers a type II hypersensitivity reaction and the graft is destroyed by vascular thrombosis. Hyperacute rejection can be prevented through careful ABO and HLA cross-matching and is now very rare.

Acute rejection
There are a number of risk factors for acute rejection, which can happen within days or weeks of transplantation. For example, a delay connecting the kidney to the blood supply activates the innate immune system, which damages the organ.

Acute rejection also takes place when there is HLA incompatibility. Recipient T cells can respond to donor peptides presented by recipient MHC or to donor MHC molecules themselves (Fig. 33.3). Although attempting

BOX 33.1
Tissue typing techniques

Tissue typing technologies are used to identify donor/recipient pairs with the lowest risk of complications (Fig. 33.2).

HLA typing
A patient being considered for a transplant is tissue typed to identify their HLA alleles. If they have suitable siblings, a family search may be made for a live related donor. Otherwise, they then go on a waiting list for a cadaveric organ. When an organ becomes available, the donor is HLA typed and a search is made in tissue typing registries for a suitable recipient.

HLA cross-matching
Cross-matching is performed to rule out preformed antibodies against donor HLA, which could cause hyperacute rejection. These antibodies could be produced by exposure to allogeneic HLA during pregnancy, blood transfusion or a previous attempt at transplantation. Donor lymphocytes are incubated with recipient serum in the presence of complement. If the recipient serum contains antibodies against donor HLA, lymphocytes are killed through type II complement-mediated cytotoxicity. The presence of antibodies to donor HLA rules out the possibility of transplantation.

Bone marrow   Thymus   Lymph node

BOX 33.1
Tissue typing techniques (*contd*.)

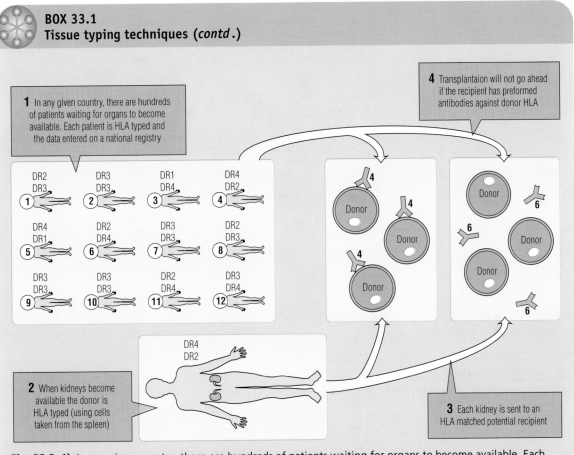

1 In any given country, there are hundreds of patients waiting for organs to become available. Each patient is HLA typed and the data entered on a national registry

4 Transplantaion will not go ahead if the recipient has preformed antibodies against donor HLA

2 When kidneys become available the donor is HLA typed (using cells taken from the spleen)

3 Each kidney is sent to an HLA matched potential recipient

Fig. 33.2 1). In any given country, there are hundreds of patients waiting for organs to become available. Each patient is HLA typed and the data entered on a national registry. **2).** When kidneys become available the donor is HLA typed using cells taken from the spleen. **3).** Each kidney is sent to an HLA matched potential recipient. **4).** Transplantation will not go ahead if the recipient has pre-formed antibodies against donor HLA.

to minimize any HLA mismatch of the donor and recipient can reduce acute rejection, the shortage of donor kidneys often means that a partially mismatched kidney is used. The survival of the kidney is related to the degree of mismatching, especially at *HLA-DR* loci (Fig. 33.4).

Alternatively, the recipient may respond to "minor histocompatibility antigens" presented by donor or recipient cells. Minor antigens are proteins that have different amino acid sequences in the donor and recipient; they are encoded by genes situated outside the HLA. Minor histocompatibility antigen mismatches are not detected by standard tissue typing techniques. The term *minor* antigens may be misleading in terms of importance; even when an HLA matched, live related donor is found, these antigens can cause graft rejection in up to one third of transplants (see Box 33.2).

Acute rejection is a type IV (cell mediated) delayed hypersensitivity reaction. Acute rejection takes several days to develop because of the time taken for donor dendritic cells to stimulate an allogeneic response and for responding T cells to proliferate and migrate into the donor kidney.

Chronic rejection
Chronic rejection takes place months or years after transplant. There is often an element of allogeneic reaction mediated by T cells in chronic rejection, which can result in repeated acute rejection. In some cases, chronic rejection may be caused by recurrence of pre-existing autoimmune disease. In other cases there is no direct evidence of damage caused by the adaptive immune system.

Tolerance
Tolerance is the state where, following exposure to an antigen, specific T and B cell responses do not occur, although responses to other antigens remain normal

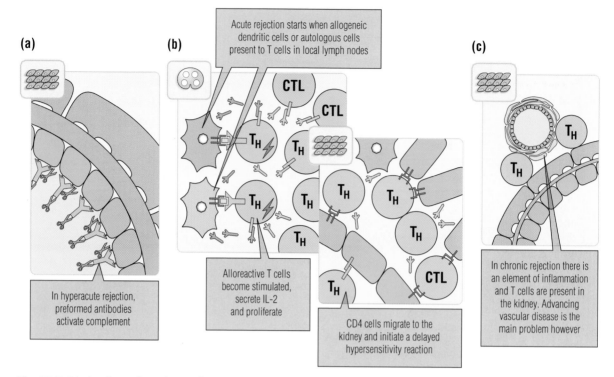

Acute rejection starts when allogeneic dendritic cells or autologous cells present to T cells in local lymph nodes

In hyperacute rejection, preformed antibodies activate complement

Alloreactive T cells become stimulated, secrete IL-2 and proliferate

CD4 cells migrate to the kidney and initiate a delayed hypersensitivity reaction

In chronic rejection there is an element of inflammation and T cells are present in the kidney. Advancing vascular disease is the main problem however

Fig. 33.3 Mechanisms of renal transplant rejection. Hyperacute (a) and acute (b) solid organ graft rejection involve different mechanisms. The mechanism of chronic rejection (c) is not clear.

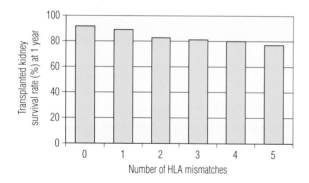

Fig. 33.4 The impressive survival rates for mismatched kidneys would not be achievable without potent immunosuppressive drugs.

(Ch. 14). In central tolerance self-reactive T and B cells are destroyed by apoptosis during negative selection in the thymus and bone marrow, respectively (Ch. 15). In peripheral tolerance, T and B cells may become **anergic**, that is, they are not killed but become unable to respond to stimulation. Peripheral tolerance has not been achieved artificially in humans. In transplantation, a state of tolerance of the foreign organ/cell is the clinical goal. Immunosuppressive drugs prevent rejection if

given at the time of transplantation but also prevent responses to infectious agents. Once the drugs are stopped, rejection can still take place. Immunosuppressive drugs lack the specificity and durability of true tolerance.

The possibility of using organs from other species (xenografts) raises several problems of tolerance: foreign proteins, which may be altered by genetic engineering, immune reactions, which will require immunosuppressive drugs, and the potential for hitherto unexperienced viruses in the transplant to grow in the human in the immunosuppressed state (Box 33.3).

STEM CELL TRANSPLANT

Stem cell transplant (SCT) is a risky procedure—even with well-matched donors and in the best of circumstances the mortality can be as high as 20%. SCT is used to restore myeloid and lymphoid cells in the following situations.

- Haematological malignancy: SCT is used after initial treatment if there is a very high chance of relapse. SCT is preceded by potent chemotherapy and irradiation to eradicate residual tumor cells. In autologous transplant, marrow is removed, frozen

Bone marrow   Thymus   Lymph node

BOX 33.2
Acute graft rejection

A 43-year-old woman with polycystic kidney disease has been on the renal transplant waiting list for 3 years, during which time she has been maintained on dialysis. Her HLA-identical brother volunteers to donate a kidney. **Live related donors** are important in kidney transplantation, provided they are not affected by the same genetic disease! The patient's serum did not react with her brother's lymphocytes during cross-match and following transplantation there was no evidence of hyperacute rejection. Transplant was followed by rejection prophylaxis with ciclosporin, azathioprine and corticosteroids. Eight days later the patient develops a fever and her renal function deteriorates.

A renal biopsy showed acute rejection as a result of minor antigen mismatch (Fig. 33.5). Initial treatment with high-dose corticosteroids was ineffective. The patient was treated for 5 days with anti-CD3 (a marker on T cells), during which time renal function

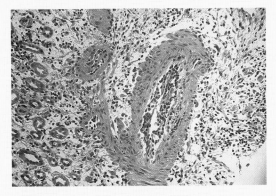

Fig. 33.5 This is a biopsy of the kidney transplant described in Box 33.2. There is a lymphocytic infiltration in the graft consistent with acute rejection.

improved and there were no further episodes of rejection.

BOX 33.3
Xenotransplanation

Between 1990 and 2000, waiting lists for transplants almost doubled, while the number of transplants carried out remained static. There are too few human organs available to meet the needs of patients. Several problems need to be overcome before xenotransplants from other species become an alternative.

- Primates assemble sugar side-chains differently from other species. Galactose–α1,3-galactose (gal–α1,3-gal) is a sugar present on the cells of most non-primate species. The immune system can recognize gal–α1,3-gal and all humans possess antibodies against gal–α1,3-gal following exposure to, for example, gut bacteria. Similar **natural antibodies** have been mentioned in Chapter 26. Antibodies against gal–α1,3-gal bind onto xenotransplanted organs, activate complement and trigger hyperacute rejection.
- Complement inhibitors from other species do not inhibit human complement. As a result of this

molecular incompatibility, xenotransplanted organs activate complement (see Ch. 19).

Transgenic pigs (see Ch. 19) are being developed with reduced gal–α1,3-gal expression to prevent natural antibody binding and with human complement inhibitors to bypass molecular incompatibility. Pigs are used because they are a similar size to humans and easy to rear in captivity. Two considerable theoretical problems remain.

- There may be acute rejection, since pig proteins elicit a T cell response.
- Even pigs reared in microbe-free conditions are infected with endogenous retroviruses; these have never been known to infect humans but they could do so following transplantation. Pig viruses are more likely to infect recipients taking immunosuppressive drugs.

and reinfused after very potent chemotherapy has been given.

- When myeloid cell production is reduced or very abnormal, for example in aplastic anemia.
- In primary immunodeficiencies, e.g., severe combined immunodeficiency (SCID).

Source of stem cells

Following transplantation, myeloid cells are regenerated from pluripotent stem cells. These can be obtained from a number of sources.

- Bone marrow is the usual source of stem cells. Harvesting requires aspiration of a considerable amount of donor marrow under general anesthetic.
- Peripheral blood stem cells are usually harvested after treating the donor with colony-stimulating factors to increase the numbers of circulating stem cells.
- Cord blood contains a large number of stem cells, which can be frozen prior to use. An advantage of cord blood is that the immature lymphocytes are less likely to cause graft-versus-host disease (GVHD; see below). Cord blood only yields enough stem cells to transplant children or small adults.

Conditioning

Conditioning consists of high-dose chemotherapy or radiotherapy, which destroy the recipient stem cells, allowing donor stem cells to engraft. Apart from creating a physical space in the bone marrow for the donor marrow cells to engraft, conditioning prevents the donor immune system rejecting the allogeneic stem cells. In this way, conditioning is similar to prophylaxis for solid organ rejection.

Graft-versus-host disease

GVHD occurs when donor T cells respond to allogeneic recipient antigens. It occurs when there are mismatches in major or minor histocompatibility antigens. All patients receiving SCT are given immunosuppressive drugs to prevent GVHD, even if donor and recipient are HLA identical. This maneuver in itself has risks of infections (Box 33.4). Acute GVHD occurs up to 4 weeks after SCT. There is widespread involvement of skin, gut, liver and lungs; when severe, acute GVHD carries a 70% mortality. Chronic GVHD occurs later and affects the skin and liver.

Removing mature T cells from the source of the stem cells, using immunological techniques, reduces the risk of GVHD. T cell depletion, however, increases the risk of graft rejection.

Donor T cells are also capable of reacting against recipient tumor cells, especially when there is a degree of HLA mismatch and mild GVHD is taking place. This beneficial **graft-versus-leukemia** effect is lost after T cell depletion of stem cell preparations (Fig. 33.7).

IMMUNOSUPPRESSIVE DRUGS

Immunosuppressive drugs are required to prevent and/or treat graft rejection and GVHD. The drugs tend to be used in combinations as part of defined regimens. For example, in renal transplant, corticosteroids, ciclosporin and azathioprine are all used from the time of transplant. Corticosteroids are withdrawn gradually after several weeks and ciclosporin after a few months. Patients may stay on azathioprine indefinitely. All of these drugs carry the risk of infection as a consequence of immunosuppression.

Many of these drugs are also used in the treatment of autoimmune disease and some familiarity with their modes of action is important (Fig. 33.8).

Corticosteroids

Corticosteroids inhibit synthesis of over 100 proteins, but at low doses they predominantly act on antigen-presenting cells, preventing some of the early stages of graft rejection. Higher doses of corticosteroids have direct effects on T cells and these are used to treat episodes of rejection (see Ch. 30).

T cell signal inhibitors

Ciclosporin and tacrolimus (discussed in Box 11.4) have improved the outcome of all types of transplant dramatically. They are used to prevent both graft rejection and GVHD.

Anti-proliferative drugs

Azathioprine, mycophenolate mofetil and methotrexate inhibit DNA production. These drugs prevent lymphocyte proliferation but they are not specific for T cells and they can cause myelotoxicity.

Monoclonal antibodies

Monoclonal anti-CD3 induces abnormal signals in T cells, which subsequently become anergic.

THE FETUS AS AN ALLOGRAFT

During pregnancy, the maternal immune system is exposed to paternal allogeneic antigen although the fetus and trophoblast are very rarely rejected. Several factors combine to prevent rejection of the fetus.

- Estrogen is a steroid sex hormone secreted by the ovaries at high levels during the middle of the menstrual cycle and persistently during pregnancy. Estrogen inhibits T cell activity for the duration of pregnancy. Estrogen has the opposite effect on B

Bone marrow   Thymus   Lymph node

BOX 33.4
Infection following stem cell transplant

A 36-year-old woman with lymphoma is at high risk of relapse following initial chemotherapy. Neither of her two siblings is HLA identical. Following an extensive search on a registry, a donor is found. Although the donor is HLA identical, there is a risk of graft-versus-host disease (GVHD) because of minor antigen incompatibility. Prophylaxis with ciclosporin is used for 6 weeks following stem cell transplant.

Fortunately, her lymphoma does not relapse and she does not develop GVHD. She does, however, have a series of infections.

Conditioning, GVHD prophylaxis and stem cell transplant itself cause severe immunosuppression and infection is the commonest cause of death in these patients. Figure 33.6 shows how immune reconstitution takes place and the specific infections likely to occur.

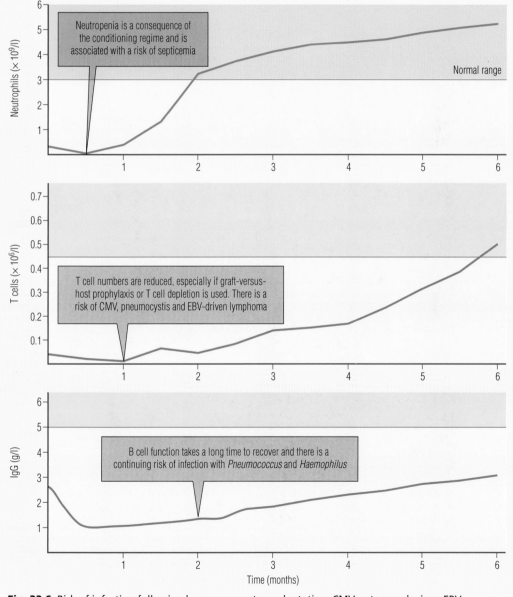

Fig. 33.6 Risk of infection following bone marrow transplantation. CMV, cytomegalovirus; EBV, Epstein–Barr virus.

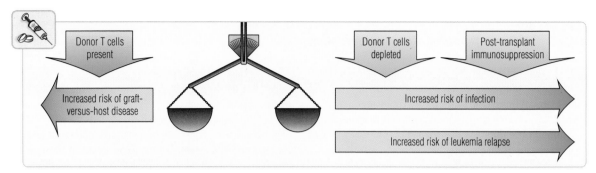

Fig. 33.7 T cell depletion has complex effects on stem cell transplant. The decision on whether or not to deplete T cells rests on the degree of donor matching and the condition being treated.

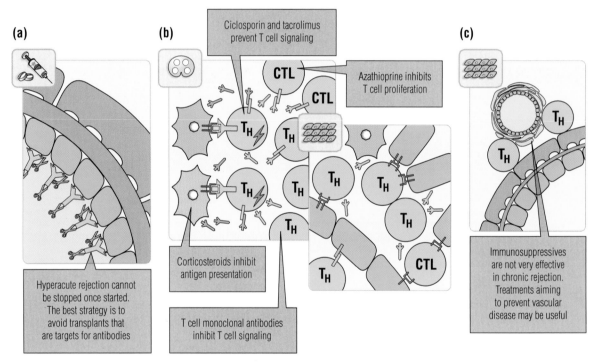

Fig. 33.8 Prevention and treatment of renal transplant rejection. An illustration of how immunosuppressive drugs work in (a) hyperacute, (b) acute and (c) chronic rejection. Similar drugs are used during stem cell transplant.

cells; consequently, there is an increase in IgG and IgA synthesis during pregnancy. This ensures that adequate amounts of IgG are transported across the placenta late in pregnancy and that IgA is available in breast milk after labor. Most pregnant women make antibodies to paternal HLA antigens, but these do not affect fetal outcome.

- The placenta secretes cytokines, which skew maternal responses towards a T_H2 pattern (Ch. 26).

- The trophoblast expresses low levels of HLA class I, which prevents recognition by maternal CD8+ T cells.
- Low-level expression of HLA class I may make the trophoblast susceptible to killing by maternal natural killer cells, which are present in high numbers. However, the trophoblast expresses high levels of HLA-G, a non-classical MHC molecule. The HLA-G appears to have the sole purpose of inhibiting natural killer cells (Fig. 33.9 and Ch. 21).

Bone marrow   Thymus   Lymph node

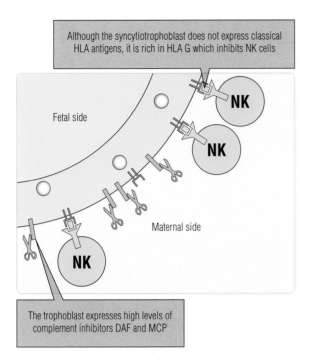

Although the syncytiotrophoblast does not express classical HLA antigens, it is rich in HLA G which inhibits NK cells

Fetal side

Maternal side

The trophoblast expresses high levels of complement inhibitors DAF and MCP

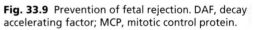

Fig. 33.9 Prevention of fetal rejection. DAF, decay accelerating factor; MCP, mitotic control protein.

LEARNING POINTS

Can you now:

- List the different types of transplant and organs which are transplanted?
- Describe the three phases of rejection of solid organs?
- Describe the two laboratory procedures designed to reduce the risk of infection?
- Explain how stem cell transplant differs from solid organ transplant?
- List immunosuppressive drugs and their modes of action?
- List the problems that need to be overcome to make xenotransplantation safe?

Tumor immunology

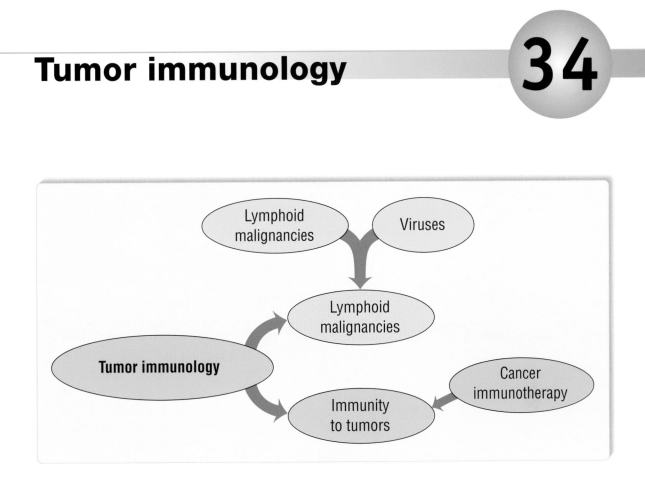

Lymphoid tumors

The malignancies affecting the adaptive immune system originate from a single lymphocyte or plasma cell. Each cell of the malignant population has undergone identical immune receptor gene rearrangements and expresses identical immunoglobulin or T cell receptor molecules. The identical nature of the cells is referred to as **monoclonality**.

The cellular origins of lymphoid malignancy are shown in Figure 34.1 and the characteristics of tumor cells in Figure 34.2. The characteristics of each type of tumor are dictated by the biology of the originating cell. For example, common acute lymphoblastic leukemia (cALL) is derived from rapidly dividing pre-B cells and is extremely aggressive. Untreated cALL can kill within weeks of diagnosis. Myeloma is derived from mature, slow-growing plasma cells, which secrete monoclonal immunoglobulin. Myeloma patients can survive for years without treatment.

Because cells from lymphoid malignancies are easy to remove and grow in vitro, we know a lot about how they arise. This is usually as a result of oncogene activation by chromosomal translocations or the effects of viruses.

Oncogenesis

Chromosomal translocations

During immune-receptor gene recombination, chromosomal breaks may not be correctly repaired. In B cells, chromosomal breaks can also occur during class switching and somatic hypermutation. Occasionally, segments of different chromosomes are brought together. This will often have lethal consequences for the lymphocyte. However, some rare chromosomal translocations have positive effects on cell survival. This may happen because translocation of an oncogene with an immunoglobulin gene promoter or enhancer may result in permanent activation of the oncogene.

In lymphoma, the oncogenes c-*myc* and *bcl-2* are commonly translocated to the immunoglobulin heavy chain gene on chromosome 8. Activated c-*myc* stimulates lymphocyte proliferation. In normal lymphocytes, proliferation is always balanced by apoptosis. Activated Bcl-2 protein protects against apoptosis and this allows unrestrained proliferation of lymphocytes (see Box 21.5).

The **Philadelphia chromosome**, seen in some cases of ALL, is a translocation of the *abl* oncogene on chromosome 9 onto a region called the break point cluster region (*bcr*) on chromosome 22. The Bcr–Abl fusion protein has anti-apoptosis effects.

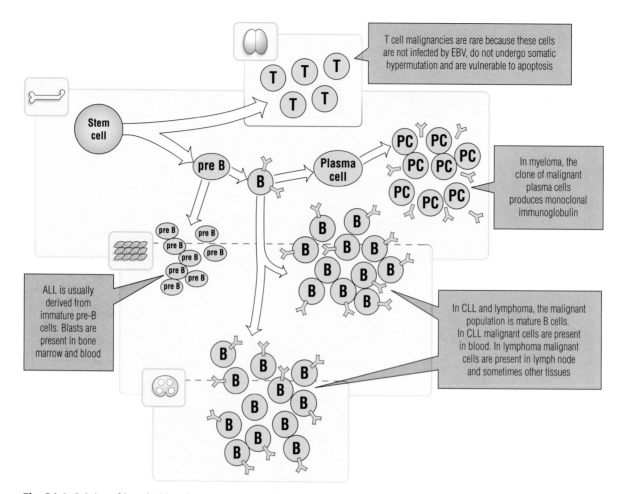

Fig. 34.1 Origins of lymphoid malignancies. Clonal populations arise in bone marrow or lymph node but they may overspill into blood or other tissues. EBV, Epstein–Barr virus; CLL, chronic lymphoblastic leukemia.

Oncogene translocations are more likely to occur after exposure to radiation: myeloma was common in survivors of the Hiroshima atomic bombings.

Viruses

Herpesvirus family members and retroviruses infect cells without killing them. It is in the interests of viruses to stimulate uncontrolled growth of these infected cells.

Epstein–Barr virus (EBV) causes infectious mononucleosis/glandular fever (Ch. 15), lymphoma and nasopharyngeal carcinoma. EBV-driven lymphoma is common in immunodeficient patients and in malarious areas. EBV produces proteins that stimulate the uncontrolled growth of infected cells and protect against apoptosis (Box 34.1).

Infection with another herpes virus, human herpes virus 8 (HHV8), can cause Kaposi's sarcoma in immunodeficient individuals.

T cell malignancy is rare, but when it occurs it is often caused by human T lymphotrophic virus 1 (HTLV1). This is a retrovirus which encodes Tax protein, which has similar effects to interleukin (IL) 2 (T cell growth factor). HTLV1 is rare in the developed world.

Cancers are usually a consequence of at least two events affecting gene expression. Figure 34.3 illustrates this principle.

Diagnosing lymphoid malignancy

Lymphoid malignancy is diagnosed by showing the presence of abnormal monoclonal cells.

In acute lymphoblastic leukemia (ALL), lymphoblasts are easily recognizable from their morphology in blood or bone marrow. The ALL cells look very different from normal mature lymphocytes. In chronic lymphocytic leukemia (CLL), however, the more mature malignant lymphocytes may look completely

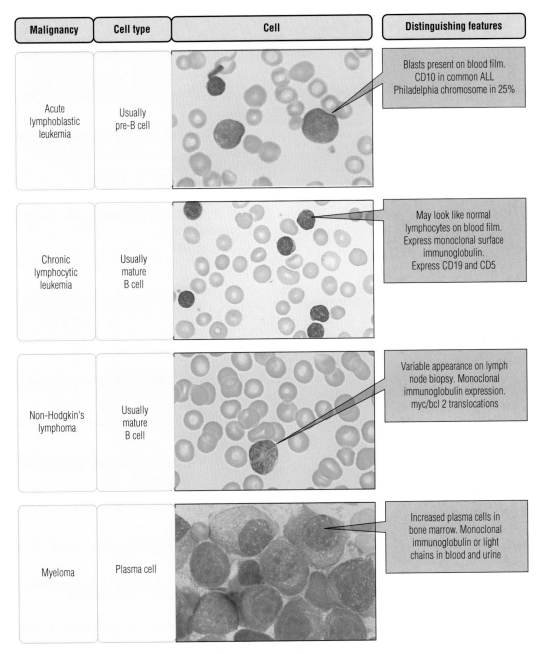

Malignancy	Cell type	Cell	Distinguishing features
Acute lymphoblastic leukemia	Usually pre-B cell		Blasts present on blood film. CD10 in common ALL Philadelphia chromosome in 25%
Chronic lymphocytic leukemia	Usually mature B cell		May look like normal lymphocytes on blood film. Express monoclonal surface immunoglobulin. Express CD19 and CD5
Non-Hodgkin's lymphoma	Usually mature B cell		Variable appearance on lymph node biopsy. Monoclonal immunoglobulin expression. myc/bcl 2 translocations
Myeloma	Plasma cell		Increased plasma cells in bone marrow. Monoclonal immunoglobulin or light chains in blood and urine

Fig. 34.2 Malignant lymphoid cells have distinctive morphology

normal and the only abnormality on the blood film may be an increase in lymphocyte numbers. This needs to be distinguished from a physiological high lymphocyte count (**lymphocytosis**) seen as a response to some infections (Box 34.2).

In lymphoma, lymph node biopsy may show diagnostic abnormal morphology. In other cases, it may be hard to distinguish lymphoma from a lymph node responding to infection. Further studies show abnormal surface molecules (for example, CD5; Ch. 14), oncogene translocations or monoclonality. Molecular techniques are used to demonstrate B cell monoclonality (Box 14.2) or abnormal gene usage (Box 14.3) in lymphoma.

Monoclonal immunoglobulins are produced in response to some infections and they are seen in some healthy elderly people: so-called **monoclonal**

BOX 34.1
Epstein–Barr virus and oncogenesis

Unlike many other viruses EBV does not convert the cellular machinery to virus production and destruction of the cell (Box 15.5). Instead, EBV immortalizes cells by producing proteins that drive B cell proliferation and inhibit apoptosis. EBV proteins also help infected cells to evade the immune response by blocking proteosome-mediated antigen degradation.

EBV causes lymphoma, particularly in two situations. In regions where malaria is endemic, Burkitt's lymphoma occurs in up to 1 in 1000 children. Burkitt's lymphoma is a consequence of polyclonal activation of B cells by both malaria and EBV. The marked polyclonal B cell proliferation increases the risk of translocations involving *myc*, leading to the growth of a malignant population.

In immunodeficient patients the normal response to EBV-infected B cells is lost and EBV is able to drive B cell growth. B cell proliferation is initially polyclonal and presents as a prolonged glandular fever-like illness with fever and lymphadenopathy. Translocations involving *myc* then occur and promote the growth of a malignant monoclonal population.

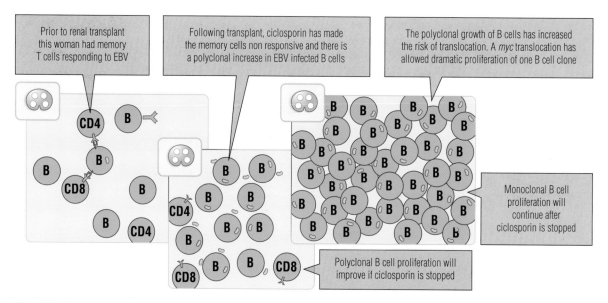

Fig. 34.3 A sequence of events is usually required in oncogenesis. In this case Epstein–Barr virus infection, post-transplant immunosuppression and then a gene translocation lead to monoclonal B cell proliferation.

gammopathy of uncertain significance (MGUS). However, monoclonal immunoglobulin is also produced by malignant plasma cells in myeloma (Box 34.3). Bone destruction (osteolytic lesions) are seen in some patients with myeloma but never in MGUS and this helps to distinguish the two conditions.

In the rarer T cell malignancies monoclonal usage of T cell receptor genes is used as a marker of malignancy.

Immunity to tumors

So far, we have discussed how cells of the adaptive immune system may give rise to tumors. However, components of the immune system may also recognize and, sometimes, kill malignancies arising in other tissues. To understand this, it is important to know how malignant cells may become antigenic, or in other words, express **tumor antigens**.

Tumor antigens

Tumor antigens are molecules produced by tumor cells that can potentially be recognized by the immune system. There are a number of different types of tumor antigen.

- Developmental proteins. These are normally only transiently expressed during development but may be re-expressed by tumor cells. For example,

 Bone marrow   Thymus   Lymph node

BOX 34.2
Chronic lymphoblastic leukemia

An elderly man presents with unusually severe shingles (herpes zoster infection), suggestive of secondary immunodeficiency. He has a raised lymphocyte count. The lymphocytes have normal morphology. Flow cytometry (Fig. 34.4) showed that the lymphocytes were abnormal B cells expressing CD5 and were monoclonal, expressing the λ light chain. The shingles was caused by immunodeficiency secondary to B cell chronic lymphocytic leukemia.

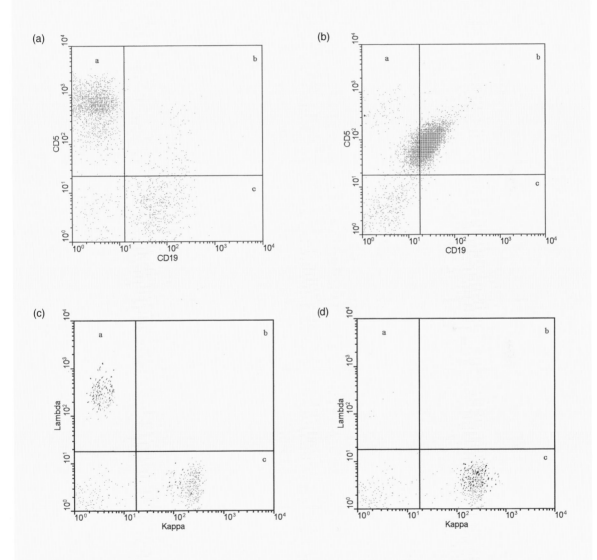

Fig. 34.4 This figure shows flow cytometry results (see Fig. 32.4 for details of flow cytometry) for a healthy control and our patient with B cell chronic lymphocytic leukemia (B-CLL). In the first two plots (a and b), the cytometric analysis has detected cells stained with CD19 (for B cells) and CD5 (usually expressed on T cells only). The patient has a population of cells that abnormally express both CD19 and CD5. The second two plots (c and d) show cells stained for κ and λ light chains. In the normal control the circulating mature B cells express a mixture of κ and λ light chains. In B-CLL, light chain expression is skewed towards either κ- or λ-chain expression.

BOX 34.3
Myeloma

A woman presents with fatigue and bone pain. Initial investigations show that she has multiple lytic bone lesions (Fig. 34.5). Electrophoresis showed a band in the serum (Fig. 4.4), which represented monoclonal IgGκ in the serum. There are also free κ light chains in the urine—referred to as **Bence Jones protein**. The presence of serum monoclonal immunoglobulin and urinary monoclonal light chains with lytic bone lesions confirm the diagnosis of myeloma. The diagnosis could also have been made by showing excessive numbers of plasma cells in the bone marrow.

The patient was started on cytotoxic chemotherapy for her myeloma and initially she made a good response. However, she developed *Haemophilus* pneumonia, a consequence of her secondary antibody deficiency, and died.

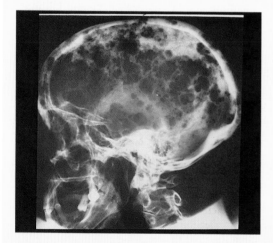

Fig. 34.5 The patient had multiple lytic lesions when a skeletal survey was done. Hypercalcemia occurs as a result of increased bone resorption and contributes to renal failure. (With permission from the Department of Medical Illustration, St Bartholomew's Hospital, London.)

carcinoembryonic antigen is normally expressed on many tissues during fetal life. Carcinoembryonic antigen can be abnormally expressed in gastrointestinal cancer.

- Lineage-specific proteins. These proteins are expressed in cancers and the normal tissues from which they arise. For example, melanoma is a skin cancer of melanocytes. Normal melanocytes and melanoma cells both express the enzyme

tyrosinase. Tyrosinase in not expressed in any other cells, normal or abnormal.
- Viral proteins. For example, EBV (see above) and human papilloma virus (in cervical cancer) produce specific proteins.
- Proteins produced through translocations. For example the Bcr–Abl fusion protein is the product of the *bcr/abl* translocation.

Developmental and lineage-specific proteins are poorly immunogenic because they are expressed on normal tissues. T cells with receptors capable of recognizing these proteins are deleted through tolerance induction. The same system that protects from autoimmunity thus impairs tumor recognition by the immune system. For example, carcinoembryonic antigen present in colon cancer does not elicit a strong immune response. None the less, tests to detect carcinoembryonic antigen are sometimes used to screen for this type of cancer.

Viral and fusion proteins tend to be more immunogenic because they are never present in the normal individual. Each of these has been investigated for its possible clinical role in diagnosing, preventing and treating cancer.

The greatest victory so far in preventing tumors is an indirect one. In some parts of the world, the risk of hepatoma caused by hepatitis B virus has been dramatically reduced following the introduction of hepatitis B vaccine. There are hopes that new vaccines based on papilloma virus and EBV antigens will decrease the incidence of cervical cancer and lymphoma.

So far, immunotherapy for cancer remains experimental. Knowledge of tumor immunity and how tumors evade the immune system is necessary to understand the problems immunologists face developing useful therapy for cancer.

Evidence for tumor immunity

The high frequency of cancers in immunosuppressed patients is often cited as evidence for tumor immunity, for example, papilloma virus-driven cervical cancer (which is 100 times more common in immunosuppressed patients). We have already discussed how common EBV-driven lymphoma is in patients with immunodeficiency. The high prevalence of these tumors in immunodeficient patients is evidence of the more effective role of the immune system in clearing viral infection than in recognizing tumors themselves. Immune surveillance for viruses is much more effective than surveillance for cancers.

However, there is also good evidence that the human immune system attempts to eradicate other types of tumor by recognizing some of the antigens mentioned above. Antibody responses are not effective at eradicating most solid tumors and T cells are required; tumors

🦴 Bone marrow   Thymus   Lymph node

that are infiltrated by T cells have an improved prognosis. These tumor-infiltrating lymphocytes (TIL) are specific for tumor antigens, for example tyrosinase in melanoma. TILs use their T cell receptors to recognize antigen presented by MHC.

Some tumors evade the adaptive immune system by decreasing expression of MHC and losing the ability to present antigen to T cells. Mutations in the MHC genes themselves are not unusual in these tumors. Cells expressing low levels of MHC make excellent targets for killing by natural killer cells, which may act as a back-up system in this situation.

Occasionally, the immune system damages the blood supply to tumors and kills them by starving them of oxygen, leading to necrosis. Very early experiments showed that tumor necrosis factor (TNF) can do this when injected at high doses into mice with cancers. Although this is how the cytokine's full name arose, it is not clear how important any of these mechanisms are in tumors in humans.

In the vast majority of tumors, the malignant cells successfully evade the immune response using various mechanisms (Fig. 34.6). Rapidly dividing malignant cells may mutate and acquire one or more of these evasion mechanisms. This will give this clone of cells an advantage over non-mutated cells.

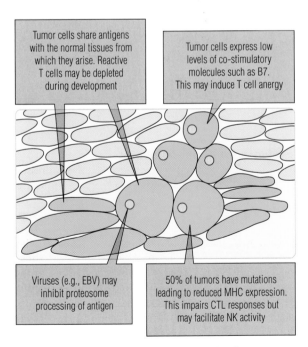

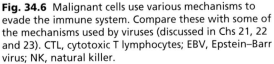

Fig. 34.6 Malignant cells use various mechanisms to evade the immune system. Compare these with some of the mechanisms used by viruses (discussed in Chs 21, 22 and 23). CTL, cytotoxic T lymphocytes; EBV, Epstein–Barr virus; NK, natural killer.

Immunotherapy

Attempts at using immunotherapy have been based on the idea that the immune system could eradicate existing tumors. Many approaches at tumor immunotherapy have been attempted and most have failed. We only mention some of the immunotherapy approaches that have been of some success.

Passive cancer immunotherapy

Passive cancer immunotherapy relies on the use of monoclonal antibodies to destroy malignant cells. Anti-CD20 is a monoclonal antibody with a variety of uses in oncology. CD20 is expressed on normal B cells and on lymphoma cells. Infusion of anti-CD20 can reduce or cure up to 50% of B cell lymphomas. Anti-CD20 destroys malignant B cells by activating antibody-dependent complement and cell-mediated cytotoxicity. Anti-CD20 also triggers B cell signaling, which induces apoptosis. Anti-CD20 has been engineered in a number of ways (Box 9.1). Anti-CD20 molecules have been conjugated to radioiodine to deliver high doses of radioactivity directly to the site of the tumor. Antibodies such as CD20 against normal antigens will damage normal cells; in this case, non-malignant B cells. Radiolabeled anti-CD20 can also be used to determine the spread of lymphoma in the body.

Active cancer immunotherapy

Active immunotherapy aims to overcome the anergy (failure to respond) of T cells. Anergy could develop if a tumor cell presents antigen to a T helper cell without the necessary co-stimulatory molecules.

The simplest way of providing co-stimulation is to infuse the patient with cytokines (Fig. 34.7a). IL-2 treatment activates T cells (and natural killer cells) directly. Unfortunately, IL-2 causes severe side-effects, the most dreaded of which is the capillary leak syndrome, in which fluid shifts to the extravascular space, causing edema and hypotension. One potential way to avoid the severe side-effects of IL-2 is to use it in vitro to stimulate peripheral blood lymphocytes. This results in the formation of a type of natural killer cell termed the lymphokine-activated killer (LAK) cell. LAK cells have a greatly enhanced non-specific cytotoxic effects on tumors in animal studies. In human trials, however, IL-2 alone was shown to be virtually as effective as IL-2 plus LAK cells (see Box 21.4).

Systemic use of interferon (IFN), both IFN-α and IFN-β, increases MHC class I expression, enabling improved tumor antigen presentation. IFNs also have direct antiproliferative effects on tumor cells, although systemic use of these cytokines also causes side-effects.

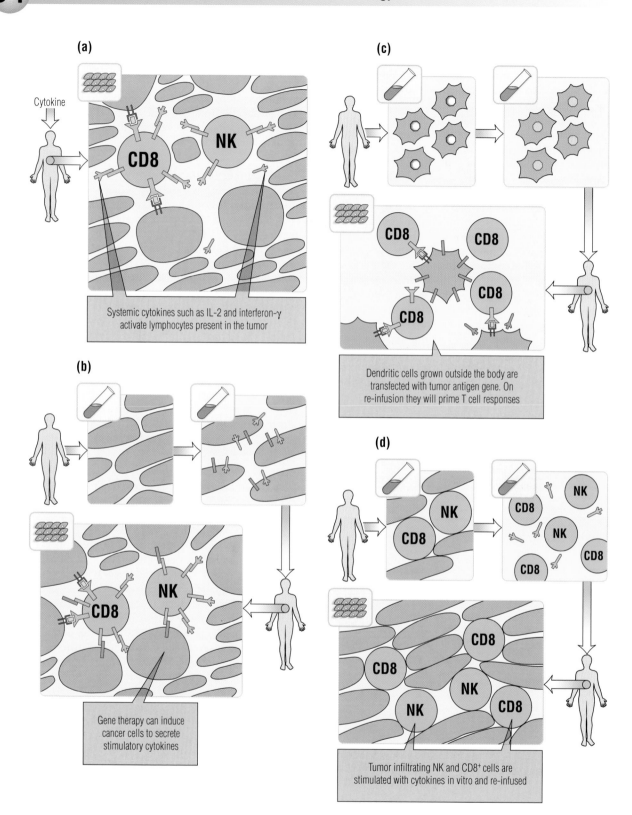

(a)

Cytokine

CD8   NK

Systemic cytokines such as IL-2 and interferon-γ activate lymphocytes present in the tumor

(b)

CD8   NK

Gene therapy can induce cancer cells to secrete stimulatory cytokines

(c)

CD8   CD8

CD8

CD8

Dendritic cells grown outside the body are transfected with tumor antigen gene. On re-infusion they will prime T cell responses

(d)

NK

CD8   CD8

NK

CD8

CD8

CD8

NK

NK   CD8

Tumor infiltrating NK and CD8⁺ cells are stimulated with cytokines in vitro and re-infused

Fig. 34.7 Active immunotherapy for cancer. IL, interleukin; NK, natural killer, CD8 indicates CD8⁺ T cells.

Bone marrow   Thymus   Lymph node

Cytokine **gene therapy** aims to localize cytokines to their desired site of action (Fig. 34.7b). If cytokines are limited to the site of the tumor, then their systemic side-effects should be reduced. Tumor cells are removed and transfected with cytokine genes. When the cells are re-infused, they secrete cytokines, such as IL-2 or IFN-γ, that overcome the block to T cell activation. Once T cells have responded to the transfected cells and become memory cells, they will acquire the ability to kill non-transfected tumor cells. Alternatively, tumor cells can be induced to express co-stimulatory molecules such as CD80(B7), the ligand for CD28, to help to stimulate T cells. The best results have been obtained (at least in mice) when therapy is used to insert genes for both cytokine and co-stimulatory molecules.

A third way of overcoming tumor cell evasion is to load tumor antigen into presenting cells, which are already equipped with co-stimulatory molecules and cytokine secretion. "Dendritic cell vaccines" (Fig. 34.7c) are made by growing dendritic cells from auto-logous blood and loading these with the relevant tumor antigen gene. These are re-infused and will then stimulate T cells in a similar fashion to the gene therapy approaches already mentioned.

A further approach is to extract TILs from the tumor and then to stimulate them in the presence of tumor antigen (for example, tyrosinase in the case of melanoma) and stimulatory cytokines. When the TILs have increased in number and become effective killers, they can be re-infused (Fig. 34.7d).

LEARNING POINTS

Can you now:

- Describe the different lymphoid malignancies?
- List the techniques used to diagnose lymphoid malignancies?
- Explain how host and viral oncogenes interact to cause cancer?
- Describe the different types of tumor antigen and explain how tumors evade the immune response?
- List several approaches to cancer immunotherapy?

Integration of the immune system with other regulatory systems

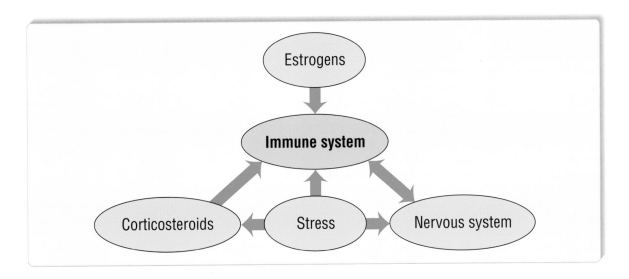

Evolution has developed ways of switching the immune system on and off in special situations, most notably during pregnancy, when the immune system may damage the fetus, and during stress and starvation, where resources are diverted elsewhere.

Rapid effects are mediated by adrenergic hormones. More delayed results are mediated by the effects of steroid hormones on lymphocytes. These cells have specific receptors for both sex hormones and corticosteroids.

THE EFFECT OF GENDER ON THE IMMUNE SYSTEM

Before puberty, the developing immune system in boys and girls is very similar. The immune system develops without the effects of sex hormones. Androgens secreted by men are broadly immunosuppresive and are secreted at a steady state throughout adult life; in men the immune response does not fluctuate until the onset of old age. In women, the immune response is integrated into the endocrine system in order to prevent rejection of the fetus during pregnancy (Fig. 35.1). As discussed in Chapter 33, the fetus expresses paternal allogeneic antigens and has the potential to be rejected by maternal T cells. The pla-

centa expresses high levels of HLA-G which helps it evade damage by natural killer cells. The placenta also secretes T_H2 cytokines which inhibit T cell responses. In addition, during pregnancy there is a systemic reduction in T cell activity, mediated by estrogen.

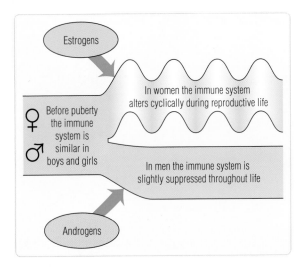

Fig. 35.1 In women between puberty and the menopause, the immune system is affected by estrogens. These have prolonged and different effects on T and B cells during pregnancy.

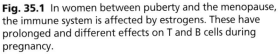

Estrogen is a steroid sex hormone secreted by the ovaries. It is secreted at high levels during the middle of the menstrual cycle and persistently during pregnancy. Estrogen has many physiological roles associated with reproduction, for example, it maintains the uterus and prepares the breasts for secretion of milk. Estrogen also inhibits T cell activity and so even in healthy women, T cell numbers in blood fluctuate during normal menstrual cycles. T cell activity is also inhibited for the duration of pregnancy, probably in order to reduce the risk of rejection of the fetus. Estrogen has the opposite effects on B cells, so that there is an increase in IgG and IgA synthesis during pregnancy. This ensures that adequate amounts of IgG are transported across the placenta late in pregnancy and that IgA is available in breast milk after labor. These immunoglobulins protect the mother from infection at a time when T cell function is impaired. The fetus is also provided with some maternal immunological memory until it is able to synthesize its own immunoglobulins. As mentioned in Chapter 33, most pregnant women make antibodies to paternal HLA antigens, but these do not affect fetal outcome. During pregnancy, estrogens have the dual effects of inhibiting T activity to protect the fetus from rejection, but increasing B cell activity to protect the fetus from infection (Fig. 35.2).

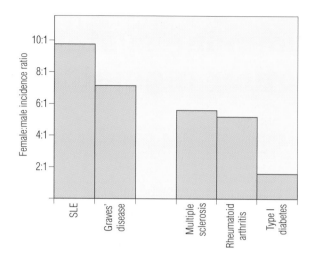

Fig. 35.3 Autoimmune diseases involving pathogenic antibodies are particularly common in women.

Women experience fewer infections throughout life than men. This may be due to the negative effects of androgens. Despite episodic T cell inhibition, women do not develop more infections than men. Even during pregnancy there is no increased risk of infection. This illustrates how important adequate immunoglobulin levels are in preventing infections.

On the other hand, women are at higher risk of developing autoimmune diseases (Fig. 35.3), at least until the menopause. The reason for the increased risk of autoimmune disease in women is not clear, but estrogens are at least partially responsible. They stimulate antibody production, whilst androgens are broadly immunosuppressive. Autoimmune diseases caused by antibodies, for example Graves' disease (type II hypersensitivity) and systemic lupus erythematosus (SLE) (type III hypersensitivity) are particularly common in women, compared with diseases mediated by T cells, such as rheumatoid arthritis (type IV hypersensitivity). This may reflect in part the stimulatory effects of estrogens on B cells.

SLE is sometimes precipitated by estrogen-containing contraceptive pills and often gets worse during pregnancy (see Box 35.1). Rheumatoid arthritis and multiple sclerosis on the other hand, improve during pregnancy and can worsen after labor (Box 15.4).

STRESS AND THE IMMUNE SYSTEM

The immune system integrates with other systems during physiological stress. The immune system can act as a sensory system early in infections, by triggering an acute phase response. In other stressful situations the immune system is inhibited by stress. The nature of the

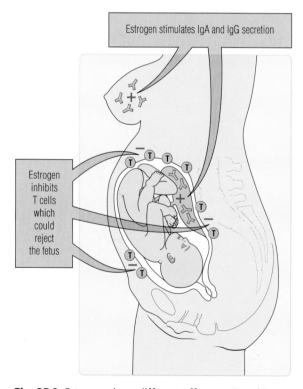

Fig. 35.2 Estrogens have different effects on T and B cells in pregnancy.

Bone marrow   Thymus   Lymph node

BOX 35.1
Effects of pregnancy on SLE

A woman known to have mild SLE presents in the 8th month of pregnancy with increasing joint pains and rashes. She has increased anti DNA antibody levels, consistent with active SLE. Despite her symptoms, she is very cheerful because she is almost to term and her previous three pregnancies have ended in miscarriages. She is treated with simple analgesics and her symptoms are brought under control.

She undergoes a normal labor at term and delivers a baby boy. The baby is noted to have a rash on his face, which looks very similar to his mother's rash. This is diagnosed as neonatal lupus and his condition improves without treatment.

This case history illustrates three important points.

- Pregnancy causes SLE to flare up.
- SLE can influence the course of pregnancy. Antiphospholipid antibodies are one of the many autoantibodies present in SLE. They can activate the clotting system and cause venous thrombosis and miscarriage.
- SLE can affect the fetus when autoantibodies can cross the placenta and cause disease in the baby. The disease improves as the antibodies disappear. Similarly, babies born to mothers with Graves' disease can develop transient hyperthyroidism.

BOX 35.2
Leptin

Leptin is a hormone produced by fatty tissues. When there are adequate fatty tissues leptin levels are high. Leptin suppresses appetite, and supports the endocrine system and the immune system. When individuals are unable to maintain adequate levels of fatty tissue, leptin levels fall. As a result, appetite increases and some endocrine systems, for example the reproductive cycle, stop functioning. The immune system is also compromised when leptin levels are low. Low levels of leptin reduce the activity of macrophages and secretion of interferon γ by T_H1 T cells. Leptin thus provides a mechanism for maintaining fat stores and switching off metabolically expensive resources, such as reproduction and the immune system, when fat supplies are low (Fig. 35.4).

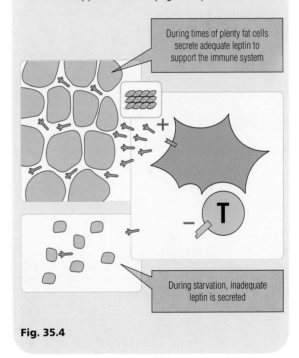

During times of plenty fat cells secrete adequate leptin to support the immune system

During starvation, inadequate leptin is secreted

Fig. 35.4

inhibitory signal differs depending on the duration of the stressful stimulation.

Acute phase response

The acute phase response is an entirely innate mechanism and is initiated by macrophages which secrete IL-1, IL-6 and TNF in response to infection. Macrophages secrete these cytokines after they have recognized pathogens using pattern recognition molecules such as Toll-like receptors. These cytokines increase production of complement and arm the adaptive immune system (see Ch. 19). TNF has direct effects on metabolism. It increases the breakdown of fat in the body's stores, possibly to increase availability of calorie supplies. However, during the acute phase response, appetite is also reduced, possibly because TNF stimulates the production of leptin (see Box 35.2). Weight loss is often a dramatic consequence of activation of the immune system.

IL-1, IL-6 and TNF also affect the central nervous system through receptors in the hypothalamus. The main response is an increase in body temperature, which is seen very rapidly after the beginning of the response to infection. The role of increased body temperature is to inhibit the replication of viruses and bacteria.

These cytokines also stimulate the secretion of corticosteroids by the adrenal glands. This is also mediated by the hypothalamus, stimulating secretion of corticotrophin by the pituitary. Corticosteroids have

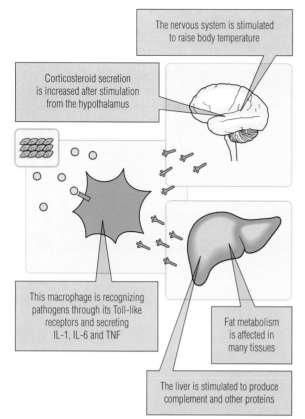

The nervous system is stimulated to raise body temperature

Corticosteroid secretion is increased after stimulation from the hypothalamus

This macrophage is recognizing pathogens through its Toll-like receptors and secreting IL-1, IL-6 and TNF

Fat metabolism is affected in many tissues

The liver is stimulated to produce complement and other proteins

Fig. 35.5 The innate immune system triggers the acute phase response. Macrophages act as sensory cells for regulatory systems.

widespread effects on metabolism and suppress the immune system if the acute phase response continues. This may act as a negative feedback control on the acute phase response.

Through the acute phase response, the innate immune system acts as a sensory system and has profound effects on the nervous system and metabolism (Fig. 35.5).

Acute responses to stress: mediated by catecholamines

The immune response also responds when the nervous system is stressed. For example, after acute stressful stimuli such as loud noises, acute anxiety or even running up several flights of stairs there is a rapid increase in the number or circulating T cells. These effects are mediated by the release of catecholamines (for example, epinephrine) by the sympathetic nervous system. Nerve fibers capable of secreting catecholamines run into lymphoid organs such as lymph nodes. Higher levels of catecholamines are also

released into the circulation by the adrenal medulla during some forms of stress. T cells express receptors for epinephrine and stimulation of these receptors causes T cells to decrease their expression of integrin molecules. Consequently, T cells are prevented from adhering to endothelium and migrating into the tissues. Hence, T cells rapidly accumulate in the blood (Fig. 35.6). T cell response to stimulation after acute stress is also reduced.

It is not yet clear why T cells are affected by adrenergic hormones during acute stress, but it appears to be part of the flight or fight response.

The sympathetic nervous system also inhibits some of the *effects* of immune system activity. This is particularly true of type I hypersensitivity, where epinephrine can reverse some of the effects of allergy. For example, epinephrine (adrenaline) should be given in anaphylaxis, where it can reverse the low blood pressure and

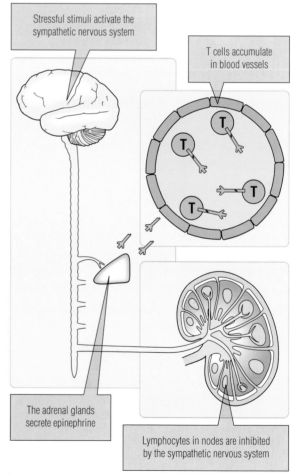

Stressful stimuli activate the sympathetic nervous system

T cells accumulate in blood vessels

The adrenal glands secrete epinephrine

Lymphocytes in nodes are inhibited by the sympathetic nervous system

Fig. 35.6 Acute response to stress. T cells are affected by epinephrine released by the sympathetic nervous system or the adrenal glands.

 Bone marrow 　　 Thymus 　　 Lymph node

reduce angioedema by reducing vascular permeability. Other β_2-adrenergic drugs are given in asthma, where they relax bronchial smooth muscle. This is discussed in Chapter 26.

Chronic effects of stress on the immune system

When stress lasts for more than a few hours, other integrated systems begin to affect the immune system. The most important of these is corticosteroids secreted by the adrenal glands. Normal secretion of corticosteroids has a range of homeostatic effects, for example, maintenance of blood pressure. Corticosteroids are secreted at varying levels during the day, for example secretion is maximal in the morning and lowest late at night. Physiological levels of corticosteroids impact on the immune system and the circadian rhythm has important consequences.

- CD4$^+$ T cell counts are often at their lowest in the morning, coinciding with the peak in corticosteroid secretion. Patients having serial CD4$^+$ T cells counts, for example during monitoring of HIV infection, should always have their counts done at the same time of day (Fig. 35.7).
- In unstable asthma, symptoms are often at their worst at night and very early in the morning after corticosteroid levels have been at their lowest. Treatment with inhaled steroids can prevent these dips (Ch. 26).

Corticosteroids are secreted at much higher levels in response to a wide range of physiological stresses,

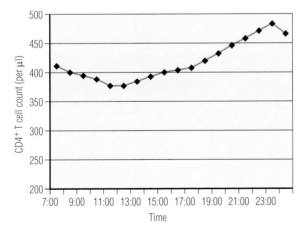

Fig. 35.7 The CD4$^+$ T cell count reciprocates serum corticosteroid levels.

including prolonged severe exercise (see Box 35.3), trauma or emotional stress such as bereavement. The innate immune system can induce corticosteroid secretion in response to infection, as mentioned above. Corticosteroids have effects on both the innate and adaptive immune systems. For example, they inhibit many aspects of macrophage function, but because they inhibit activities such as antigen presentation, T cell function is also reduced. The consequence of high level corticosteroid secretion is mild immunodeficiency. The role of corticosteroid drugs as immunosuppressive drugs has been mentioned in Chapter 33.

Although the effects of stress on the immune system are often very subtle, it makes good sense to ensure that patients with compromised immunity have ways of avoiding or dealing with stressful situations.

Another possible consequence of prolonged stressful situations is weight loss, because of poor access to food or inability to eat. This has negative effects on the immune system, aside from the effects of depletion of some of the nutrients mentioned in Chapter 32. The immune system requires adequate levels of leptin to function normally (see Box 35.2) and loss of fatty tissue may thus cause mild immunodeficiency. These effects may also be subtle, but maintaining fat stores is important in immunodeficient patients.

In response to prolonged stress or weight loss the immune system is switched off. This mechanism has presumably evolved because at times of stress there is a need to conserve resources for systems that are more immediately important (Fig. 35.8).

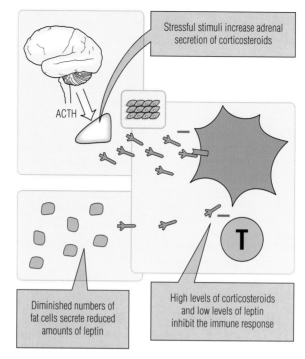

Stressful stimuli increase adrenal secretion of corticosteroids

ACTH

Diminished numbers of fat cells secrete reduced amounts of leptin

High levels of corticosteroids and low levels of leptin inhibit the immune response

T

Fig. 35.8 The immune system in chronic stress.

LEARNING POINTS

Can you now:

- Describe how estrogens protect the fetus from immunological rejection whilst maintaining maternal antibody levels?
- Explain how estrogens may affect the risks of autoimmune disease?
- Describe how catecholamines affect the immune system?
- Explain the effect of corticosteroids and leptin?
- List the clinical and therapeutic aspects of stress responses?

Bone marrow   Thymus   Lymph node

Review of immunity in health and disease

In this chapter, we review the contents of this last section, which covered vaccines and clinical problems involving the immune system.

To illustrate the kinds of problem the immune system can cause, we follow the life of a physician born in 1942. None of the problems she experiences is particularly rare.

The vast majority of infections can be dealt with by the innate and adaptive immune systems working in unison. Some infections, for example measles (Box 36.1), are usually cleared by the immune system and only cause trivial problems in the vast majority of cases. But even measles can be life threatening in some individuals. Other infections (for example hepatitis B) are much harder for the immune system to clear and can cause life-long infection. Either type of infection can be prevented by the use of vaccines.

Vaccines stimulate components of the adaptive immune system to produce immunological memory (Ch. 24). Specific antibodies either prevent infection from taking place or bind to toxins produced by pathogens, reducing the severity of the disease.

Vaccines produced from killed pathogens or recombinant proteins are very safe but tend to produce weak responses. Adjuvants are often used to boost the effects of killed or subunit vaccines. Other vaccines use live pathogens that have been attenuated. Live vaccines are often more effective than killed or subunit vaccines, but there is a higher risk of side-effects.

Newer technologies aim to stimulate the immune system in novel ways, for example by inserting the gene for an antigen using DNA vaccines.

Hypersensitivity reactions are an important cause of disease and are caused by the immune system reacting to a range of antigens (Ch. 25). These antigens can include peptides produced by microbes. It is possible that in some infections (for examples, forms of leprosy) the immune response causes at least as much damage as the pathogen itself.

Atopy is an immediate hypersensitivity reaction to environmental antigens, mediated by IgE (type I hypersensitivity; Ch. 26). We use the term allergy synonymously. Allergic diseases are one of the commonest forms of hypersensitivity and are thought to be increasing in prevalence in the developed world. This increase in allergy is occurring although immunity mediated by T helper 2 (T_H2) cells, IgE and mast cells, which was originally developed to fend off worm infestations, is less required as these are now rare in the developed world. There is also a decline in bacterial infections in developed countries; the hygiene hypothesis suggests that this may skew the immune system towards T_H2 responses.

The most widely recognized forms of allergy occur immediately after patients have been exposed to allergens and are caused by the effects of mast cell degranulation after IgE crosslinking (Box 36.2). Allergy can also have a late phase, mediated largely by eosinophils. The late phase accounts for many of the symptoms of diseases such as asthma.

Apart from infections and allergens, hypersensitivity can also occur in response to autoantigens (Ch. 27). Although a degree of autoimmunity is normal, autoimmune mechanisms can cause disease through three mechanisms: direct effects of antibodies (type II hypersensitivity; Ch. 28), immune complexes (type III; Ch. 29) or delayed hypersensitivity (type IV; Ch. 30). Autoimmunity has complex genetic and environmental origins and reflects the breakdown of normal self tolerance. It is not unusual for these diseases, especially organ-specific autoimmune disease, to run in families.

In type II hypersensitivity, antibodies bind to cells, causing a number of effects. In Chapter 27 we described how antibodies binding to red cells can fix complement or stimulate opsonization. In either instance, hemolytic anemia is the result. Antibodies

BOX 36.1
Infancy

At the age of seven, our patient developed a widespread blotchy rash and high fever. Her family recognized the characteristic rash of measles. However she deteriorates over the next 2 days and develops signs of pneumonia. Luckily, she gradually improves without specific treatment.

Measles pneumonia is an unusual complication of this viral infection. Measles also causes brain inflammation (encephalitis) from time to time. A vaccine for measles has been in routine use in the developed world since the 1970s and has largely prevented these infrequent, but potentially life-threatening, complications. In the developing world, measles remains a major cause of death of young children.

 Blood vessel   Gut   Peripheral tissue

BOX 36.2
Childhood

As an 11-year-old, our subject goes on a family picnic. A few minutes after eating a peanut butter sandwich, she develops swelling of the face and breathlessness. Luckily her symptoms improve spontaneously. Relatively little was known about peanut-induced anaphylaxis in the 1950s and skin prick and specific IgE testing were not widely available. The experience put her off peanuts for life, and she never had the same experience again. It is also possible she "grew out of" her allergy. This case illustrates how it is possible to have anaphylaxis to specific allergens without any background of allergy.

BOX 36.4
Life as a student

Our subject is successful in getting into medical school. At the age of 24 while training she is infected with hepatitis B virus. Effective vaccines were not available in the 1960s. She becomes jaundiced and she is also found to have kidney disease. Glomerulonephritis sometimes complicates hepatitis B infection; this is caused by circulating immune complexes of viral antigen and antibodies. Once again she is very lucky and her condition improves gradually. A year later her kidney and liver function is normal and she is thought to have successfully eradicated the hepatitis virus.

BOX 36.5
The family

Our subject's younger sister has been unwell with fatigue for several weeks. On a visit home, our subject decides her sister may have diabetes, remembering that organ-specific autoimmune disease tends to run in families. The sister's blood sugar is high, confirming the diagnosis.

can also mimic the effects of trophic hormones, as in Graves' disease (Box 36.3). Detection of these autoantibodies, using a variety of techniques, is used to help make the diagnosis.

Type III hypersensitivity is caused by immune complexes. These can form in the tissues (for example farmer's lung) or circulate in the blood. Although circulating immune complexes can be the consequence of autoimmune disease, they can also be the result of exogenous antigens, usually from infections, as in Box 36.4. Immune complexes activate the innate immune system and cause inflammation. The kidneys are very often the targets for this process.

Type IV hypersensitivity can also be the result of infection (for example tuberculosis, leprosy) or autoimmunity. In the autoimmune diseases insulin-dependent diabetes, rheumatoid arthritis and multiple sclerosis, T cells infiltrate the target organs and cause chronic inflammation (Box 36.5). The damage in each case is mediated by cytokines. Tumor necrosis factor is

probably the most important of these. Each of these autoimmune diseases is associated with specific autoantibodies. Although these may be useful in making the diagnosis, they are not strongly implicated in damaging the target organs.

Transplantation is used to replace diseased organs. In all types of allogeneic transplant, except for corneal transplant, rejection is a major problem (Ch. 33). At its most severe, hyperacute rejection takes place when antibodies bind allogeneic HLA antibodies, destroying the transplanted organ within minutes. Acute rejection is caused by T cells responding to allogeneic antigens in the donor organ. These two types of rejection are similar to type II and type IV hypersensitivity, respectively. The fetus resembles a transplanted organ but it is not rejected by the mother because T cell responses are dampened down by systemic factors (estrogens and cytokines), and natural killer cells are inhibited by local factors in the uterus.

Bone marrow transplant is a special case because T cells arising from the donor can attack the recipient, giving rise to graft-versus-host disease. The risks of graft rejection and graft-versus-host disease are minimized by tissue typing techniques (Box 36.6).

BOX 36.3
Adolescence

Our subject has now progressed to high school, but her family begins to notice weight loss and irritability. At first her family thinks she is simply studying too hard in her efforts to get a place at medical school. Her condition deteriorates and eventually she goes to see a physician. He finds she has hyperthyroidism and a diagnosis of Graves' disease is made (Ch. 28). She responds very well to drug treatment.

 Bone marrow · Thymus · Lymph node

BOX 36.6
The family

After a further 15 years, our subject's sister has developed chronic renal failure as a result of the diabetes. Our subject is unable to act as a donor because of the history of viral hepatitis. One of her siblings is found to be an exact HLA match and donates his kidney. The transplant goes ahead without any signs of rejection. This is lucky, because even in the early 1980s, many of the potent anti-rejection drugs, for example ciclosporin, were not available.

BOX 36.7
Retirement

Our subject is now 55 and planning her retirement. Unfortunately, she has had two very painful bouts of shingles, caused by reactivation of the chickenpox virus, herpes varicella zoster. She has also suffered from a series of chest and sinus infections. An immunodeficiency state is considered and her T cell, IgG and IgA levels are found to be low. Her blood also contains a monoclonal IgM protein. A sample of bone marrow is taken and shows multiple myeloma. A diagnosis of immunodeficiency secondary to myeloma is made.

Immunodeficiency can occur as a result of primary defects within the immune system or secondary to external factors. Primary immunodeficiencies usually have genetic components (Ch. 31). Severe secondary immunodeficiencies occur in patients infected with HIV, malignancies or after specific drug treatments (Ch. 32). Mild secondary immunodeficiencies occur in patients with poor nutrition and during physiological stress.

Immunodeficiencies cause either recurrent infection or opportunist infections with low-virulence organisms. They need to be recognized because, if left untreated, infections can cause irreversible damage or death. The type of infection often gives important clues to the severity and type of immunodeficiency operating (Box 36.7).

Cells of the innate immune system quite often form malignancies (Ch. 34). This is especially true of B cells because they can be infected with Epstein–Barr virus and because they undergo somatic hypermutation. Much is known about the genetic basis of these lymphoid malignancies.

The immune system also has a role in fighting cancers, although, more often than not, the immune system recognizes oncogenic viruses rather than tumor antigens themselves. Many tumors have developed molecular mechanisms for evading the immune system. Tumor immunotherapy aims to reverse some of these mechanisms.

Index

Abbreviations: Ig, Immunoglobulin; MS, multiple sclerosis; SLE, systemic lupus erythematosus.